Clinical Management of Patients in

SUBACUTE
and LONG-TERM
CARE SETTINGS

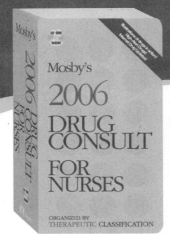

Clinical Management of Patients in

SUBACUTE
and LONG-TERM
CARE SETTINGS

TERRY MAHAN BUTTARO, MS,
 APRN-BC, ANP, GNP, CEN, CCRN
Assistant Clinical Professor
Simmons College
Boston, Massachusetts

SUSAN AZNAVORIAN, MS, APRN-BC
Adjunct Clinical Faculty
Simmons College
Boston, Massachusetts

KAREN DICK, PhD, RN
Coordinator of Adult and Gerontological Nursing
  Practitioner Program
University of Massachusetts
Boston, Massachusetts

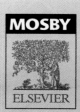

MOSBY
ELSEVIER

11830 Westline Industrial Drive
St. Louis, Missouri 63146

CLINICAL MANAGEMENT OF PATIENTS IN SUBACUTE AND LONG-TERM CARE SETTINGS
Copyright © 2006, Elsevier Inc.

ISBN-13: 978-0-323-01862-3
ISBN-10: 0-323-01862-9

NOTICE

Knowledge and best practice in this field are constantly changing. As new research and experience broaden our knowledge, changes in practice, treatment and drug therapy may become necessary or appropriate. Readers are advised to check the most current information provided (i) on procedures featured or (ii) by the manufacturer of each product to be administered, to verify the recommended dose or formula, the method and duration of administration, and contraindications. It is the responsibility of the practitioner, relying on their own experience and knowledge of the patient, to make diagnoses, to determine dosages and the best treatment for each individual patient, and to take all appropriate safety precautions. To the fullest extent of the law, neither the Publisher nor the Authors assumes any liability for any injury and/or damage to persons or property arising out or related to any use of the material contained in this book.

ISBN-13: 978-0-323-01862-3
ISBN-10: 0-323-01862-9

Executive Publisher: Barbara Nelson Cullen
Publishing Services Manager: Jeff Patterson
Project Manager: Clay S. Broeker
Designer: Julia Dummitt

Printed in the United States of America
Last digit is the print number: 9   8   7   6   5   4   3   2   1

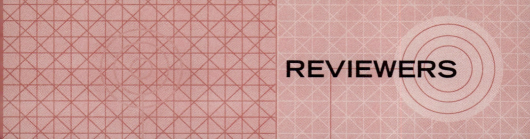

REVIEWERS

Kathryn A. Blair, RN, PhD, FNP
Professor
University of Northern Colorado
Greeley, Colorado

Pamela Z. Cacchione, PhD, RN, GNP, BC
Assistant Professor
School of Nursing
Saint Louis University
St. Louis, Missouri

Julie P. Fago, MD
Geriatrician
Bethel, Vermont

Barbara Toni Hudson, MSN, RN, CS
Family Nurse Practitioner
Ash Grove Family Care Clinic
Citizens Memorial Hospital
Ash Grove, Missouri

Susan Neary, PhD, RN, CS
Assistant Professor of Nursing
Nursing Department
Simmons College
Boston, Massachusetts

Carmen T. Ramirez, EdD, RN, CPC, ACNP
University of Arkansas for Medical
 Services
Little Rock, Arkansas

Valerie K. Sabol, RN, MSN, ACNP, CCNS
Clinical Instructor
School of Nursing
University of Maryland
Baltimore, Maryland

Joanne Sandberg-Cook, MS, APRN-BC, ANP, GNP, PM, CRRN
Dartmouth-Hitchcock Medical
 Center
Lebanon, New Hampshire

Sharon E. Swain, MN, FNP-C
Western Carolina University
Asheville, North Carolina

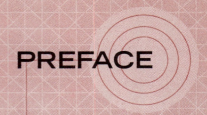

PREFACE

Today, patients are often discharged from acute care facilities to rehabilitation, subacute, and long-term care settings for skilled nursing and rehabilitation services. Healthcare providers in these settings require specific skills and expertise to care for these patients. Many texts address patient care in the primary care and acute care setting, but there are a limited number of reference tools that address the complex needs of patients cared for in skilled nursing and long-term care facilities. Internet accessibility provides national guidelines and medical studies that direct care, but unfortunately, these resources are not always readily available in postacute settings. These facts influenced the authors to create a pocket-sized guide for the experienced practitioner. In these clinical areas, practitioners need a readily accessible reference to provide guidance in the assessment and management of patients recovering from acute illness or surgery. The majority of patients in these settings are older; thus the care of older adults with multiple comorbidities is emphasized. However, younger patients are also admitted to both subacute and long-term facilities, so the reader may find specific references to pregnancy or other issues that impact decisions for care. Because the focus of this text is the management of the more acute disorders encountered in skilled nursing and long-term care facilities, some of the more common geriatric issues are not discussed.

FORMAT

Experienced rehabilitation and long-term care nurse practitioners recommended a format designed to permit quick access to information describing components of the history, physical exam, and management plan. Bullets were chosen to direct the clinician to analyze essential information efficiently.

Chapters 1 and 2 of this text describe the changes in healthcare delivery and the admission process for a patient transferred to the rehabilitation, subacute, or long-term care setting. Regulatory and reimbursement issues also are discussed.

Subsequent segments are organized by system, and there is a consistent format for each chapter. Each disorder is first briefly described. Risk factors; history and physical examination; diagnostics; differential diagnosis; treatment plan; complications; considerations for consultation and hospitalization; and nursing, patient, and family education follow.

Possible history and physical examination findings are detailed to assist providers in determining the assessment. Diagnostic recommendations list appropriate tests, recognizing that in some facilities diagnostic evaluation may be limited. Categories of diagnostic evaluation include laboratory evaluations and other clinically indicated tests. An asterisk (*) placed beside a diagnostic test signifies that while a specific diagnostic test may not be necessary for every patient, it may be indicated for some patients. Clinical presentation, patient preference, and the provider's knowledge of the patient may also render some diagnostics unnecessary.

The differentials list both probable and possible diagnoses, encouraging the reader to consider potential causes for the patient's signs and symptoms. Treatment recommendations are based on research findings and empirical data, recognizing that many decisions for care are based on the provider's knowledge of the patient and prevailing practice. It is important to appreciate, however, that medical research is ongoing and that treatment recommendations can and do change. Providing adequate information to patients and families, allowing patients to choose, and respecting that choice is always the primary goal in any treatment plan; thus the importance of the patient's and family's wishes are emphasized, as some patients and families choose minimal intervention.

Although provider practice in these settings is often autonomous, recommendations for consultation and hospitalization are included to encourage communication and collaboration, as well as to assist the provider in determining the need for immediate consultation. The reader should be aware, however, that every situation requiring hospitalization and referral might not be included in this section. In addition, state practice statutes may dictate more specific consultation and referral regulations, thus, pre-empting the consultation and hospitalization guidelines described in this text.

The importance of education for patients and families is widely acknowledged and reiterated in this text. Education for the staff nurses and medical assistants is also addressed as we consider this an essential element of collaborative care.

As clinicians, we appreciate the difficulties associated with providing care to patients in subacute and long-term facilities. Hopefully this text will stimulate interest in the care of this growing population and facilitate the medical and nursing management of these patients.

Terry Buttaro
Susan Aznavorian
Karen Dick

ACKNOWLEDGMENTS

We wish to thank our colleagues and the reviewers who encouraged this endeavor. They understood our vision for a textbook that addressed the increasing complexity of post-hospital care and the importance of providing ongoing education for the staff caring for our patients.

Barbara Cullen, our Executive Publisher at Elsevier, recognized the importance of providing quality care in rehabilitation, subacute, and long-term care facilities and directed this publication. Her guidance and the assistance of Elsevier's editing and production staff are very much appreciated.

Throughout this project, our families and friends have been enthusiastic and understanding. They recognize the commitment we feel for our patients and the nursing profession. There are not words enough to thank them for their patience.

Lastly, we must thank our patients and their families.

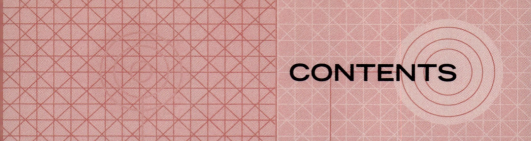

CONTENTS

CHAPTER 1

General Considerations for Care in Long-Term Care and Subacute Settings

The utilization of nursing home beds for patients in need of substantial skilled care after or instead of acute hospitalization occurred as a result of other changes in the healthcare system. A site for care was sought as payers looked to deliver services away from costly inpatient acute care facilities. Day surgery and ambulatory intravenous centers were opened, and patients were discharged from the hospitals "sicker and quicker." Home care agencies, family caregivers, and traditional nursing care facilities (skilled nursing facilities [SNFs] or nursing homes) were not prepared to provide the appropriate level of care. These financial concerns along with the change in philosophy of care coincided with an increased emergence of assisted living facilities and senior housing developments, leaving unfilled beds in existing nursing homes. In 1981 in Massachusetts, Fallon Community Health Care, a managed care plan with specific utilization criteria for specific services, negotiated a bed lease arrangement with a SNF. Fallon wanted to provide appropriate care for their patients in need of some rehabilitation before returning to prehospitalization living arrangements utilizing the least costly site for those patients. Healthcare providers looked at clinical needs, not provider location, provider convenience, or patient/family choice for site of care.

Subacute beds can be housed in skilled nursing facilities, transitional care units or step down units within an acute care hospital, in specialty hospitals, or in free standing facilities. The focus in subacute care is always on goal achievement, managing the consequences and cause of the current problem along with the previous health care conditions.

1

The Joint Commission on Accreditation of Health Care Organizations (JCAHO) has defined subacute care as:

"...the comprehensive inpatient care designed for someone who has an acute illness, injury, or exacerbation of a disease process. It is goal oriented treatment rendered immediately after, or instead of acute hospitalization to treat one or more specific active complex medical conditions or to administer one or more technically complex treatments, in the context of a person's underlying long-term conditions and overall situation. Generally, the individual's condition is such that the care does not depend heavily on high technology monitoring or complex diagnostic procedures. Subacute care requires the coordinated services of an interdisciplinary team that includes physicians, nurses and other relevant professional disciplines trained to assess and manage specific conditions and perform necessary procedures. Subacute care is given as part of a specifically defined program, regardless of the site. It is generally more intensive than traditional nursing facility care and less than acute care. It requires frequent (daily or weekly) recurrent patient assessment and review of the clinical course and treatment plan for a limited (several days to several months) time period, until the condition is stabilized or a predetermined treatment course is completed."

Care in subacute units requires an increased presence of medical providers as well as an increase in skilled staff. As well as professional expertise, providers must be aware of the regulations, requirements, and reimbursement systems in place in the subacute system.

Government regulations have impacted the changes in practice in nursing homes. In 1987, the Omnibus Budget Reconciliation Act (OBRA) improved quality of care in nursing homes through the standardization of staffing, documentation, restraint use, medication use, and physician/nonphysician provider requirements for patient evaluations. The enactment of the Balanced Budget Act (BBA) in 1997 was an effort by the government to control costs by reducing Medicare payments to nursing homes and eliminating fraud and abuse. The implications of the BBA of 1997 have been monumental. Medicare's case mix concept with prospective payment system (PPS) has been in effect since 1998. Payment to nursing facilities participating in Medicare and Medicaid programs is based on an episode of care. This prospective payment system assumes that care is driven by a patient's functional dependence and the utilization of rehabilitation services. Per diem payment for therapies, along with ancillary and capital costs, is bundled and based on each patient's classification into one of 44 resource utilization groups (RUGS) similar to the hospital's diagnosis-related group (DRG). However, the RUG is based on care needs and utilization rather than diagnosis. The RUGS have seven major categories: rehabilitation, extensive services, special care, clinically complex care, impaired cognition, behavior only, and physical function. These RUGS are based on the MDS-PAC (post-acute care MDS). The minimum data set (MDS), which consists of more than 400 items, is the assessment, care planning, and quality assurance tool regarding a patient's functional status, psychosocial status, medical condition, cognitive patterns, communication and hearing patterns, physical function, structural problems, continence, skin condition, special treatments, and procedures. The information from the MDS establishes a beneficiary's eligibility for Medicare services and for the level of reimbursement based on the patient's acuity during the 14 days prior to admission to a subacute bed.

CRITERIA FOR ADMISSION

As a rule, patients admitted to an SNF subacute unit must require 4 to 6 hours of skilled nursing care in a 24-hour period or be able to tolerate a minimum amount of therapy each day: up to 3 hours a day, 6 days a week, from 2 or 3 therapeutic rehabilitation disciplines. Most patients are admitted directly from the hospital (approximately 4% to 16% of acute care hospital admissions are potential candidates for a subacute unit) and need significant skilled medical treatment, monitoring, and/or rehabilitation related to the acute care stay. Medicare reimburses subacute care as long as the patient has stayed in the hospital for 3 nights and has met the skilled criteria for admission (within 30 days of hospital discharge). Insurance will only reimburse for the subacute stay when the patient has a skilled nursing need or rehabilitation needs. Managed care patients may or may not have been hospitalized before admission to the subacute unit. Managed care organizations may have contracts with a subacute unit as well as specific expectations for their patient's subacute stay, and their patients may be admitted directly from the emergency department or home as long as there is a skilled need.

Some subacute units have screeners who seek out appropriate patients for the unit. These screeners communicate with the admissions person on the subacute unit regarding bed availability and schedule a date to transfer a patient to the unit. The nonphysician provider (nurse practitioner [NP], physician assistant [PA], or clinical nurse specialist [CNS]) may be asked to review a patient's screen to determine the potential for improvement or problems, as well as to examine discharge planning issues and the estimated length of stay. It is important that the subacute unit be able to manage specific patients properly based on a patient's medical condition, acuity, and behavior, as well as the skills of the unit staff.

The patient's finances and insurance may be an issue should such a patient need or want long-term care. Before the patient is admitted, discharge planning needs must be considered. Does the patient have a living situation that will be safe and available for him or her? Will the patient be able to manage independently again? Can the patient stay on the unit long term if necessary? Is the family supportive and involved?

PATIENT PROFILE

A typical patient may require intravenous antibiotic therapy for an infection, rehabilitation after a fall or cerebrovascular accident, anticoagulant regulation for a deep vein thrombosis (DVT), pain management, or extensive skin treatments or specialized dressings for skin breakdown. Exacerbations of heart failure, chronic obstructive pulmonary disease (COPD), or other chronic conditions may also be well managed on a subacute unit.

Surgical patients may be recovering from thoracic or abdominal surgery, joint replacement or orthopedic injury, lower limb amputation, post operative wound infection, or post operative weakness. They may also need teaching or adjustment to a new colostomy. Medical problems include but are not limited to tube feedings, diabetic teaching, weaning from oxygen, medication titration, change in mental status, functional decline, deconditioning after hospitalization, or exacerbation of an existing condition or injury.

DOCUMENTATION

Thorough documentation is essential to satisfy the requirements of the MDS, state regulations, medical necessity, coding, billing, and regulatory and certifying organizations. The history and physical examination must be completed and documented by the physician within 48 hours of the patient's admission to the subacute unit (see Chapter 2). Each patient encounter should be documented in the patient's record using the standard SOAP format. The documentation should reflect the level of skill involved in the encounter (see Chapter 2). The patient's weight, vital signs, current laboratory values, mental status, progress with rehabilitation, response to medications and interventions, current functional status (including eating, sleeping, and bladder and bowel patterns), and pertinent physical findings should all be addressed in the patient's record. Rationales for decisions regarding patient care should be evident. Specific wound dimensions and changes in the healing of a wound should be carefully documented. Clinical guidelines, clinical pathways, and protocols should be utilized. Evidence of practice to continually move the patient along the continuum of care should appear as goals are addressed. What is written in the patient's record is the documentation for regulations, reimbursement, litigation, and quality of care.

ADMISSION PROCESS

The patient should arrive on the subacute unit with a discharge summary and/or a three-page referral form, depending on the referral source. Medicare requires that a physician perform the admission history and physical examination (see Chapter 2). The patient can subsequently be seen by an NP, PA, or CNS, who should also review the discharge summary and referral forms and examine the patient. Additional information should be elicited from the patient and/or family, because changes in medications during a recent acute illness can impact the subacute progress. For example, diuretics may have been discontinued in the acute care setting, but they may become necessary as the patient's condition changes.

Any questions or concerns about the discharge orders from the referral source should be addressed to enhance continuity of care. Often care has been started in the hospital and needs to be completed during the subacute admission. Communication with the providers from the referral site, whether it is the case manager, nurse, or physician promotes continuity and good interagency relationships.

ADVANCED DIRECTIVES

If the patient does not have a healthcare proxy, it is prudent to have a practical conversation with the patient and family discussing the need for a decision maker in the event the patient becomes incapacitated. It is also very important to clarify the "do not resuscitate" status (and have the appropriate paperwork signed by the patient or responsible party). Once signed, the healthcare proxy and "do not resuscitate" documents should be placed in the chart. A copy should be given to the healthcare proxy and primary care physician.

HISTORY AND PHYSICAL EXAMINATION

Medicare will not reimburse the nonphysician provider for the initial patient history and physical examination because current regulations require these be performed by a physician. However, it is essential that the nonphysician provider review the history and obtain additional history as is necessary from the patient, family, referring facility, or physician.

In addition, the nonphysician provider should also perform a thorough physical examination. Often thrush, athlete's feet (dermatophytosis), a breast mass, skin breakdown, cerumen, or impacted or guaiac positive stool may be found. All dressings should be removed to carefully examine all skin areas. The assessment should include information on eyes, hearing, and teeth, as well as medical, nursing, and functional diagnoses. These should all be included in a detailed problem list in the patient's chart with a list of allergies and current medications.

NURSING CARE AND ORDERS

Goals should be established for a patient plan of care that is inclusive and reasonable. The more specific the care that the patient requires (for example, special foot care for all diabetics), the more reimbursement the facility receives. Careful documentation is required for reimbursement. Staff may also need education regarding specific orders. It is also necessary to remember that each facility usually has standing orders and expectations, which may require special written orders. All facilities are required to administer the tuberculosis (TB) diagnostic (PPD) and clarify flu and pneumonia vaccine status on admission. Tetanus immunization should also be updated. Patients on warfarin (Coumadin) should have parameters placed in a Coumadin book. It is crucial to try to anticipate problems and address them in the orders. This will facilitate patient care for the staff nurses and minimize problems for covering medical providers.

In addition to orders received on page one from the referring physician/ hospital, orders should reflect the patient's needs and best interests. Orders are individualized for each patient and intended to promote well-being, safety, and comfort. Issues that should be considered include, but certainly are not limited to, the following:

- Regularly scheduled weights and vital signs
- Diet and nutritional considerations
    - Multivitamin with minerals daily
    - Fortified foods, supplemental feedings, and/or between meal snacks if indicated
    - Assistance with feeding if necessary
- Safety issues
- Intravenous fluids or medications
- Skin care
    - Bathing routine (if daily showering is indicated)
    - Routine sacral and heel care to prevent skin breakdown
    - Regularly scheduled positioning changes in bed and wheelchair for patients at risk for skin breakdown
    - Special mattresses if indicated
- Eye care
    - Twice daily eye wash with half-strength baby shampoo to control blepharitis
- Mouth and dental care
    - Dental consultation is necessary for patients with broken, decayed teeth, and/or gingivitis.
    - Specific directions are needed for mouth care each morning, evening, and PRN (to help decrease the incidence of aspiration pneumonia and promote oral health).
- Foot care
    - Cream to lower extremities daily
    - Diabetic foot care if indicated
    - Linard boots to prevent heel ulcers in susceptible patients
- Dressing orders and consultations with wound specialists if indicated
- Mobility (e.g., ambulate independently, bed to chair)
- Physical and occupational therapy referral
- Bowel management program
    - If incontinence has been a problem, a bladder and bowel program is necessary.
- Pain and sleep medications if indicated
- Accuchecks and sliding scale regular insulin orders if indicated

- Warfarin (Coumadin) orders and parameters if indicated
- Endocarditis prophylaxis: for patients with prosthetic heart valves, mechanical bioprostheses, homografts, complex congenital heart disease or congenital defects, surgically constructed pulmonary shunts, acquired valvular dysfunction, hypertrophic cardiomyopathy, mitral valve prolapse with regurgitation and/or thickening of the leaflets, or previous history of infective endocarditis)
- Osteoporosis prevention regime
- Other therapeutic medications, always considering allergies, comorbidities, cost, as well as the facility formulary
- Appropriate initial laboratory diagnostics as indicated by history, physical examination, medications, and comorbidities
  - Common practice includes ordering CBC/diff, glucose, electrolytes, BUN, creatinine, and PT/INR if indicated. Consider TSH and LFTs.
- Flu vaccine, pneumovax, and tetanus immunization if indicated

DISCHARGE PLANNING

The discharge plan starts during the admission process. The patient's social situation as well as patient and family concerns must be addressed and considered. Orders should reflect education needs for the patient and family addressing the need for information and techniques, which will affect the patient's independence for discharge.

The name, address, and phone number of the primary care provider and any agencies or services used by the patient prior to the illness should be determined and documented in the patient's chart. Communication with previous healthcare providers and agencies providing care, whether it was a home care agency or day care, is often indispensable. This information will assist with discharge planning. In addition, open communication with members of the nursing and rehabilitation staff, social worker, and of course, the attending physician facilitates effective, collaborative patient care.

FAMILY ISSUES

Patients and families especially may need assistance in coping with a new diagnosis, a decline in function, placement issues, or terminal illness. Whenever possible, it is necessary to obtain the patient's permission to speak with the family, not only to share information, but also to establish goals for care and a therapeutic relationship. (Always be cognizant of HIPPA regulations.) This is also a good time to orient patient and family to the facility and the system, establish realistic patient and family expectations, discuss discharge plans, if appropriate, and identify one family member as the spokesperson for providers to communicate with. Encourage patients and families to first communicate problems with the bedside nurse who, in turn, will communicate with the healthcare provider. Families need to know how the system works so they feel comfortable with the care and feel part of the team.

Bibliography

Burl, J.B., & Campbell, I. (1997). Impact of a paradigm change in the management of HMO patients admitted for subacute care. *Annals of Long-Term Care, 5*(12), 426-432.

Dajani, A.S., et al. (1997). Prevention of bacterial endocarditis: Recommendations by the American Heart Association. *Journal of the American Medical Association, 277*(22), 1794-1801.

Dimant, J. (1998). PPS and other recent federal regulatory developments: A paradigm change needed in the roles of physician and medical director. *Annals of Long-Term Care, 6*(13), 434-438.

Heist, K.K. (1998). SNFs, RUGS, and PPS. *ADVANCE for Providers of Post-Acute Care, 2*(5), 39-41.

Joint Commission for the Accreditation of Healthcare Organizations. (1996). *Accreditation protocol for subacute programs.* Oakbrook Terrace, IL. JCAHO.

Levenson, S.A. (1996). *Subacute and transitional care handbook: Defining, delivering, and improving care.* Beverly-Cracom Publications.

Ouslander, J.G., et al. (1997) *Medical care in the nursing home.* New York. McGraw-Hill.

Rantz, M.J., et al. (1999). The minimum date set: No longer just for clinical assessment. *Annals of Long-Term Care, 7*(9), 354-359.

Stahl, D.A. (1997). Balanced Budget Act of 1997: What it means for subacute care. *Nursing Management, 28*(11), 28-29.

Tomosa, N., & Morley, J. (2000). *Clinics in Geriatric Medicine: Subacute Care for Seniors, 16*(4), entire issue.

CHAPTER 2

Regulations and Reimbursement

As the population ages and healthcare costs are shifted, more patients are being cared for in skilled nursing and long-term care facilities. Care in these facilities consists of two levels: (1) routine or basic custodial care and (2) skilled nursing rehabilitation services. Usually, Medicare-eligible patients will be admitted for skilled care or rehabilitation under Medicare Part A, after being hospitalized for a minimum of 3 days. The goal of skilled nursing or rehabilitation care is to return the patient to the community. Some patients are unable to return to the community and become permanent residents in the nursing home.

Federal and state regulations require physician presence in acute rehabilitation, skilled nursing, and long-term care settings. Medicare, Medicaid, and state regulations establish specific requirements for patient visits (Box 2-1). In July 2003, The Center for Medicare and Medicaid Services (CMS) reiterated that a nonphysician provider (nurse practitioner [NP], clinical nurse specialist [CNS], or physician assistant [PA]) in a skilled nursing or routine nursing facility may perform any required physician task as long as the nonphysician provider has a collaborative relationship with the physician (MD or DO), is not employed by the nursing facility, and the task is not prohibited by state law. NPs must be certified by the American Nurses Credentialing Center (ANCC), the American Academy of Nurse Practitioners, or other national credentialing organization, and, as of January 1, 2003, must have graduated from an accredited program with a master's degree. CNSs also must have a graduate degree and be certified by the ANCC or other credentialing organization, PAs attend accredited educational programs and are certified by the National Commission on Certification of Physician Assistants. In addition, the NP, CNS, or PA must be licensed by the state, and the care provided to the patient must be within the nonphysician provider's scope of practice as described by state law.

BOX 2-1   CMS Physician/Nonphysician Requirements in Skilled Nursing and Long-Term Care Settings

Acute Rehabilitation

1. Initial comprehensive visit must be performed by physician within 48 hours of admission.
2. After initial visit, physician and nonphysician provider may alternate visits.
3. Patient should be seen every 7 days.

Skilled Nursing Care in Non-Acute Settings

1. Initial comprehensive visit must be performed by physician within 30 days of admission.
    a. Nonphysician provider can see patient for medically necessary visits prior to physician's initial comprehensive visit.
2. Patient visit is required every 30 days for the first 90 days; after 90 days, visits can be extended to every 60 days (but Medicare requires physician visit every 120 days). Physician and nonphysician provider visits may alternate.
3. Nonphysician provider can make additional visits as medically necessary.

Long-Term Care Facility

1. Initial comprehensive visit by physician or nonphysician provider. Attending physician may waive initial history and physical if performed 5 days prior to admission or during hospital stay.
2. Patient visit required every 30 days for the first 90 days after admission; after 90 days, patient visits can be extended to once every 60 days (but Medicare requires physician visit every 120 days). Nonphysician provider can make additional visits as medically necessary.

- State regulations determine the performance of physician tasks by nonphysician providers, if the delegation of tasks is permitted by state law or facility policy.
- Nonphysician provider visits are subject to scope of practice laws in each state.
- Nonphysician provider cannot be employed by the facility and must have a collaborative relationship with the physician. NPs, PAs, and CNSs employed by the facility *can* see a patient (and write orders) for a medically necessary visit. The orders must be verified and signed by the physician.
- NP or clinical nurse specialist can sign Medicare and Medicaid certifications and recertifications if permitted by state regulations and not employed by the facility. At this time, a PA cannot sign certifications and recertifications in a SNF, but if permitted by state regulations, he or she may sign certifications in the long-term care facility.

For patients in skilled nursing facilities, as well as for patient in long-term care in a Part A Medicare stay, the CMS regulations require that the initial comprehensive visit be made by the physician. (Nonphysician providers cannot be reimbursed for the initial comprehensive visit.) The history, physical examination forms, and certification documentation for skilled care are completed by the physician at this visit. CMS has specified that the nonphysician provider may visit the patient before the patient is seen by the physician (and be reimbursed), but only if the visit is medically necessary (a new medical problem necessitating medical evaluation before the physician is able to see the patient). The nonphysician provider and physician may then alternate visits to the patient. The nonphysician provider can also make visits when medically necessary. In long-term care facilities, the nonphysician provider, if not employed by the facility, can perform the admitting history and physical examination on these patients as long as these patients do not require skilled nursing or rehabilitation care and the visits are not reimbursed by Medicare.

Healthcare providers are reimbursed by Medicare, Medicare managed care organizations, Medicaid, and/or private health insurance. For eligible patients, Medicare Part B reimburses visits by nonphysician providers at 85% of the payment made to physicians, or 80% of the lesser of the actual charges. Medicare requires the healthcare provider to obtain a Medicare PIN (individual's billing number) and UPIN (number for ordering goods or services) from the local Medicare carrier. In some cases, the PIN is reassigned to a group number to allow the employer to receive reimbursement from Medicare. Reimbursement is based on the complexity of decisions involved in each encounter. Payment is related to the level of acuity based on Current Procedural Terminology (CPT) codes determined by the American Medical Association (AMA) and the federal government (Box 2-2). SNF and long-term care facility visits are classified as problem focused (examination of one body area/ organ system), expanded problem focused (examination of two body areas/organ systems), detailed (examination of two body areas/organ systems), or comprehensive (examination of eight organ systems) (Box 2-3). The CPT and International Classification of Diseases (ICD-9) codes submitted for billing must be well supported by the documentation in the patient's record. While the history, physical examination, and the extent of medical decision-making usually determine the correct level of billing, time spent during the encounter establishes the proper billing for counseling, coordination of care, and meeting with families. (The amount of time spent on these aspects of care should be documented in the patient's record.) The provider's documentation should support the level of complexity involved in medical decision-making (including differential diagnoses, number of diagnostics, risk for complications, and management choices). To comply with reimbursement requirements, the documentation for each visit must be able to stand on its own without depending on unwritten information. Visit documentation should begin with the date and reason for the visit and include pertinent family, social and past medical history. The chief complaint, history of present illness, review of systems, physical examination, previous diagnostics, assessment and treatment

---

BOX 2-2   Billing Codes for Nursing Facility Services

New or Established Patient Comprehensive Nursing Facility Evaluations Requires Detailed Interval History, Comprehensive Examination, and Straightforward Medical Decision-Making

99303—High complexity: complex admission or readmission (50 minutes); must be performed by a physician, can involve counseling, coordination of care; may also be used for established patient with a significant, permanent change in status that necessitates a new plan of care *or* if taking over care from another provider and new problems are identified and addressed in care plan

99302—Moderate complexity: simple admission or readmission or complex; annual assessment (40 minutes); also may be used for new problem or change in status (i.e., myocardial infarction, stroke, or other significant new problem treated in facility)

99301—Low complexity: stable or recovering patient requiring simple annual assessment (30 minutes)

Subsequent Nursing Facility Evaluations Requires Two of the Following: History, Physical Examination, or Medical Decision-Making

99313—High: major medical event or major new problem requiring extensive evaluation, diagnostics, and treatment (35 minutes)

99312—Moderate: new complaint, change in treatment, not responding to previous treatment at follow-up; requires examination of several organ systems/body areas (25 minutes)

99311—Low: routine, recertification, or follow-up visit, to a stable, recovering, improving patient (15 minutes)

Nursing Facility Discharge

99316—Discharge: more than 30 minutes
99315—Discharge: 30 minutes or less

Procedure Codes for Common Procedures in Nursing Facilities

43760—Change gastrostomy tube
43761—Reposition gastrostomy tube
T7010—Suture removal
53670—Foley catheterization: simple urethra

---

plan must reflect the patient's condition. Visits to patients who are unstable, need immediate treatment, or require close monitoring are considered high-complexity visits. Visits to patients who are stable are considered to be low-acuity visits. Failure to document appropriately might result in payment denial as well as accusations of billing fraud.

Reimbursement from insurers other than Medicare can vary from state to state and does not necessarily have the same healthcare provider restrictions regarding patient visitation and reimbursement. NPs, CNSs, and PAs should

---

BOX 2-3 **Recognized Body Areas and Organ Systems for Evaluation and Management Services**

Body Areas	Organ Systems
Face and head	Constitutional
Neck	Eyes
Chest, breasts, and axilla	Ears, nose, mouth, and throat
Abdomen	Cardiovascular
Genitalia, groin, and buttocks	Respiratory
Back and spine	Gastrointestinal
Extremities	Genitourinary
	Musculoskeletal
	Skin
	Neurologic
	Psychologic
	Hematologic and lymphatic

---

obtain a Medicaid provider number from the state in which they practice and be empaneled by private healthcare insurance plans to ensure reimbursement.

NPs and other nonphysician providers can assist physicians and improve patient care in these facilities. However, it is essential that nonphysician providers discuss federal and state regulations with their collaborating physicians as well as the nursing facility to ensure that patients admitted to acute and long-term care settings receive timely, appropriate assessment and consistent quality care. Knowledge of regulations and relevant legislation is necessary for all healthcare providers to ensure compliance with Medicare guidelines and ensure appropriate reimbursement, particularly because Medicare policies are often amended. Proper documentation and billing practices must also be reviewed with the collaborating physician and practice manager to ensure that services are billed correctly.

RESOURCES

For information regarding state practice acts: */www.ncsbn.org/public/regulation/ nursing_practice_acts.htm*

For information about the CMS: *www.cms.hhs.gov/medlearn/matters* or *www.cms.hhs.gov/providerupdate/january2004/nonphys.asp*

Bibliography

American Medical Association. (2003). *Current procedural terminology 2003.* Chicago: AMA.

Buppert, C. (2002). Billing for nurse practitioner services: Guidelines for NPs, physicians, employers, and insurers. *Medscape Nurses, 4*(1). *www.medscape.com/viewarticle/422935*. Accessed June 30, 2004.

Laporte, M. (2003). CMS clarifies physician use of midlevel practitioners. *Caring for the Ages, 4*(9), 4,11.

Lusis, SA. (2004). Medicare reimbursement in long-term care. *Medscape Nurses*. Accessed May 7, 2004.

Skin Disorders

SKIN LESIONS

People of all ages are affected by skin disorders. However, older people are at increased risk because of a diminished immune system; increased exposure to sun, smoke, and pollutants; and the physiologic skin changes associated with aging (aged skin is dryer, more fragile, and less elastic). In addition, drug reactions are common in the elderly population because they consume so many medications.

The most common skin problems include contact dermatitis, xerosis (dry skin), atopic dermatitis (eczematous dermatitis), psoriasis, warts, fungal infections, herpes simplex or zoster, and cancers. Complications from illnesses such as diabetes and peripheral vascular disease can also present as skin disorders. Skin symptoms may also indicate a systemic or metabolic disease and can require an emergency response.

Risk Factors

- Aging causes dryness, increased fragility, thinning, decreased elasticity, changes in pigment cells, and a decrease in cellular immunity, which contributes to bullous pemphigoid and zoster.
- Extra skin folds associated with obesity increase the risk for infection and rashes.
- Medications may cause allergic reactions or contact dermatitis and increase the risk for fungal infections.
- Poor hygiene and institutionalization increase the risk for scabies, lice, yeast, and skin infections.
- Immunocompromised persons have increased risk for scabies, herpes zoster, fungal infections, skin ulcers, and other dermatoses.

15

- Radiation treatment may compromise the lymphatic system and lower skin immunity.
- Environmental influences such as heat or humidity increase the risk for dry skin and fungal infections.

History

It is important to elicit the patient's allergies (i.e., a sulfa allergy will prohibit using Silvadene cream), current medications (including ointments and over-the-counter, herbal, and prescribed medications), and past medical history. Medications can cause rashes, and several will exacerbate psoriasis or other skin disorders. A personal history of hypercholesteremia can explain xanthomas. Immunocompromised patients (i.e., patients with diabetes or receiving chemotherapy) are more prone to herpes zoster, yeast, or fungal infections. A family history is necessary, as some skin disorders are familial.

A careful symptom analysis is essential as information regarding the onset and progression of the skin lesion aids in diagnosis. A review of systems to determine associated symptoms, exposures, or related illness is also important and may suggest possible diagnosis. For example:

- Psoriasis may have a gradual onset or be exacerbated by recent stress, injury, or streptococcal infection.
- Recent injury, stress, fever, malaise, pain, and pruritus frequently precede a herpes zoster eruption.
- Exposure to medications, toxins, new clothing, cosmetics, and soaps may cause contact or allergic dermatitis.
- Recent antibiotic use may result in *Candida* or *Tinea*.
- An explosive onset of rash may indicate a streptococcal infection.
- Travel history is important because stasis dermatitis may occur after sitting for long periods in a car or plane.
- Associated symptoms, such as fever, may accompany cellulitis or herpes zoster; pruritus is associated with xerosis, contact dermatitis, seborrheic dermatitis, allergic reactions, psoriasis, renal failure, and cholestasis.
- Pruritus that increases in severity at night suggests scabies.
- Bleeding, nonhealing lesions suggest malignancy.

Physical Examination

A careful skin examination of hair, scalp, mouth, under breasts, intergluteal folds, groin, nails, and feet (including plantar surfaces) noting and documenting the size, location, and characteristics of the lesions is necessary. Accompanying physical findings are important to determine. Lymphadenopathy may suggest infection or malignancy; fever and malaise are common with herpes zoster and skin infections. The distribution of the lesions is also significant. Unilateral lesions that occur along a dermatome without crossing the midline are indicative of herpes zoster. The following factors should be considered when examining the lesion and surrounding skin.

Characteristics
It is important to determine both the size and features of a lesion.
- Macules: nonpalpable, flat, and less than 1 cm
- Papules: small, palpable, and raised less than 1 cm
- Plaques: large, flat, and superficial; can be grouped papules greater than 1 cm
- Vesicles: small, fluid-filled papules (as in herpes zoster)
- Nodules/tumors: large, palpable, and often hard
- Cysts: soft, well-defined, and palpable
- Pustules: small papules filled with purulent fluid
- Bullae: large vesicles
- Wheals: irregular, elevated skin areas with well-defined borders
- Telangiectasis: dilated, superficial blood vessels; frequently seen with malignant lesions, cirrhosis, and rosacea
- Fissures: deep crevices; seen in xerosis and athlete's foot
- Erosion: shallow open area (as opposed to an ulcer, which is deeper)
- Scales: dead cells cast off; seen with xerosis and psoriasis
- Excoriation: erosion from scratching
- Edema: fluid retention
- Atrophy: thinning, shrunken appearance
- Lichenification: increased thick skin markings associated with psoriasis and other chronic skin disorders
- Crust: dried exudate, including eschar
- Hypopigmentation/hyperpigmentation
- Burrows: tracks under the skin; associated with scabies

Consistency
- Soft, hard, or fluctuant

Margins
- Defined, raised, and regular or irregular

Condition of Surrounding Skin
- Scratch marks, lichenification, hypopigmented/hyperpigmented, erythema, or edema

Location
Location often will suggest the type of skin lesion.
- Scalp: skin cancers, herpes zoster, lice, and psoriasis
- Face: basal cell carcinoma, squamous cell carcinoma, rosacea, seborrheic dermatitis, and lentigos (age spots)
- Ears: psoriasis, seborrheic dermatitis, carcinomas, and tophi

- Lips: herpes simplex, carcinomas, and perlèche (corners of lips)
- Mouth: leukoplakia, aphthous ulcer, thrush, and cancers
- Tongue: candidiasis, leukoplakia, or painless lesions; also a common site for carcinomas, especially in smokers
- Nails: onychomycosis, psoriasis, and melanoma
- Hands: xerosis, allergic dermatitis, scabies (between fingers, wrist folds), and lentigo
- Elbow: psoriasis (extensor surface)
- Axilla: folliculitis, contact dermatitis, and candidiasis
- Trunk/torso: tinea versicolor, keratoses, and carcinomas
- Knees: psoriasis
- Under breasts: intertrigo/candidiasis
- Back: psoriasis, herpes zoster (along dermatome), and carcinomas
- Abdomen: bullous pemphigoid
- Groin: yeast, psoriasis, and infections
- Lower extremities: xerosis, arterial/venous ulcer, tumors, and melanoma
- Feet: tinea, xerosis, melanomas, and tophi (on toes)

Differential Diagnosis

Skin disorders are differentiated by the appearance of the lesion. For example, macules may suggest some disorders, while papules, plaques, or vesicles suggest other skin conditions. Distinguishing between lesions aids in the differential diagnosis. However, many disorders have more than one type of lesion.

Macules

- Drug reaction: a macular, papular, occasionally vesicular, erythematous, pruritic rash that usually starts 1 to 10 days after a drug is started. The reaction is often accompanied by systemic symptoms and may last up to 2 weeks after the drug is stopped. Occasionally, reaction has a delayed response.
- Purpura: flat, discolored, purplish lesions; common in elders
- Stasis dermatitis or varicose eczema: acute and chronic, but usually a persistent, pruritic inflammation of the lower extremities associated with increased pigmentation, venous disease, and edema. The skin may develop ulcerated areas if not treated. Skin is often dry, scaly, erythematous; occasionally bullae may be present. Often confused with contact dermatitis, cellulitis, or cancer. Common in obesity; more common in women than in men.

Papules

- Scabies: contagious, pruritic papules or vesicles with burrows caused by mites; found in finger/toe webs, wrists, axillae, areolae, hairline, abdomen (belt line), scrotum, groin, and buttocks fold. Transmitted by close contact. Incubation period is 4 to 6 weeks. Itch is worse at night. May have associated lymphadenopathy, excoriations from scratching, and superimposed infection. Frequently confused with contact dermatitis, seborrheic dermatitis, or psoriasis.

- Pediculosis: very pruritic lesions often noted on scalp, body, or pubic areas. Scales not easily removed.
- Actinic keratosis: flat or elevated macule or papule that may be erythematous, white, gray, or yellow with adherent scale and may occur on sun-exposed skin. May develop into a horn or squamous cell carcinoma.
- Basal cell carcinoma: slow-growing, painless lesion often noted on the face. Lesion has ill-defined borders and may have a rolled edge or central ulceration. Lesions are nonhealing and bleed easily.
- Keratoacanthoma: a smooth, nodular lesion with a central keratin plug that occurs rapidly and is locally destructive. The lesion is benign but may resemble a squamous cell carcinoma.
- Squamous cell carcinoma: firm, hard, irregular fleshy pink lesion that can increase in size rapidly or ulcerate. It is locally invasive with potential to metastasize and may involve lymph nodes.
- Melanoma: asymmetric brown, black, or multicolored lesion that can be macular, papular, nodular, or even plaquelike. The lesion grows rapidly and has irregular margins and may have several shades of colors (pink, red, black, or blue on surface). Lesion may occur in mouth, eye, nails, soles of feet, or elsewhere on body.
- Seborrheic keratoses: black to brown raised lesions with rough, waxy surface usually found on the face and body
- Acne rosacea: symmetric inflammatory papules and pustules with telangiectasia and flushing on nose, cheeks, forehead, and chin; may cause rhinophyma and conjunctivitis.
- Cutaneous horn: usually occurs above the neck and often on an ear.
- Psoriasis: thickened epidermis with silver, white, scaly, well-demarcated, adherent, bright papules and plaques that occur on scalp, ear canals, behind ears, elbows, knees, buttocks, intergluteal cleft, nails, palms, and soles of feet. A chronic disease more common in women and characterized by remissions and exacerbations, psoriasis is pruritic and may be precipitated by stress, anxiety, drugs, illness, or trauma.
- Cherry angiomas: small, harmless, erythematous papules related to dilated blood vessels

Vesicles, Pustules, and Bullae
- Drug reaction: see Macules.
- Herpes zoster: a reactivation of the chicken pox virus, zoster occurs 10 times more often in those older than age 60. The rash (grouped vesicles on an erythematous base) develops after 1 to 3 days of malaise and/or fever accompanied by numbness or pain along one or more dermatomes (frequently, but not always, a cranial, facial, or thoracic dermatome) unilaterally without crossing the midline. A vesicle on the nose or near the eye requires particular attention as it may be indicative of ophthalmic involvement.

Vesicles become pustules in 3 to 4 days and crust in 7 to 10 days. Initial pain may be confused with angina or renal colic, but zoster may also be confused with urticaria or caruncles.

- Herpes simplex: tingling, burning, itching 24 hours before outbreak, the herpes vesicle usually occurs on lip and heals in 8 to 10 days.
- Burns: vesicles on any area exposed to an electrical, chemical, or thermal agent.
- Bullous pemphigoid: intact, tense, pruritic, subepidermal vesicle on lower abdomen, groin, or flexor surfaces of extremities; an autoimmune disorder that is common in elders. Differentiate with pemphigus lesions, which are flaccid bullae with ulcers or erosions.
- Contact dermatitis: erythematous areas with papules, vesicles, erosions, and crusting (with occasional oozing); develops after direct skin exposure to a substance. May be allergic or irritant induced. Common irritants include poison ivy, bleach, alcohol, jewelry, fragrances, nail polish, and topical medications such as neomycin, bacitracin, silver sulfadiazine, or lanolin.
- Toxic epidermal necrolysis: occurring usually on the lower extremities, the initial presentation is an erythematous area that rapidly progresses to a vesicular eruption. Often drug related or confused with cellulitis, toxic epidermal necrolysis is an acute emergency, requiring immediate attention.
- Intertrigo: plaques, patches, papules, pustules with well-defined borders; occurs in moist skin surfaces, such as the inframammary folds, inner thighs, axilla, or perianal area, where skin is in close contact with skin. Caused by *Candida*, intertrigo is sometimes confused with psoriasis, seborrheic dermatitis, contact dermatitis, or bacterial folliculitis.

Erosions/Ulcers
- Perlèche/angular cheilitis: moist, cracked, inflammatory fissures with deep folds at corners of mouth, caused by mixed bacterial and *Candida* infection. Associated with retention of saliva and food particles, poorly fitting dentures, or lack of dentures.

Plaques
- Tinea infections: pruritic, malodorous lesions with sharply demarcated borders caused by dermatophyte (fungal) infection; found in moist skin folds such as groin, axillae, and inframammary folds (particularly in women), or between fourth and fifth toes. Can cause hair loss or maceration. Onychomycosis is manifested as thick, yellow nails.
- Tinea versicolor: white, pink, hypo/hyperpigmented scaly papules and plaques that are occasionally pruritic; affects trunk, neck, and upper extremities during periods of high heat. Confused with pityriasis rosea, seborrheic dermatitis (usually in hairy areas), vitiligo, psoriasis, and nummular eczema.
- Psoriasis: see Papules
- Seborrheic dermatitis: pruritic, erythematous, scaling in areas of sebaceous glands (scalp, auricular area, eyebrows, face, nasal bridge, lateral sides of

nose, nasolabial folds of upper lip, and under a mustache); a chronic disorder that may be confused with psoriasis, atopic dermatitis, impetigo, rosacea, contact dermatitis, pityriasis versicolor or rosea, and scabies. Dandruff is seborrheic dermatitis of scalp.

- Thrush (*Candida* of mucous membranes): white or gray plaques that are difficult to scrape away. Oral thrush may be confused with aphthous ulcers or leukoplakia and extend down esophagus. Occurs frequently in patients on steroids or antibiotics.

Diagnostics

Diagnosis is usually made clinically and is based on lesion and symptoms. When diagnosis is unclear and/or treatment is not successful, a dermatologist should be consulted. Dermatologists might use a potassium hydroxide (KOH) preparation for fungal lesions, allergy skin tests, mineral oil scabies preparation, Tzanck preparation for evaluation of herpes simplex or herpes zoster, or biopsy or excision of lesion. Other diagnostics to consider include:

- Serum B_{12} level should be considered in the case of recurrent perlèche.
- A Doppler ultrasound may be warranted to exclude arterial disease in patients with stasis dermatitis or varicose eczema.

Treatment Plan

Treatment is individualized for each patient. Any new rash requires that all medications and dressing ointments be reviewed. Dry skin and pruritus are fairly prevalent, particularly in colder, winter climates, and, therefore, it is important to recognize and manage xerosis to promote patient comfort and prevent dry, cracked skin. General principles of skin care include:

- Adequate hydration and good hygiene decreases skin problems. Use tepid water and mild soaps (unscented Dove, Basis) to help prevent dry skin. Clean nails well to prevent secondary infection from scratching.
- Moisturizing creams should be applied daily (to damp skin) immediately after skin is patted dry after bath to prevent xerosis. Ammonium lactate 12% cream is suitable for patients with severe xerosis.
- Pruritus must be controlled to prevent scratching and superimposed infection. Creams containing menthol or phenol help relieve pruritus and, in elderly patients, should be tried before using antihistamines.
- The potency of topical corticosteroid depends on location, extent of involved area, length of use. Mild corticosteroids should be used on face and in skin folds. Overuse of topical corticosteroids can cause striae, thinning of skin, and systemic absorption.
  - Limit use of high-potency topical corticosteroids to 4 weeks of twice daily use.
  - Chronically use triamcinolone cream or 2.5% hydrocortisone sparingly and with caution.

- Treat fungus infections 2 weeks beyond clearance of rash, and continue with preventive measures.
- Topical creams and ointments should be applied sparingly and only to involved area.
- Expose skin to air (especially feet and areas covered by diapers) and keep skin off of skin in skin folds (e.g., under the female breast, in the groin area, on the feet).
- Consider environmental impact on skin. Maintain room temperature at approximately 68° F. Humidified air is often recommended, especially during winter months, although the benefit has not been proven.
- Cotton clothing absorbs moisture best.
- Protective clothing, sunscreen, and wide-brimmed hats should be worn when going out in the sun.

Macules

Drug reaction
- Identify and remove offending agent; may take 2 to 4 weeks for rash to resolve
- Symptom reduction: cool compresses, calamine, or Sarna lotion for pruritus
- Pharmacologic therapy
  - Severe reactions
    - Epinephrine 1:1000 (0.3 mL intramuscularly [IM]/subcutaneously [SQ] every 15 to 30 minutes) if systemic symptoms. Monitor for cardiovascular side effects.
    - Oral antihistamines
      - First generation antihistamines (must be used with caution in some patients, particularly elders, because of side effects)
        - Diphenhydramine (Benadryl) 25 mg q6h PRN, *or*
        - Hydroxyzine HCl (Atarax) 10 mg PO TID PRN, *or*
        - Cyproheptadine (Periactin) 2 to 4 mg PO tid
      - Second generation antihistamines
        - Fexofenadine (Allegra) 30 to 180 mg PO daily, *or*
        - Loratadine (Claritin) 10 mg PO daily, *or*
        - Cetirizine (Zyrtec) 5 to 10 mg PO daily (also associated with somnolence; use cautiously in elders)
    - Oral corticosteroids
    - **Emergency department (ED) evaluation if necessary or if initial response is poor**
  - Mild reactions: consider topical antihistamines and/or topical corticosteroids; consider Medrol dose pack for quick steroid taper

Stasis dermatitis
- Decrease edema to prevent skin ulceration and promote wound healing when lower extremity ulcers are present.

- Improve lower extremity venous return: elevate legs at least 30 minutes, four times daily, above level of heart. Discourage standing idle or sitting without elevating lower extremities.
- Rule out arterial disease: compare ankle blood pressure with brachial blood pressure. If ratio is less than 0.7, compression therapy is contraindicated.
- Compression stockings or ACE wraps (if not contraindicated): should be put on first thing in the morning before patient gets out of bed and removed at bedtime. Pneumatic compression may be indicated for severe edema.
- If the wound is oozing or the patient is unable to apply compression stockings: apply dressing, Kling, and then ACE wraps with even compression. Consider Unna boot with zinc oxide and gelatin, applied with even pressure, starting at foot (may need assistance, if unfamiliar with application). Initially change Unna boot every 2 to 3 days. Once oozing stops and/or edema decreases, may leave Unna boot on for 7 days.
- Use mild soap or mineral oil to clean/hydrate skin. Avoid trauma and hot water baths.
- Pharmacologic therapy
  - Diuretic therapy if indicated to reduce edema
  - Antibiotic therapy if indicated for infection
  - Lubricate dry, pruritic areas with a thin film of mild corticosteroid ointment (hydrocortisone 2.5% [Hytone]) BID for 1 to 2 weeks

Papules

Scabies
- Topical corticosteroids for pruritus
- Second generation H_1 blocker fexofenadine (Allegra), 60 mg PO tid prn *or* cetirizine (Zyrtec), 5 to 10 mg PO at bedtime *or* hydroxyzine (Atarax), 10 mg PO tid to qid (use Atarax cautiously in elders) for pruritus
- Permethrin 5% (Elimite) cream from neck down with special care to axillae, umbilicus, interdigital webs, gluteal cleft, under nails, and along hairline. Apply under nails and in umbilicus using cotton swabs. Wash off in 8 to 12 hours. Repeat treatment in 1 week.
- Wash all linens and clothes in hot water. Dry in commercial dryer on hot cycle.
- Vacuum area.
- Reevaluate in 3 to 6 weeks.
- Treat asymptomatic contacts once.
- Monitor for secondary infection.
- Consult dermatology if considering use of ivermectin 200 mcg/kg in single dose (usually 12 to 18 mcg).

Pediculosis
Head and pubis
- White vinegar rubbed into scalp and pubic hair may loosen nits.
- Shampoo with regular shampoo or soap, then rinse. Apply permethrin (Nix 1% crème rinse) or pyrethrins 0.33% (Rid). Leave for 10 minutes, then rinse out and vigorously comb hair with fine-toothed special nit comb. (Soak combs and brushes in Rid for 1 hour after use.) Repeat shampoo and combing in 10 days.
- Machine wash or dry clean all personal items.
- Disinfect environment.
- Treat controls only once.
Eyelashes
- Apply Vaseline to eyelashes BID for 5 days. Remove nits manually.
Body
- Treat with 5% permethrin (as for scabies), with retreatment after 1 week.
- Disinfect environment.
- Treat contacts only once.

Actinic keratosis
- Refer patient to dermatology for liquid nitrogen (necrosis will occur in 10 to 14 days with formation of new epidermis) or, using gloves, apply fluorouracil 1% (Efudex cream) BID and cover with DSD for 2 to 4 weeks. Skin will become intensely inflamed, crust, and dry.

Basal cell carcinoma, keratoacanthoma, melanoma, cutaneous horn, and squamous cell carcinoma
- Refer to dermatology for biopsy and/or complete excision.

Seborrheic keratoses
- No treatment unless they become irritated, annoying, or disfiguring. Pruritic keratoses require further evaluation for internal malignancy.

Acne rosacea
- Eliminate extrinsic causes of vasodilation, such as heat, stress, sun exposure, spicy foods, alcohol, hot beverages.
- Pharmacologic therapy
  - Metrogel (metronidazole 0.75%) lotion or cream BID after washing and gently patting skin dry. Use alone for 2 months until clear, then once daily or
  - Clindamycin lotion 1% BID (after careful washing and drying) for 2 months until clear, then once daily
  - If severe case rosacea, oral antibiotics in conjunction with topical treatment may be beneficial. Consider using one of the following oral antibiotics for 2 months, then taper off oral antibiotics and maintain topical therapy.
    - Tetracycline 500 mg PO BID, *or*

■ Erythromycin 500 mg PO BID, *or*
■ Doxycycline 50 mg PO BID for 2 months

Psoriasis

- Provide emotional support.
- Encourage relaxation and meditation.
- Scalp lesions: tar shampoo (tazarotene 0.05%) thin film daily and applied with gloves. Use cautiously with broken skin and if pregnancy is a consideration. Avoid facial area. Very drying.
- Mild disease
  - Gently remove scale with Aveeno bath. Apply moisturizers, lubricants to limit dryness and cracking.
  - Use topical steroids (hydrocortisone 1% to 2.5% lotion or gel) on hairy sites once or twice daily.
- During exacerbation
  - Consult dermatology.
  - Use corticosteroid cream 0.05% (Temovate) two to three times a day for 2 to 3 weeks (do not use on facial area).
  - Occlusion with moist wrap (Saran) or DuoDerm (leave on 5 to 7 days) over steroid cream might be helpful to soften plaque.
  - Consider Dovonex (calcipotriene 0.005%), a vitamin D_3 derivative; apply a thin layer of cream to affected areas (and rub in completely) BID for 5 days.
    - Avoid face and mucous membranes.
    - Contraindicated in hypercalcemia or Vitamin D toxicity (use with caution in at-risk patients).
    - Reevaluate use after 8 weeks.
    - Causes burning, itching, and erythema.
- For extensive psoriasis or if unresponsive to treatment, consult a dermatologist for:
  - UVB: risk for sunburn and skin cancers
  - PUVA: psoralens plus UVA; risk for skin cancers
  - Intralesional injection of corticosteroid 3 to 5 mg
  - Methotrexate: 7.5 to 22.5 mg PO weekly. Monitor liver function tests (LFTs), platelets, folate, white blood count (WBC). Consider a daily folic acid supplement.
  - Oral retinoids
  - Cyclosporine: nephrotoxic; long-term safety risk; can cause hypertension.

Vesicular, Pustular, and Bullous Disorders

Herpes zoster

- **Immediate consultation/referral if there is ophthalmic involvement.**
- Antiviral therapy must begin within 48 to 72 hours of onset of rash
  - Acyclovir 800 mg PO five times a day for 7 to 10 days (appropriate for patients with diminished renal function)

- Famciclovir 500 mg PO TID for 7 days (appropriate dose based on renal function and must be calculated for each patient)
- Valacyclovir 1000 mg PO TID for 7 days (appropriate dose based on renal function and must be calculated for each patient)
- Prevent complications of local infection, dissemination, and chronic pain (post-herpetic neuralgia: pain lasting longer than 1 month after episode of zoster).
- Encourage rest.
- Relieve acute symptoms.
  - Cool compresses with Domeboro's solution (one package in pint of water, use paper towels or gauze pads wet with solution, leave on for 30 minutes) QID or normal saline wet dressings
  - Calamine lotion for pruritus
  - Acetaminophen (Tylenol) with around-the-clock dosing for pain (no more than 4 g Tylenol PO daily [preferably 3 g]; if patient is on Coumadin (a blood thinner), maximum dose of Tylenol is 2500 mg PO daily
  - Cautious use of antihistamines for pruritus; consider Allegra or Zyrtec
  - Narcotics if pain is severe
- Keep staff and children who have not been immunized and those who have not had chicken pox away until lesions are dry and crusted.
- Use universal precautions.
- In a long-term care facility, keep patient with herpes zoster away from immunocompromised patients until lesions crust and dry.
- Monitor for dissemination (lesions outside affected dermatome) and ophthalmic involvement. Consult with physician if suspected dissemination or ophthalmic involvement.

Herpes simplex
- Prevent with sunblock to lips.
- May use docosanol 10% cream (Abreva), an over-the-counter product, on affected skin lesions five times daily at the first sign of herpes simplex outbreak.
- May need intermittent acyclovir 200 mg PO five times a day for 5 days (prophylactically at first symptom or before dental work or oral surgery in patients with a history of severe outbreaks).

Burns
- Pain management
- Clean with mild soap and water or normal saline, then apply a thin layer of Silvadene (if patient is not sulfa allergic), Bactroban (if patient is sulfa allergic), or Aquaphor dressing. Cover with tefla, then with a dry, sterile dressing.
- Keep debris and eschar from accumulating in the wound.
- May be able to use second skin (Tegaderm) if the area is small (monitor

every 8 hours for fluid buildup or infection). Depending on wound appearance, may leave Tegaderm in place 3 days to 1 week. Remove Tegaderm cautiously to avoid skin trauma.
- Some burns can be left open, washed with normal saline, have Aquafor applied, and then be left open to air.
- Keep patient well hydrated.

Bullous Pemphigoid
- If it is a localized lesion, use topical corticosteroid (see Contact Dermatitis) cream alone or after Domeboro solution soak (apply wet dressing to affected lesions for 30 minutes as often as four times a day) to desiccate lesions.
- Generalized, widespread: Consult physician and/or dermatologist regarding prednisone therapy (initially 40 to 60 mg PO daily, then taper slowly once disease is under control with no new lesions). Dermatologist may prescribe methotrexate or azathioprine (Imuran), which requires specific laboratory monitoring.

Contact Dermatitis
- Remove offending agent.
- If severe reaction, consider epinephrine (see Drug Reaction) and ED evaluation.
- Use Calamine, Sarna lotion, or cool compresses for pruritus.
- Antihistamines (see Drug Reaction) should be used cautiously in elders.
- If oozing, desiccate with Domeboro solution for 1 to 2 days (see Herpes Zoster).
- For mild to moderate eruption, use a topical corticosteroid (betamethasone 0.05% or triamcinolone 0.025% BID). Consider preventing evaporation with corticosteroid ointment under plastic wrap, cotton gloves, telfa, or Vaseline. Leave on overnight.
- May require oral steroids with quick taper (Medrol dose pack).
- Monitor for superimposed infection.

Toxic Epidermal Necrolysis
- **Acute care/emergency room evaluation**
- Prompt withdrawal of possible causative agent; any drug started within past 2 months should be stopped if possible
- Treated as if second-degree burn: moist dressing, keep hydrated, and manage pain

Intertrigo
- Keep area dry (air-dry frequently), treat inflammation, and prevent recurrence.
- Use cool compresses with Domeboro solution (30 minutes, up to four times a day) until skin is dry.
- Avoid tight clothing.

- Use nystatin (Mycostatin) cream or powder, 100,000 units/g, three to four times a day for 2 weeks after gently washing, rinsing, and patting the affected areas dry.
- Use tolnaftate (Zeasorb) powder to prevent recurrence after inflammation subsides and after treatment with nystatin.

Erosions/Ulcers (See also Wound Care)

Perlèche/Angular Cheilitis

- Nystatin (Mycostatin) cream, 100,000 units/g three times a day to affected skin area for 1 week
- Nystatin lozenge or suspension if indicated
- Soaking of dentures in nystatin (Mycostatin) suspension, 100,000 units/mL overnight
- Dental consult for better dentition

Plaques

Tinea Infections

- In patients with recurrence or patients at risk, special antifungal soaps once a week
- Zeasorb AF powder each day to areas prone to *Tinea*
- Active infections: dry well after bath; miconazol (Lotrimin) 1% or ketoconazole (Nizoral) 2% cream BID for 2 to 4 weeks to affected areas
- If ambulatory, patient should wear white socks; use lambs' wool between toes
- *Tinea capitis*: may need oral agent such as Nizoral 200 mg PO daily for up to 6 weeks; must be used cautiously because of drug interactions and side effects

Tinea Versicolor

- Selenium sulfide (Selsun or Pert Plus) 2.5% lotion or shampoo; leave on for 10 minutes, then follow with shower; use daily for 2 weeks, then once a week
- Pharmacologic therapy
  - Lamisol solution (terbinafine 1%); apply to affected areas BID for 7 days, *or*
  - May consider single-dose Nizoral 200 mg to 400 mg PO each day for 7 days (use cautiously, as noted earlier)

Seborrheic Dermatitis

- Requires vigilant care
- Prevention: for scalp hair, face, and beard, Head and Shoulders shampoo daily for 2 weeks, then twice a week
- Mineral oil rubbed into scalp and left on overnight (with shower cap on) will loosen scale
- Acute exacerbation: shampoo with selenium sulfide shampoo, massage well into scalp, wait 2 to 3 minutes, rinse, and repeat *or* shampoo with Nizoral

shampoo (2% ketoconazole) daily; discuss with patient cutting hair and shaving beard.
- If pruritus: hydrocortisone cream 1% to 2.5%; thin film to affected areas twice a day until improved, then taper slowly
- If on eyelids: remove crusts in the morning with ½ strength baby shampoo, then apply Blephamide ophthalmic ointment daily for 2 weeks

Thrush
- Good oral hygiene
- Mycostatin mouthwash (Nystatin 100,000 U/mL) 5 mL QID; swish and swallow for 10 days

Complications

- Systemic absorption of steroids a possibility if high-potency topical steroids are used for long periods of time
- Atrophy of skin from steroid use
- Superimposed bacterial infection may occur, especially with pruritic lesions and *Tinea*
- Post-herpetic neuralgia in patients with herpes zoster
- Sleep deprivation from pruritus

Consultation/Hospitalization

- **Immediate emergency room evaluation is indicated for suspected anaphylaxis and toxic epidermal necrolysis.**
- **Immediate** consultation with an ophthalmologist or acute care facility is indicated for suspected ophthalmic involvement associated with herpes zoster.
- Dermatology consultation is recommended for:
  - Intractable pruritus
  - Zoster lesions present on the cheek or nose and for lesions that cross dermatomes
  - Any lesion that worsens with initial treatment or does not respond to initial therapy
  - Persistent skin ulcer
  - Any questionable lesion requiring biopsy or excision
- Occupational therapy consult is indicated to assist with application of compression hose.
- Dental consultation is indicated for poor dentition or if dentures cause perlèche.

Nursing Home/Rehabilitation Staff and Patient/Family Education

- Staff, pregnant women, or people without history of chicken pox should not provide care to patient with herpes zoster until lesions are dry and crusted. Emphasize the importance of universal precautions.

- Explain the necessity of avoiding excessive bathing (which may dry skin), rubbing alcohol, and hydrogen peroxide.
- Demonstrate to nurses, families, and patients the proper way to apply a thin coat of moisturizer on damp skin. Explain rationale for avoiding cornstarch.
- Discuss the importance of preventing patient scratching to avoid super-imposed infection and safety measures to prevent trauma to fragile skin.
- Explain the importance of avoiding diapers at night and constrictive clothing.
- Explain the importance of good oral care. Teeth and dentures should be brushed well at least two times a day and good oral hygiene encouraged after inhalers are used. Cleaning inhalers, humidifiers, and nebulizers to avoid thrush or infection should be promoted.
- Discuss and demonstrate the application of compression stockings as well as the importance of carefully laundering and adequately rinsing compression stockings.
- Although there is no clear evidence to support the use of daily yogurt while on antibiotic therapy, it may be helpful to encourage patients to eat plain yogurt with lactobacillus (if there is no indication of lactose intolerance) daily while on antibiotic therapy to decrease fungus overgrowth.
- Explain the importance of adequate hydration.
- Explain the side effects associated with steroid therapy (e.g., infection, gastrointestinal bleeding, hyperglycemia).
- Encourage staff and families to be emotionally supportive to patients with skin lesions. Discuss stress reduction techniques with patients, families, and staff.

Bibliography

Arndt, K.A., et al. (1997). *Primary care dermatology*. Philadelphia: W.B. Saunders.

Buttaro, T.M., et al. (2003). *Primary care: A collaborative practice* (2nd ed.; pp 190-272). St. Louis: Mosby.

Chotzen, V., et al. (1998).Aging skin: Best approaches to common problems. *Patient Care Nurse Practitioners*, July, 28-40.

Goodheart, H.P. (2004). Skin problems in the elderly woman: Dry skin and eczematous conditions. *Women's Health in Primary Care*, 7(5), 215-218.

Goolsby, M.J. (1998). The elusive itch. *Advance for Nurse Practitioners*, November, 61-64.

Habif, T. (2001). *Skin disease: Diagnosis and treatment*. St. Louis: Mosby.

Kucera, K.J. (2004). Managing common skin problems in the elderly. *The Clinical Advisor*, 7(6), 23-30.

Seavolt, M.B., & Tomecki, K. (2003). Treatment of common cutaneous infections in the long-term care setting. *Annals of Long-Term Care*, 11, 48-52.

WOUND CARE

Wounds can be acute or chronic. Acute wounds include lacerations, abrasions, avulsions, crush injuries, puncture wounds, insect or mammalian bites, traumatic or surgical wounds, burns, and skin tears. Pressure ulcers (which affect 1.5 to 3 million Americans at any given time), arterial ulcers, venous ulcers (present in 3.5% of people over the age of 65), diabetic foot ulcers, and nonhealing surgical or traumatic wounds are considered chronic wounds.

Preventing wounds and avoidance of complications are important for all patients and essential for patients who are immunocompromised by age, diabetes, peripheral vascular disease, and other illnesses. Because wound healing is affected by internal and external factors, special diligence is required in managing wound care. Early attention and appropriate care can decrease costs and enhance quality of life. Management of wound care as well as assessing and managing underlying factors contributing to the wound should be the goal of care.

Risk Factors

- Immobility/bedridden/chairbound: if unable to change position, patient is at risk for pressure ulcer.
- Gait abnormalities, positioning devices, and braces: increase risk for pressure ulcers.
- Advanced age: increases risk for prolonged wound healing (frail skin is susceptible to skin tears; polypharmacy, sensory deficits, skin changes related to age, and impaired mobility increase risk for skin breakdown).
- Trauma: frequent cause of skin tears, lacerations, avulsions, or open wounds.
- Diabetes mellitus with/without neuropathy: increases risk for arterial/neuropathic ulcers. Poor glycemic control impacts healing.
- Peripheral vascular disease: increases risk for venous and arterial ulcers.
- Surgery: fractured hips increase risk of skin shearing and pressure ulcers; surgical wounds require care.
- Autoimmune disease, chemotherapy, and radiation therapy: may weaken immune system and impact healing.
- Increased exposure to moisture (urine and perspiration): weakens tissue.
- Obesity: impacts mobility, reduces tissue perfusion, impacts wound healing, and increases risk for infections (e.g., *Candida* in skin folds, lower extremity ulcers).
- Medications (e.g., steroids) and poor nutritional status: impact the healing process.
- Smoking: delays wound healing and increases risk for arterial ulcers.

History

History aids in establishing the type of wound and contributing factors in order to facilitate treatment. Determining past medical history, current medications, risk factors, allergies (sulfa is an active component in Silvadene, often used in dressing care), tetanus status, history of substance abuse (associated with poor nutritional status), and previous history of skin breakdown are also necessary. Additional information to consider includes:

- How long has breakdown been present? Is the wound acute or chronic?
- Causative/contributing factors: pressure, shear, and incontinence of urine or stool
- Nutritional history
- Pain assessment (venous ulcers usually not painful, arterial ulcers are painful, diabetic ulcers may be painless if patient has neuropathy)

Physical Examination

A complete physical examination is necessary to determine the extent of the skin breakdown as well as the underlying cause. Wound characteristics, the condition of the skin surrounding the wound, and the patient's general health help to determine the appropriate treatment.

- Vital signs
  - Temperature: fever suggests infection
  - Hypoxia: decreased oxygen saturation may be a sign of decreased tissue perfusion
- Skin
  - Wound location
    - Most pressure ulcers occur on the sacrum, greater trochanter, ischial tuberosities, heels, lateral malleolus, and back of the head.
    - Venous ulcers commonly occur below the knee (often in the area of the medial malleolus) and are poorly differentiated.
    - Arterial ulcers are very painful and generally found on the pretibial area, tips of toes, and lateral malleolus. The borders are well-distinguished from the surrounding areas, and the wound bed is usually dry rather than exudative. Thickened nails also suggest arterial disease.
    - Diabetic ulcers are usually dry, often found on the plantar surface of foot; a black eschar is possible. Patient may be unaware of ulcer.
  - Size: what is seen on surface is often smallest part of the wound because tissue damage may be substantial. Wound measurements, including length, width, and depth (obtained with a sterile cotton swab), are necessary for documentation and to determine response to treatment.
  - Wound characteristics
    - Presence of necrotic tissue: black and yellow slough must be débrided.
    - Presence of sinus tracts, undermining, and tunneling: must be documented and measured.
    - Presence or absence of granulation tissue
      - Red is healthy granulation tissue; healing wounds are pink and robust with pink/red healing edges.

- Pale wounds with little or no color suggest lack of oxygenation from poor circulation; nonhealing tissue is flat with raised, hard edges.
  - Condition of surrounding skin: stasis dermatitis with increased pigmentation and edema are associated with venous ulcer disease; skin is shiny, hairless in arterial ulcer disease
  - Exudate: note drainage quantity, color, odor, and consistency.
  - Signs of infection: note erythema, warmth, tenderness, edema, and purulent drainage.
- Peripheral vascular system
  - Absent or diminished pulses suggest occlusion (may need referral for revascularization).
  - Peripheral edema (wounds cannot heal until edema is eliminated)
- Neuromuscular
  - Gait: inappropriate shoes or inappropriate pressure exerted
  - Neurologic: decreased sensation especially with diabetes mellitus

Differential Diagnosis

Acute Wounds
- Surgical
  - Primary intention: wound surgically closed with sutures, staples, or glue.
  - Secondary intention: wound is left open, wound edges are not approximated, healing is prolonged, and scar formation is likely. The wound is often infected and may be surgically closed after some healing (tertiary intention).
- Burns
  - First degree: superficial, erythematous, and painful
  - Second degree: partial thickness skin destruction; erythematous with vesicles; painful
  - Third degree: painless with full thickness tissue destruction extending into subcutaneous tissue (or deeper into muscle); usually dry with pale, erythematous, or black, necrotic tissue
- Skin tears: often noted on hands, arms, or legs; may be no tissue loss with a skin tear (Payne-Martin category I), or may be partial (Payne-Martin category II) or full thickness (Payne-Martin category III) tissue loss
- Abrasions/lacerations: will heal in 2 to 3 days in a well-nourished person with minimal intervention

Chronic Wounds
- Pressure ulcer: occurs in 66% of older adults with hip fractures; frequently found over bony prominences, sacrum, greater trochanter, back of head, ischial tuberosity, and lateral malleolus; must remove eschar to stage wound correctly.

- Stage 1: nonblanchable erythema of intact skin; difficult to assess in darkly pigmented skin; no loss of epidermis; inflammatory response with vasodilation; bogginess/induration beneath intact skin may indicate extensive tissue damage beneath skin (patient is at risk for rapid deterioration to stage 3 and stage 4 decubiti).
  - Stage 2: injury is through dermis and epidermis, but not into subcutaneous tissue; often called an abrasion, opened vesicle, or shallow crater/ulcer.
  - Stage 3: extends into subcutaneous tissue, but does not involve underlying fascia.
  - Stage 4: full thickness destruction, necrosis, and damage to muscle, bone or supporting structures, tendons, and joints; may have sinus tract(s).
- Arterial ulcers are associated with abnormalities in blood flow. Ulcers are painful, flat, and dry, with well-defined margins, and are found over pretibial area, tips of toes, lateral malleolus, or heel. Limb may be cool, thin, pale, shiny, and hairless with decreased or absent pulses and thick nail growth. Necrosis and gangrene are common.
- Venous ulcers are less painful and usually located below the knee in the area of the medial malleolus. Ulcers are exudative, with irregular edges and a beefy base. Peripheral pulses are palpable, and surrounding skin is edematous and hyperpigmented. Venous ulcers are associated with dermatitis, varicosities, and poor venous circulation.
- Diabetic ulcers usually occur on feet and are often related to trauma, neuropathy, and arterial disease. They are usually painful but may be painless if neuropathy is present.
  - Appearance: frequently full thickness ulceraton with pale wound bed, dry edges, and necrosis; associated with diabetic deformities, such as plantar callous, Charcot's foot, and atrophy of pedal arch and metatarsal footpad.
- Other: basal cells cancers, squamous cells cancers, and melanomas, often on sun-exposed areas.

Diagnostics

- Braden Scale or Norton Score to predict pressure sore risk (available in facilities)
- Oxygen saturation: < 94% not adequate for wound healing

Laboratory Evaluation

- CBC/differential: to determine immune response (leukopenia/neutropenia), infection (elevated WBC with left shift suggests sepsis), or anemia (decreased tissue oxygenation deters wound healing)
- Albumin < 3.5 g/dL: associated with poor nutritional state and poor wound healing
- Pre-albumin: < 30 mg/dL associated with malnutrition

- Fasting serum glucose/HgbA1C: monitor diabetes/hyperglycemia (wound healing enhanced by tight glycemic control)
- Serum iron and transferrin*: low transferrin and normal serum iron suggest protein-calorie malnutrition
- Blood cultures*
- Wound culture*

Imaging
- Radiograph*: if acute or traumatic injury; to determine fracture, infection, or soft tissue injury
- Bone scan or magnetic resonance imaging (MRI)*: if there is concern regarding osteomyelitis in stage 4 pressure ulcers

Other Diagnostics
- Bone biopsy: if bone affected and wound not healing; often in stage 4 pressure ulcer
- Vascular studies: consider if patient is a candidate for surgical revascularization; without adequate arterial flow, there is little hope of healing

Treatment Plan
General Principles of Wound Healing
- Psychosocial issues and quality of life should be addressed.
- All wounds are contaminated but not necessarily infected.
  - Look for infection in chronic wounds: pain, erythema, warmth, edema, purulent exudate, delayed healing, discoloration of granulation tissue, pocketing of wound base, and wound breakdown.
  - Use systemic antibiotics only if cellulitis, osteomyelitis, bacteremia, or sepsis is present. Consider cephalexin (Keflex) 500 mg PO every 6 hours for 7 to 10 days *or,* if patient is allergic to penicillin, consider clindamycin (Cleocin) 150 to 300 mg PO every 6 hours for 7 to 10 days.
- Healing occurs if patient is well nourished, wound bed is moist with good perfusion, and infection, debris, and pressure are not present.
  - Manage moisture: change diapers frequently, cleansing the skin with gentle cleaner. The skin should be gently patted dry and barrier creams applied. Remove diapers at night.
  - Manage tissue load: change position in bed every 2 hours and raise heels off bed. Position patient properly to remove pressure on bony prominences: special low-air loss or air-fluidized mattress, especially for stage 3 and stage 4 ulcers; head of bed should be at lowest degree of elevation possible for medical condition; special cushions (RoHo or Gel cushion) when sitting (position should still be changed hourly). Doughnuts should not be used.

* If indicated.

- Patients with decubitus ulcers should not be sitting for longer than 1 hour, even after decubitus is healed.
- Risk for recurrence: healed area is only 80% the strength of normal tissue.
- Avoid friction or shear: use transfer device if necessary.
- Manage temperature to improve blood flow to wound bed: maintain patient body temperature at 98° F.

- Manage comorbid conditions (e.g., hyperglycemia, anemia) and reduce risk factors. Smoking cessation should be encouraged and frequently addressed.
- Control factors that impair healing (e.g., spasticity, incontinence of urine and stool). Suprapubic catheter or referral for urinary diversion may be necessary. Initiate a bowel regimen or referral for diversion (colostomy).
- Manage wound pain and pain related to dressing changes. (Document patient's response to interventions and adjust as necessary.)
- Wound and dressing care
  - Remove dressings before showering. (Showering helps débride wounds, even decubiti, and should be encouraged.)
  - Dressings should be lightly fluffed and placed only in wound bed. (Light, loose packing decreases risk of sinus tracts.) Protect surrounding tissue with A&D ointment or other barrier cream.
  - In patients with multiple wounds, the most contaminated area should be dressed last.
  - Protect surrounding skin from tape irritation with 3M skin prep.
  - Avoid tape on sensitive skin (3M tape is usually least traumatic). Use Kling, stockinette, or Tubex to hold dressing in place.
  - Assess healing and response to dressing care: a clean pressure ulcer should exhibit evidence of healing within 2 to 4 weeks. Change dressing care as the wound changes.
- Take photos of wound progression and/or make weekly wound measurements or drawings for documentation.
- Improve nutrition/hydration.
  - Nutrition: 30 to 35 calories per kg daily: 1.25 to 1.5 g protein per kg daily
  - 1.5 to 2 liters fluid daily
  - If hypoalbuminemia, consider Procel, 1 scoop daily, or Promod, 1 scoop three times a day
  - Vitamin supplementation: multiple vitamins with minerals 1 PO daily. Vitamin C, 500 mg PO daily, and zinc sulfate, 220 mg PO BID, are frequently added, although there is no evidence that proves efficacy.
- Manage edema: elevate lower extremities and treat heart failure and edema with diuretics, if appropriate. Graded compression with edema: 30 to 40 mm Hg at ankle, 12 to 17 mm Hg below knee (thromboembolic disease stockings [TEDS] are only 18 mm Hg). Compression stockings are contraindicated in arterial disease.
- Povidine iodine, acetic acid, and Dakin's solution are used judiciously in ½ or ¼ strength.

- When applied to dry eschars, ¼ or ½ strength povidine iodine aid in drying the eschar and seem to promote wound healing. However, povidine iodine, acetic acid, and Dakin's solution, although frequently prescribed by physicians, are not recommended by the Agency for Health Care Policy and Research, as these substances are considered cytotoxic.
- Hydrogen peroxide should never be used in packing.
- Telfa does not enhance epithelialization.
- Débridement
    - Heel ulcers should not be débrided.
    - Remove callus gently from around foot ulcers.
    - Necrotic areas must be débrided before dressing care can promote healing.
        - Consider referral for surgical débridement with sharp, sterile blade.
        - Mechanical débridement: normal saline irrigation with high-pressure syringe or normal saline wet to dry dressing loosely packed in wound bed
        - Enzymatic débridement: initially scratch or crosshatch eschar with sterile needle or scalpel to create area for enzyme to penetrate; Santyl or Accuzyme in thin layer on wound bed, covered by a dressing
        - Autolytic débridement: moist, retentive dressing left on to soften or dissolve necrotic tissue

Dressing Care

- Acute wounds
    - Surgical: primary intention; dry sterile dressing (DSD) after washing area gently with normal saline (N/S) wash, then gently patting dry
    - Secondary or tertiary intention: for wounds with profuse drainage, irrigate wound with N/S, gently pat wound bed dry, and apply calcium alginate product to wound bed (not appropriate for wounds with dry eschar); absorbent DSD
        - If wound drainage is profuse, use calcium alginate with absorbent DSD after N/S irrigation (using 35-mm syringe with a 19-gauge angiocath) × 3, then gently dry wound bed.
        - If wound drainage is serous and minimal, irrigate wound with N/S, gently pat dry, and apply hydrogel to wound. Cover with loosely packed, damp N/S fluffed gauze, then cover with DSD.
        - If wound has odor and exudate, irrigate wound with N/S, then apply cadexomer iodine gel, followed by absorbent topper (DSD).
        - If wound margins are macerated, use zinc/lanolin, A&D ointment, other barrier cream, or DuoDerm to margins, or wipe healthy skin with prep pads. Use Montgomery straps for frequent dressing changes on sensitive skin.
        - Sutures are usually removed in 5 to 15 days depending on the surgeon's preference and the location of the wound. Facial sutures are removed sooner (in 3 to 5 days).

- Burns
  - First degree: cool compresses every 4 hours as needed. Wash with normal saline, gently pat dry, and then apply Silvadene or Bactroban (if sulfa allergy) for 14 to 21 days. Cover with DSD or use transparent film (Tegaderm) dressing (change Tegaderm every 3 days after cleaning wound as described earlier).
  - **Second- or third-degree burns or burns on face, hands, feet, or perineum require physician evaluation.**
- Skin tears: wash with normal saline. Pat dry. Approximate skin. Use steristrips, DSD, and Kling or DuoDerm, alone (changing DuoDerm every 3 days). May also use transparent film (Tegaderm) alone (changing every 3 days), or xeroform/Vaseline gauze/adaptic covered by DSD and Kling. Kling or elasticized tubex is used on arms and legs to avoid using tape. Use DuoDerm or other occlusive dressings cautiously on lower extremities.
- Abrasions/lacerations: wash with normal saline; pat dry. Approximate margins with steristrips. Cover with xeroform and DSD as for skin tear. If no drainage, may leave open to air.
- Chronic wounds
  - Pressure ulcers
    - Relieve pressure.
    - Keep wound bed clear of debris with débridement or frequent dressing changes.
    - Keep head of bed (HOB) as low as possible.
    - Suspend heels off bed with special boots.
    - Maintain turning schedule (patient should be turned every 1 to 2 hours).
    - Use Hoyer lift if there is risk of shearing.
    - Incontinence care: consider Foley catheter or suprapubic catheter if urinary incontinence is affecting wound care; minimal diaper use and proper hygiene.
    - Use airflow mattress/Roho cushion on chair.
    - Initially, out of bed for meals only; after healing begins, back to bed 1 hour after meals.
    - Stage 1: BID wash with normal saline, dry, dermogram cream; or every 72 hours: wash with N/S, dry, and apply duoderm with instructions to check each shift for duoderm placement.
    - Stage 2: BID wash with normal saline, dry, and apply xeroform/adaptic, then DSD, *or* wash with N/S, dry, apply duoderm, and change every 72 hours, as in stage 1.
    - Stage 3 and stage 4: BID wash with normal saline, dry, and apply N/S damp (wet to dry) fluffed dressing in base of wound covered with DSD. Use a barrier cream to the wound edges to prevent maceration.

- Wounds may be irrigated with shower or irrigated with N/S (use a 35-mm syringe with 19-gauge angiocatheter) × 3, then gently pat dry.
- Liberal amounts of A&D ointment or barrier cream to skin around wound edges to protect skin from dampness and exudates, *or* paint surrounding skin with 3M No Sting Barrier Film.
- For wound beds with thick, tough fibrous tissue or black eschar: consider Accuzyme (to débride wound), $\frac{1}{8}$-inch thick to wound bed and cover with gauze moistened with N/S, then dry or rolled gauze and dry dressing.
- For wound beds with red granulation tissue, fibrous tissue, and black eschar, may use Panafil (less irritating than Accuzyme, indicated for wound healing and enzymatic débridement, $\frac{1}{8}$-inch thick to wound bed and cover with gauze moistened with N/S, then dry or rolled gauze and covered with dry dressing or transparent dressing.
- For wounds with minimal yellow exudate/fibrous tissue, may use Santyl, $\frac{1}{8}$-inch thick to wound bed and covered with dry gauze or gauze moistened with N/S. Cover with dry dressing.
- Change dressings every 12 to 24 hours (wound bed should not be dry).
- If continued eschar, refer for sharp débridement.
- Use 3M No Sting Barrier Film to surrounding skin (do not use in infected areas) and 3M tape to prevent further skin breakdown.
- Consider negative pressure wound treatment (vacuum assisted closure [VAC] dressing) for exudative stage 3 or 4 wounds.

- Arterial wounds
  - Wound requires moisture. Elevate HOB with lower extremities dependent. Keep lower extremities warm. Avoid compression stockings.
  - Perform daily foot care with attention between toes.
  - If there is eschar, consider $\frac{1}{4}$- to $\frac{1}{2}$-strength Betadine (painted on eschar only once or twice daily).
  - If wound bed is dry, wash with N/S, then use a damp N/S dressing and DSD.
  - If dry gangrene, leave open to air.
  - If wet gangrene with odor, consider $\frac{1}{2}$-strength Dakin's solution wash. Follow with DSD. Use Dakin's solution cautiously with intact skin. Consult vascular surgeon for specific dressing and/or revascularization.
  - Consider cilostazol (Pletal), an antiplatelet/vasodilator, 50 to 100 mg PO BID (contraindicated if there is a history of heart failure).
  - Encourage walking.
  - Manage pain.
  - Seek referrals for revascularization.

- Venous wounds
  - Decrease edema with elevation of lower extremity, compression stockings, and diuretics if appropriate, *or*
  - Consider multilayer compression bandage system (Profore), changing every 5 to 7 days. This is contraindicated if there is a latex allergy, an ankle brachial index < 8, or severe diabetic vascular disease.
    - Contraindicated if ankle-brachial index < 0.8
  - Consider an Unna boot, changing it every 3 to 7 days.
    - Use gloves. Wash leg well with N/S; dry; remove loose skin, and then wrap with Unna boot from toes to below knee. Cover with Ace wrap. Wrap must not be too tight. Check circulation, sensation, and movement (CSM) in toes every 8 hours. Kling under boot may be applied if there is a skin reaction, but not recommended if no reaction. Keep Unna boot dry and protected from urine.
  - If Unna boot is not indicated, most venous ulcers can be healed with N/S wash, damp normal saline dressing covered by DSD and Kling.
- Diabetic ulcers
  - Daily foot care
  - Provide glycemic and infection control.
  - If ulcer on foot, patient must be non–weight bearing. Refer to podiatry for care and special shoes.
  - Diabetic ulcer care: wash with N/S, dry, then cover with N/S damp dressing and DSD. (Some vascular surgeons prefer 0.25% povidone iodine solution.)
  - Patients may need hospitalization for limb-threatening infection, bone involvement, or severe ischemia.
  - For a nonhealing wound, consider growth factor dressing with Regranex gel 0.01%.
    - Clean wound with normal saline. Dry. Wound should have adequate blood supply and minimal necrotic base.
    - Daily: apply thin coat ($^1/_{16}$-inch) of Regranax gel with cotton swab to ulcer only. Top with moist saline dressing only on wound.
    - 12 hours after Regranex dressing applied, remove. Wash with saline, dry, apply moist saline dressing, again ONLY on wound itself.
- Adjutant therapy for ulcers
  - Provide surgical referral for direct surgical closure or skin grafts or skin flaps.
  - Consult a physical therapist or skin specialist for pulse ultrasound, electric stimulation, and ultraviolet light.
  - Consider Vacuum-Assisted Wound Closure (VAC®) Granufoam Dressing to remove exudates and improve circulation to the wound.
  - Hyperbaric oxygen (if indicated) is used for necrotizing fasciitis, refractory osteomyelitis, and diabetic ulcers.

Consultation/Hospitalization

- Surgical referral is indicated for full thickness burns or burns on the face, feet, hands, or perineum; wounds with deep lacerations/puncture wounds; and wound débridement.
- Consider surgical referral for colostomy if stool incontinence is affecting wound healing and scheduled stooling and bowel regimen do not control problem of stool contamination (often done in paraplegia).
- Orthopedic referral is indicated for fractures, suspected tendon injury, or suspected osteomyelitis.
- Referral to a bed specialist is indicated for patients with stage 3 and 4 decubitus ulcer.
- Consider referral to urology for urinary diversion if urinary incontinence is affecting wound healing.
- Podiatry consultation is indicated for padded hosiery, foot ulcers, callous care, and special shoes to redistribute weight, or to make a special shoe insert or cast.
- Physical therapy referral is recommended for gait training as well as for ultrasound or electric stimulation to aid in healing.
- Enterostomal referral is indicated for special skin care problems.
- Dietary consultation is recommended for nutrition evaluation.
- Neurology consultation is recommended if indicated.
- Referral to pain clinic should be considered for wound pain not responsive to pain management interventions.
- Referral to a vascular surgeon is indicated for revascularization if pulses are not present, if amputation is a consideration, or if vascular ulcer is not improving in 3 to 4 weeks.
- Hospitalization is indicated for any limb-threatening infection, for amputation, or for bone involvement.

Complications

- Endocarditis
- Cellulitis
- Osteomyelitis
- Fistulas
- Septic arthritis
- Sinus tract or abscess
- Maggot infestation (although a potential complication, maggots are used for wound débridement in some centers)
- Wound dehiscence
- Scarring
- Amputation
- Sepsis

Education for Nursing Home/Rehabilitation Staff

- Measure and document wounds weekly (or more frequently, if indicated), and notify healthcare provider if wound is deteriorating.
- Discuss with physical therapy and nursing staff transfer techniques and how to position and move patients without causing skin injury.
- Explain to nurses the importance of packing wounds loosely.
- Educate nursing staff about good foot care.
- Reinforce universal precautions and how to dispose of soiled dressings.
- Discuss with nurses individualized bowel regimen and good hygiene with diapers.
- Educate nursing staff on how to prevent shearing.
- Discuss with nurses the necessity of removing dressings before patient showers.
- Stress the importance of patient ambulation to improve circulation.
- Educate nurses about regular weekly skin checks (including feet and areas between toes).
- Discuss the principles of good hygiene, nutrition, extremity elevation, and good skin care to prevent skin breakdown. Explain the consequences of inadequate wound care.
- Involve nursing staff in pain management issues.
- Educate staff about the importance of washing, rinsing, and drying TEDS. Demonstrate how to apply TEDS correctly.
- Explain the necessity of weekly weights, wound measurements, monitoring blood sugars, and reporting changes as well as signs and symptoms of infection to healthcare provider.
- Stress with the nursing staff the necessity of turning patients in bed every 1 to 2 hours and repositioning patients in chairs every 20 minutes.

Patient/Family Education

- Discuss with patient and family:
  - Importance of good hygiene, ample nutrition, adequate hydration, and exercise
  - Pain management to control discomfort
  - Diabetic teaching to control hyperglycemia and enhance wound healing
- Encourage patient and family participation/learning during dressing changes.

Bibliography

Akbari, C.M., & Pompaselli, F.B. (2000). Understanding and managing diabetic foot disease. *Internal Medicine, 21*(3), 10-17.

Buttaro, T.M., et al. (2003). *Primary care: A collaborative practice* (2nd ed.). St. Louis: Mosby.

Cervo, F.A., et al. (2000). Pressure ulcers: Analysis of guidelines for treatment and management. *Geriatrics, 55*(3), 55-60.

Doughty, D.B., et al. Lower extremity ulcers of vascular etiology. In R.A. Bryant (Ed.), *Acute and chronic wounds: Nursing management*. St. Louis: Mosby.

Gardner, S.E., et al. (2001). A tool to assess clinical signs and symptoms of localized infection in chronic wounds: Development and reliability. *Ostomy/Wound Management, 47*(1), 40-47.

Houghton, P.E., & Campbell, K.E. (1999). Choosing an adjunctive therapy for the treatment of chronic wounds. *Ostomy/Wound Management, 45*(8), 43-52.

Miller, M.S. (2002). Wound care: Out on a limb. *The Clinical Advisor*, May, 149-152.

Miller, M.S. (2002). No pressure wound care. *The Clinical Advisor*, January, 83-86.

Skidmore-Roth, L. (2004). *Mosby's 2004 nursing drug reference*. St. Louis, Mosby.

Wiersma-Bryant, L.A. (2001). Management of edema. In Sussman, C., & Bates-Jensen, B., (Eds.), *Wound care: A collaborative practice manual for physical therapists and nurses*. Gaithersburg, MD: Aspen Publishers.

PRURITUS

ICD9: 698.9

Pruritus is an itch elicited by chemical or physical stimulation of cutaneous nerve receptors from internal or external sources, resulting in the need to scratch. Pruritus can be a symptom of an internal problem or a local dermatologic condition. It is a common complaint in the elderly that is often attributed to xerosis, although the cause may be related to a medication, endocrine disorder, iron-deficiency anemia, malignancy, or other pathology. The scratching itself may lead to a rash or superimposed disease.

History

The history of the current complaint (HPI) and symptom analysis are useful in determining the source. The sudden onset of severe pruritus suggests an underlying pathology. Additional history includes medications, insect bites, skin care habits, shaving routine, use of fragrances, and environmental exposures to heat, humidity, or pets. Family history and any past medical history of mental illness, diabetes, alcohol use, or metabolic/endocrine disease should also be elicited.

Physical Examination

The skin examination should determine the presence of jaundice, rashes, dry skin, or scratch marks. Any evidence of anemia, lymphadenopathy, organomegaly, or neurologic changes must be noted.

Differential Diagnosis

The differential diagnosis is extensive, although the history and physical examination aid in determining the cause. Common causes (and associated signs and symptoms) of pruritus are listed as follows:

- With skin lesion: see skin rashes
  - Allergic response: urticaria
  - Sunburn: erythema (with/without vesicles)
  - Insect bite
  - Infestations
    - Scabies: burrows with small vesicle at end (may also be associated with erythematous papules/nodules or crusted lesions) commonly located in web spaces, flexor aspects of wrists, nipples, axillae, genitalia; pruritus worsens at night
    - Lice: common in institutionalized patients; itching severe, possibly with visible nits or lice on hair, body, genitalia
  - Drug reaction: symmetric macular, papular eruption
  - Contact/irritant dermatitis
  - Seborrheic dermatitis: dry, flaky skin around scalp, eyebrows, eyelids, nose, bearded areas
  - Bullous pemphigoid: tense vesicles on erythematous or normal skin associated with pruritus before vesicular eruption
  - Psoriasis: well-demarcated erythematous plaques with silvery scale
  - Fungal infection: commonly located in warm, moist areas; maceration of skin
  - Folliculitis: infection of hair follicles
  - Lichen simplex dermatitis: thickened areas on ankles, legs, or forearms associated with repeated scratching
- Without skin lesion
  - Xerosis: most common; worse on extremities; related to internal and environmental factors, dehydration, diuretics
  - Psychogenic: neurotic scratching, worse at night, usually scratch marks on opposite side of body from dominant hand
  - Systemic illness: consider if pruritus undiagnosed after 2 weeks
  - Endocrine disorder
    - Hypothyroid: usually dry skin
    - Hyperthyroid: frequently moist skin
    - Diabetes: neuropathy or skin infection
    - Estrogen withdrawal in postmenopausal women
    - Carcinoid
  - Hematologic
    - Polycythemia vera
    - Iron deficiency anemia
  - Malignancies
    - Lymphoma and leukemia: from increased histamine

- Multiple myeloma
- Other malignancies
- Liver disease: obstructive biliary or chronic liver disease
- Renal disease: chronic renal failure, secondary to excess urea or dialysis
- Parasitic infections

Diagnostics

If there is no response after 2 weeks to initial treatment with skin care and creams, diagnostic testing should be considered. Diagnostics are individualized and based on the history and physical findings.

- CBC/differential with eosinophil count will reveal anemia, allergies, polycythemia
- Erythrocyte sedimentation rate (ESR)
- Iron studies if indicated
- LFTs
- Thyroid-stimulating hormone
- Serum glucose and electrolytes, blood urea nitrogen (BUN), and creatinine; determine elevated blood sugar, renal dysfunction
- Serum calcium, phosphate: if suspected kidney disease

If diagnosis is still elusive, consider:

- 5-Hydroxy indoleacetic acid (5HIAA), a 24-hour urine test for carcinoid
- Chest radiograph: assessment for pulmonary malignancy
- Skin biopsy
- Stool: for occult blood, ova, and parasites
- Serum protein electrophoresis (SPEP): for myeloma

Treatment Plan

Treatment is individualized, and it is very important to determine the underlying cause. Whatever the pathology, however, it is important to treat the symptoms to promote patient comfort.

Treat first for xerosis, utilizing the principles of skin care.

- Hydrate.
- Decrease frequency of complete bath and use warm, not hot, water.
- Use Cetaphil on face and a mild soap (e.g., Dove, Basis, Neutrogena) on body.
- Skin lotions and creams such as Eucerin, Vaseline, and Lac-Hydrin 12% (which draws moisture into skin) should be applied immediately after bathing.
- Ask family to do laundry and explain to nursing staff the importance of using unbleached linen.
- Prevent evaporation of moisture.
- Humidify air.
- Room temperature should be approximately 68° F.

Also treat pruritus.
- Phamacologic therapy
  - Zonalon topical cream (doxepin Hcl 5%): thin film applied four times a day topically for up to 8 days (do not occlude)
  - Hydroxyzine (Atarax) 10 mg PO TID as needed, while monitoring for anticholinergic side effects
  - If inflammation, hydrocortisone 1% to 2.5% BID for 1 week
  - If infection is present, antibiotic therapy
  - If appropriate, cholestyramine 4 g TID to decrease bile salts
  - Aspirin for polycythemia vera
  - Doxepin 25 mg PO at bedtime for sleep (used cautiously in elderly patients because of associated side effects)
- Nonpharmacologic therapy
  - Oatmeal baths, cool lotions (e.g., calamine, menthol, sarna), and cool compresses may be used for comfort.
  - Use an air conditioner if necessary.
  - Trim nails.
  - Reduce stress.
  - Eliminate suspicious agents (e.g., new fragrances, scented soaps).
  - Wear cotton clothing.

Consultation/Hospitalization

- Hematology/oncology
- Acupuncture for pruritus or stress
- Psychiatry
- Endocrine
- Nephrology
- Dermatology (see Skin for biopsy)
- Massage therapy for stress reduction
- Activities to divert attention

Patient/Family Education

- Provide special teaching related to the specific illness if cause is not related to a skin disorder.

CELLULITIS

ICD-9: 682.9

An acute spreading infection of the deep dermis and subcutaneous tissue, cellulitis commonly occurs on the lower extremities, but can occur anywhere. The cause is usually beta-hemolytic streptococci (often group A) or *Staphylococcus aureus*. A portal of entry is often not found. The elderly are particularly at risk because of associated systemic illness, dry skin, and skin diseases.

Risk Factors

- Previous cellulitis
- Lymphedema: tight, weeping skin predisposes to infection
- Obesity
- Poor hygiene
- Venous insufficiency/stasis, peripheral vascular disease
- Recent coronary artery bypass graft (CABG) with saphenous vein venectomy
- Immunocompromised: steroid use or lymphatic compromise (e.g., mastectomy, radiation therapy)
- Diabetes mellitus: elevated blood sugars may suggest infection
- Chronic skin irritation
- Intravenous lines and medications: irritating to veins
- Tinea pedis/onychomycosis: compromises skin integrity
- Heart failure with edema
- History of falls, fractures, or trauma: compromises skin integrity

History

In elderly patients, a change in mental status may be the first sign of illness, but patients may also be asymptomatic. Common complaints include fatigue, fever, chills, pain, edema, and myalgias. A history of rash, ulcer, wound, insect or animal bite, recent dental work or surgery, ear infection, or sinus infection also may be significant. Time of onset, associated symptoms, medication, allergies, and medical history should also be reviewed.

Physical Examination

The cardinal skin signs include edema, erythema, warmth, pain, and possibly a vesicular eruption and red streaking (lymphadenitis). A careful examination searching for a portal of entry; associated infection, such as sinus infection (if facial cellulites); joint erythema, edema, or tenderness; *Tinea pedis;* or lymphadenopathy is necessary. Additional examination includes:

- Vital signs: determine presence of fever, tachycardia, tachypnea, hypotension
- Cardiopulmonary examination: determine cardiovascular response to infection

Diagnostics

- CBC/differential: determine if leukocytosis is present
- Serum electrolytes, BUN, and creatinine
- ESR: if concerns about associated bone involvement

- Blood culture: if rigors, recurrence, or no response to therapy
- Radiograph: especially if hand or foot involvement
- Wound cultures: usually unnecessary
- Uric acid: if gout is suspected

Differential Diagnosis

- Necrotizing fascitis: erythema, edema with development of black eschar, rapidly spreads with systemic toxicity; may be associated with leukocytosis, hyponatremia, and elevated creatinine
- Folliculitis: superficial infection of hair follicles (erythematous papules, pustules) associated with friction, perspiration, occlusion of follicles associated with lack of aeration, and restrictive clothing
- Erysipelas: more superficial infection of dermis and upper subcutaneous
- Deep vein thrombosis (DVT): usually, but not always, in lower extremity with possible calf tenderness; related to immobility, hypercoagulation, or intravenous therapy
- Ruptured Baker cyst: cyst in popliteal space; can rupture
- Gout: warm, tender, red, joint; pain with mobility
- Local reaction to bite
- Vasculitis

Treatment Plan

Antibiotic therapy is based on patient presentation and the probable bacterial agent. For uncomplicated infections in patients without fever or systemic symptoms, the following antibiotics are appropriate:
- Dicloxacillin (Dynapen) 500 mg PO every 6 hours for 14 days
- If penicillin (PCN) allergy, consider:
  - Cephalexin (Keflex) 250 to 500 mg PO every 6 hours for 14 days, *or*
  - Levofloxacin (Levaquin) 250 to 500 mg (dose dependent on renal function) PO daily for 14 days, *or*
  - Erythromycin 500 mg PO every 6 hours for 14 days; azithromycin (Zithromax) or clarithromycin (Biaxin) if unable to tolerate erythromycin, *or*
  - Clindamycin (Cleocin) 300 mg PO every 6 hours for 14 days (use cautiously if patient has history of *C. difficile*)

For patients with diabetes, consider:
- Amoxicillin/clavulanic acid (Augmentin), *or*
- Ciprofloxacin (Cipro) 500 mg PO BID combined with clindamycin 300 mg PO every 6 hours for 14 days

For patients with a high fever, chills, or systemic symptoms, or if a patient is unable to tolerate oral medications, consider:
- Cefazolin (Ancef) 1 to 2 g IV every 8 hours for 14 days, *or*

- Clindamycin (Cleocin) 600 mg IV every 8 hours for 14 days (appropriate if PCN allergy), *or*
- Nafcillin (Unipen) 2 g IV every 4 hours for 14 days

If methicillin-resistant *Staphylococcus aureus* (MRSA) is suspected:

- Vancomycin (Vanocin) 1g IV every 12 hours for 14 days (adjust dose for elderly and altered renal function)

Additional treatment:

- Rest
- Application of moist heat for 15 minutes every 30 minutes (cautiously, to avoid further skin damage)
- Elevation of affected extremity
- Hygiene
- Dressing care if appropriate
- Tetanus prophylaxis if appropriate

Consultation/Hospitalization

- Hospitalization is indicated for patients with suspected bacteremia, sepsis, hypotension, orbital cellulitis, or necrotizing fasciitis.
- Urgent consultation with hand specialist is needed if there is hand involvement.
- Orthopedic consultation is recommended for suspected joint infection and osteomyelitis.
- Physician consultation is indicated for patients who do not respond to treatment within 24 to 48 hours. Hospitalization may be indicated, particularly for diabetic or immunocompromised patients.

Complications

- Bacteremia and sepsis
- Joint infections/osteomyelitis
- Hand cellulitis may invade joint spaces.
- Diabetics require close monitoring for development of ulcerations and osteomyelitis.
- Be alert for patients at risk for infective endocarditis.

Education for Nursing Home/Rehabilitation Staff

Discuss the following with nursing staff:

- Notify the healthcare provider if glycemic control in diabetic patients becomes unstable.
- Perform IV site care if applicable.
- To prevent recurrence, avoid trauma with wheel chairs, transporting patient, and transferring patient.

- Educate in fall prevention.
- Ensure good nail, skin, and foot care.
- Protect vulnerable skin with wraps and padding.
- Clear pathways of obstructions.

Patient/Family Education

- Explain to patients and families the diagnosis and treatment.
- Discuss prevention of injuries and importance of hygiene, as well as the need to keep skin well moisturized.

Bibliography

Cohen, P.R., & Kurzrock, R. (2004). Community-acquired methicillin resistant *Staphylococcus aureus* skin infection: an emerging clinical problem. *Journal of the American Academy of Dermatology, 50*(2), 277-280.

O'Donnell, J.A., & Hofman, M.T. (2001). Skin and soft tissues: Management of four common infections in the nursing home patient. *Geriatrics, 56*(10), 33-38, 41.

Wall, D.B., et al. (2000). Objective criteria may assist in distinguishing necrotizing fasciitis from non-necrotizing soft tissue infection. *American Journal of Surgery, 179*(1), 17-21.

Pulmonary Disorders

EXACERBATION OF COPD

ICD-9: 491.21

The fourth most common cause of death in North America, chronic obstructive lung disease (COPD), is characterized by airflow limitation that is not fully reversible. The disease is associated with an abnormal inflammatory response of the lungs to noxious particles or gases. Inability to completely exhale is significant.

An acute exacerbation of COPD is characterized by a 2-day history of increased cough, dyspnea, and purulent sputum accompanied by wheezing, pharyngitis, upper respiratory disease, chest tightness, fever, or impaired pulmonary function. The cause of an exacerbation is not always readily recognizable, except that the patient may not be responding as well to usual therapy. Most exacerbations are related to a viral or bacterial infection, although other precipitants may be implicated. The most common bacterial organisms involved are *Streptococcus pneumoniae, Haemophilus influenzae,* and *Moraxella catarrhalis.* All patients with COPD are at risk for a mild to severe exacerbation. The risk for an exacerbation requiring hospitalization increases with age.

Risk Factors

- Recent oral or respiratory infection
- Smoking
- Toxic inhalation of pollutants, noxious agents, or smoke
- Alpha$_1$-antitrypsin deficiency
- Immunologic deficiency
- Chronic oral corticosteroid use: patient immunocompromised

- Excessive sedation from medication: patient unable to properly clear secretions
- Winter months: dry air may result in thickened secretions and dehydration
- Dehydration: moist secretions are easier to clear
- Nonadherence with medication regimen
- Incorrect use of inhalers

History

Pertinent information that should be obtained includes family history of alpha$_1$-antitrypsin deficiency or premature COPD, medication history (particularly those associated with increased cough/bronchospasm [β-blocker, angiotensin-converting enzyme [ACE] inhibitor]), drug allergies, recent upper respiratory infection [URI], history of COPD exacerbation (including therapy, emergency department treatment, hospitalization, intubation), drug/substance abuse, decreased exercise tolerance, and adherence to previously prescribed treatment plan. Onset of current symptoms, presence of dyspnea, cough, purulent sputum, and/or other symptoms should also be elicited.

Some of the signs and symptoms associated with an exacerbation of COPD are similar to those related to other cardiac or pulmonary conditions, especially cough and dyspnea. The severity of exacerbation is determined by the presence of the following cardinal symptoms:

- Increased cough
- Increased sputum production and increased purulent sputum
- Worsening dyspnea
- Wheeze
- Fever
- Anorexia
- Mental status change, anxiety, or somnolence: secondary to hypoxemia

Physical Examination

Some patients will not appear in acute distress. Aspects of the physical examination that suggest disease exacerbation and/or complications of COPD (i.e., cor pulmonale) may include the following:

- General appearance: often restless, uncooperative; usually sitting up, hunched forward with hands on knees, + air hunger; note any pursed lip breathing
- Vital signs: temperature, pulse, respirations, pulse oximetry, forced expiratory volume (FEV), spirometry; fever, tachycardia, tachypnea, or hypoxemia may be present; FEV may be reduced
- Skin: may be dry or diaphoretic; cyanosis may be present (bluish color to lips, mucous membranes, extremities, and nailbeds)
- Lungs: use of accessory muscles; reduced respiratory excursion; AP diameter >2:1 (usual barrel chest in COPD is an AP diameter 1:1); decreased diaphragmatic excursion; hyperresonant percussion; decreased

breath sounds; presence of rhonchi/wheezes indicates secretions in large airways; absence of rhonchi/wheezes may indicate poor respiratory excursion (common in acutely ill and elderly patients) and/or inability to move air

- Cardiac: determine presence of right-sided heart failure (i.e., jugular vein distention [JVD], right ventricle heave, displaced point of maximum impulse (PMI), loud S_2 of pulmonic valve closure, tricuspid murmur).
- Abdomen: hepatojugular reflux, hepatosplenomegaly, and ascites indicates right-sided failure.
- Extremities: lower extremity edema may indicate right-sided heart failure.

Differential Diagnosis

The etiology of the patient's cough or dyspnea should always be determined, even in patients with known COPD. Disorders that should be included in the differential include the following:

- Asthma
- Congestive heart failure (CHF) and pulmonary edema: associated with weight gain, orthopnea, jugular venous distention (JVD), ascites, and edema
- Pulmonary embolus (PE); can be difficult to exclude; symptoms include dyspnea, hemoptysis, and chest pain; patient may have low systolic blood pressure and low oxygen saturation in spite of high-flow oxygen, as well as pleural rub; consult with the medical director (MD) concerning the need for D-dimer assay and spiral computed tomography (CT)
- Pneumothorax
- Pleural effusion
- Arrhythmia
- Pneumonia: infiltrate on radiograph; also consider if unable to correct hypoxemia
- Malignancy
- Medication induced cough: β-blockers, ACE inhibitors, Amiodorone
- Tuberculosis
- Bronchiectasis
- Alpha$_1$-antitrypsin deficiency: should be suspected in younger patients with COPD and positive family history alpha$_1$-antitrypsin deficiency
- Gastroesophageal reflux disease (GERD): frequent, dry cough
- Differentiation of mild, moderate, and severe exacerbation: based on three diagnostic criteria: increased sputum production, increased sputum purulence, and worsening dyspnea

Diagnostics

- Oxygen saturation: nail polish should be removed and hands warmed; oxygen saturation should be > 90% on room air

- Spirometry
    - Bedside evaluation of forced expiratory time (FET) is accomplished by having the patient maximally inhale, then maximally and forcefully exhale while the provider auscultates over the trachea measuring the time between the beginning of inspiration and the end of expiration. An FET $\geq$ 6 seconds indicates airflow obstruction.
    - Peak expiratory flow (PEF) < 1 L/min or FEV_1 < 1 L indicates a severe exacerbation.
- For mild, moderate, or severe exacerbation, consider the following:
    - Chest radiograph: to exclude pneumonia, pneumothorax, and heart failure
    - Stat arterial blood gases*: moderate to severe exacerbation; PaO_2 should be > 60 mm Hg.
    - Electrocardiogram (ECG)*: to exclude right ventricular hypertrophy, arrhythmias, or ischemia
    - Complete blood count with differential (CBC/diff): monitor leukocytosis as well as an increased hemoglobin/hematocrit (especially hematocrit [Hct] > 55%), indicating severity of hypoxemia
    - Serum glucose, serum electrolytes, blood urea nitrogen (BUN), and creatinine*: to monitor fluid and electrolyte balance
    - Theophylline level*
    - D-dimer assay, spiral CT, or ventilation/perfusion quotient (VQ) scan: if PE is a consideration
    - Alpha$_1$-antitrypsin level if alpha$_1$-antitrypsin deficiency is suspected
    - Purified Protein derivative (PPD)*: PPD testing usually required on admission to facility
    - Sputum cultures usually not recommended, but they may be considered if there is a poor response to initial antibiotic therapy

Treatment Plan

Treatment is individualized for each patient and past response to intervention is an important consideration. Hospitalization should be considered for some patients (see Consultation/Hospitalization), but it is partially dependent on patient and family wishes and the facility's ability to care for the patient.

Recent evidence suggests that patients with a COPD exacerbation improve with early treatment. Critical interventions include the following:

- Give oxygen at 2 to 4 L by mask or nasal cannula to maintain oxygen saturation above 90% (PaO_2 < 60 mm Hg) for moderate or severe exacerbations to correct tissue oxygenation (may take 20 to 30 minutes to achieve steady state). Increase oxygen, if necessary, but monitor for signs of carbon dioxide retention.

---

* If indicated.

- Monitor nocturnal oxygen saturation. Patients with an oxygen saturation of 88% or lower during the night will benefit from continuous oxygen therapy at night.
- Continuous oxygen therapy has been proven beneficial for patients with polycythemia (Hct > 55%), pulmonary hypertension, increased $PaCO_2$ (> 45 mm Hg), decreased oxygen saturation (< 88% awake or asleep), and right-sided heart failure.
- Bronchodilators are the first pharmacologic agents indicated for an exacerbation of COPD. They relax smooth airway muscle in mild, moderate, or severe exacerbations. A handheld nebulizer (HHN) is often easier for acutely ill or elderly patients, but a multiple dose inhaler (MDI) can also be used (and if used properly, medication deposition in the lungs may be better).
  - Albuterol: short-acting beta agonist, 500 mcg by HHN every 1 to 2 hours (in acute exacerbation). Do not exceed recommended daily dose (1 to 2 puffs QID) without MD consultation or 180 mcg (2 puffs) with spacer MDI every 1 to 2 hours in acute exacerbation. Monitor heart rate, as albuterol has been associated with tachycardia and ischemia. Oral albuterol (4 mg PO BID) is not usually used in acute exacerbation, but patients with chronic COPD may be on oral albuterol. Inhaled albuterol may be used alone *or with*
  - Ipratropium: anticholinergic (Atrovent), 500 mcg QID HHN or 36 mcg (2 puffs) MDI QID with spacer: decreases smooth muscle tone by blocking muscarinic receptors; also reduces sputum volume; maximum of 12 puffs/day
  - Duonebs for HHN contain both albuterol and atrovent.
  - Combivent via MDI, two inhalations QID, contains both albuterol and atrovent.
- Glucocorticosteroids
  - Although its use is controversial in COPD, methylprednisolone sodium succinate (Solu-Medrol) may aid in decreasing inflammation in acute exacerbations and should be started immediately for severe exacerbation. Usual dosage: 60 to 125 mg intravenous (IV) (0.5 mg to 2 mg/kg) every 6 hours for 3 days, then changed to oral prednisone for 2 week taper. Some patients, however, may need longer IV corticosteroid therapy (up to 2 weeks). The hazards of steroid therapy preclude treatment for mild COPD exacerbations.
    - Oral prednisone taper (to be started after IV steroids): 60 mg PO on days 4 to 7, 40 mg on days 8 to 12, 20 mg on days 12 to 15; to shorten recovery time and help restore lung function for moderate to severe exacerbation
- Oral prednisone 40 to 50 mg daily for 5 to 10 days *or* prednisone taper for mild to moderate exacerbation not requiring IV glucocorticosteroids
- Monitor blood sugars (Accuchecks BID to QID) and control hyperglycemia (see Chapter 9).

- Inhaled steroids may also be beneficial in acute exacerbations, although the benefit of long-term therapy is controversial.
- Antibiotic therapy: adjust dose appropriately for renal impairment and maintain sufficient fluid intake. Duration of treatment should be guided by patient response; some patients may require 14 days of antibiotic therapy.
  - For mild exacerbations:
    - Amoxicillin (Amoxil) 500 mg PO every 8 hours × 10 to 14 days (may be associated with higher rate resistance) *or*
    - Doxycycline (Vibramycin) 100 mg PO BID × 10 to 14 days *or*
    - Trimethoprim-sulfamethoxazole 160/800 mg (Bactrim DS), 1 tablet PO BID for 10 to 14 days
  - For moderate to severe exacerbation or if patient does not improve on above regimen, consider:
    - Amoxicillin/clavulanate (Augmentin), 500 mg PO every 8 to 12 hours for 10 days with food *or*
    - Clarithromycin (Biaxin), 500 mg PO BID for 10 days with food or Azithromycin (Zithromax), 500 mg PO on day 1, then 250 mg PO daily for 4 days *or*
    - Ceftriaxone (Rocephin), 1 g IV every 24 hours for 10 days, or other third-generation cephalosporin *or*
    - Levofloxacin (Levaquin), 250 to 500 mg IV/PO every 24 hours for 10 days
- Methylxanthines
  - Aminophylline, 0.9 mg/kg IBW IV, or theophylline, 150 to 450 mg PO BID, can be considered (in consultation with MD) for severe exacerbations. Aminophylline aids in lowering pulmonary artery pressure. Drug levels must be carefully monitored (therapeutic level 10 to 20 mcg/mL) to prevent toxicity, and the drug should be avoided if ectopy develops. Use is controversial because of side effects and unclear benefit.
- Additional management recommendations:
  - Tiotropium bromide (Spiriva), a longer acting anticholinergic, can be used once daily for stable patients (should not be used concurrently with ipratropium). Both Spiriva and salmeterol (Serevent), a long-acting bronchodilator are not appropriate for acute exacerbations, but have been associated with a decreased number of COPD exacerbations when used for long-term management.
  - Identify and treat associated problems (e.g., CHF, arrhythmia, anxiety).
  - Avoid respiratory depressants (e.g., sedatives, hypnotics).
  - Begin respiratory therapy if available.
  - Monitor fluid balance and nutrition: intake and output (I&O), encouragement of fluids, and nutritional supplements and small, frequent feedings to provide adequate fluids/proteins/calories to prevent weight loss and muscle wasting.

- Consider mucolytic agents for patients with thick, tenacious sputum. However, the benefit of mucolytic agents is unproven.
- Once patient is stable, review prevention strategies: vaccination, exercise, proper use of medications and devices (i.e., HHN, MDI) fluid intake, hygiene with MDI and HHN, use of spirometry. Consider long-lasting β-agonist along with anticholinergic MDI, nocturnal, or continuous oxygen therapy (if indicated).
- Prevent complications of immobility, such as thromboemboli, deconditioning.
- Consider subcutaneous heparin to prevent DVT, especially if patient has polycythemia.
- Monitor vital signs, weight, and blood sugar while on steroid therapy.
- Encourage smoking cessation for patients who still smoke. (Smoking cessation has been proven to decrease vulnerability to infection.)
- Consider osteoporosis prevention. (Osteoporosis is more common in COPD patients, especially with long-term or frequent steroid therapy [oral or inhaled].)
- Immunize: Pneumovax × 1, then every 5 years (if patient unaware of previous Pneumovax status, vaccine should be given); influenza immunization yearly.
- If indicated, monitor blood gases to determine presence of hypercapnia.

Consultation/Hospitalization

- Hospitalization is indicated if patient has severe exacerbation (sudden onset resting dyspnea), new onset peripheral edema, previous history of acute exacerbation (particularly if hospitalization within past year), newly occurring arrhythmia, diagnostic uncertainty, confusion, lethargy, coma, is unable to clear airway, or does not respond to initial medical management.
- Consult with pulmonologist for:
  - Suspected alpha$_1$-antitrypsin deficiency for alpha$_1$-antitrypsin replacement therapy
  - Continuous positive airway pressure (CPAP) if appropriate and available (Use cautiously with patient with low BP, arrhythmia, myocardial infarction [MI], cognitive changes, aspiration, extreme obesity, or facial abnormalities.)
  - Pulmonary function tests
  - Consideration for lung volume reduction surgery or lung transplantation
  - Pulmonary rehabilitation to learn proper breathing techniques and improve exercise tolerance
- Consult Dietary in regard to meeting the patient's increased nutritional needs. Consider a feeding tube for the short term if patient is unable to eat secondary to increased respiratory distress.

- Consult Respiratory Therapy (if available) for chest percussion, and to teach proper breathing techniques.
- Consult Physical Therapy (PT) to emphasize strength training and aid in preventing illness-related deconditioning.
- Consult Occupational Therapy (OT) to teach patient energy conservation.

Complications

Complications of delay in treatment: need for intubation, deteriorating mental status, aspiration, and disease progression. Additional complications include sepsis, shock, hypercapnia, acute respiratory arrest, and death.

Education for Nursing Home/Rehabilitation Staff

- Explain to staff the importance of reporting any fever, anorexia, change in sputum, or increased sputum production or increased respiratory distress, increased shortness of breath (SOB), or mental status changes.
- Teach nursing staff the importance of good mouth care and the need to observe for thrush.
- Stress the importance of accurate I&O and weights.
- Teach staff how to use oxygen saturation machine correctly, importance of monitoring oxygen saturation routinely during the day and periodically at night to detect hypoxia.
- Encourage fluids at room temperature; cold liquids can constrict airway.
- Encourage activity. Patients should be encouraged to get out of bed periodically throughout the day and for meals.
- Staff should understand how to teach patients correct use of MDI and nebulizers.
- Staff should be taught to use spirometer.
- Discuss with staff the importance of cleaning nebulizers and MDIs.
- Explain to staff importance of yearly influenza immunization.
- Discuss with staff importance of psychologic support for patients and families.

Patient/Family Education

- Explain disease process, pharmacologic therapy, and importance of good nutrition, adequate sleep, fluid intake, and participating in pulmonary rehabilitation.
- Discuss importance of avoiding allergens, smoke, and other respiratory irritants.
- Encourage smoking cessation for patients and family members.
- Emphasize importance of Pneumovax immunization and yearly influenza immunization (if no allergy).

Bibliography

Adams, S.G., et al. (2000). Antibiotics are associated with lower relapse rates in outpatients with acute exacerbations of COPD. *Chest, 117*, 1345-1352.

Calverly, P.M.A., Barnes, P.J. (2000). Are inhaled steroids beneficial in COPD? A pro/con debate. *American Journal of Respiratory Critical Care Medicine, 161*, 341-344.

Cydulka, R. (2002). COPD management in the emergency department. *Journal of COPD Management, 3*(3), 10-13.

Gross, N. (2002). Treatment of COPD in the veterans' affairs patient. *Journal of COPD Management, 3*(3), 4-9.

Hunter, M.H., & King, D.E. (2001). COPD: Management of acute exacerbations and chronic disease. *American Family Physician, 64*, 603-612, 621-622.

Manda, W., & Rennard, S.I. (2003). COPD: New treatments. *Consultant, 43*(8), 953-965.

National Heart, Lung and Blood Institute: Morbidity and Mortality. (2002). *Chart book on cardiovascular, lung and blood diseases*. Baltimore, MD: National Institutes of Health.

Pauwels, R.A., et al. (2001). Global strategy for the diagnosis, management and prevention of chronic obstructive pulmonary disease. NHLBI/WHO global initiative for chronic obstructive lung disease (GOLD) executive summary. *Respiratory Care, 46*(8), 798-825.

Sinn, D.D., et al. (2003). Contemporary management of chronic obstructive pulmonary disease; clinical applications. *Journal of the American Medical Association, 290*(17), 2301-2312.

Snow, V. (2001). How to manage acute COPD exacerbations: New guidelines. *Consultant 41*(7), 1171-1173.

Snow, V., et al. (2001). Joint expert panel on chronic obstructive pulmonary disease of the American College of Chest Physicians and the American College of Physicians—American Society of Internal Medicine. Evidence base for the management of acute exacerbation of chronic obstructive pulmonary disease. *Annals of Internal Medicine, 134*, 595-599.

Stoller, J.K. (2002). Acute exacerbation of chronic obstructive pulmonary disease. *New England Journal of Medicine, 346*(13), 988-994.

Wilkinson, T.M.A., et al. (2004). Early therapy improves outcomes of exacerbations of chronic obstructive pulmonary disease. *American Journal of Respiratory Critical Care Medicine, 169*, 1298-1303.

PNEUMONIA

ICD-9: 486

An acute lower respiratory tract infection involving the gas-exchanging units of the lungs, pneumonia is a major source of morbidity and mortality in all age groups, but particularly in elders and those with co-morbid illness. Pneumonia occurs more often in nursing homes than in other locations. The most common infectious pneumonias affecting elders in the nursing home include the community-acquired pneumonias as well as *Streptococcus pneumoniae, Haemophilus influenzae*, and gram-negative bacilli (*Klebsiella, Pseudomonas aeruginosa*, *Serratia*, *Enterobacter*, and methicillin-resistant *Staphylococcus aureus* [MRSA]). However, aspiration, anaerobes, viral, mycoplasma, and fungal etiologies should also be considered.

Risk Factors

- Age > 70 years
- Alcohol: diminishes immune system
- Altered mental status/dementia: increases risk of aspiration
- Chronically ill or immunocompromised
- COPD
- Cough deficit
- Lack of influenza/pneumococcal vaccination
- Malnutrition
- Medications: sedatives or anticholinergics
- Nasogastric (NG) tube: increases risk of aspiration
- Poor dentition or oral hygiene
- Smoking history
- Swallowing deficit

History

A change in mental or functional status is often the first symptom noticed by the nursing staff. Further information should include the history of the present illness (HPI), allergies, current medications, past medical history, and advanced directives.

- Anorexia, tachypnea (respiratory rate > 25), increased weakness or falls, lethargy, or a change in functional or mental status may be the only sign of illness.
- Cough (new or increasing in severity), dyspnea, fever, malaise, chills, pleuritic pain, and purulent sputum production are significant symptoms, although in elderly or immunocompromised patients, the common signs and symptoms of pneumonia or an infectious process may be absent.

Physical Examination

The physical examination can be variable. An alteration in mental or functional status is an important clinical finding, especially when combined with abnormal vital signs.

- Vital signs
  - Fever may be absent.
  - Oxygen saturation may be normal or decreased.
  - Blood pressure: hypotension is possible and suggests dehydration or infection.
  - Heart rate

- Cardiac: determine rate and rhythm. Heart rate > 120 suggests systemic illness.
- Lungs: respiratory rate > 28 is significant, as tachypnea is considered to be a sensitive indication of pneumonia. Other significant pulmonary signs include dyspnea, fremitus, bronchophony, egophony, dullness to percussion, unilateral crackles, and/or wheezes that do not clear with cough.
- Abdomen: check for distention and bowel sounds, as hypoxia may cause ileus.
- Neurologic: change in mental or functional status is also an important clinical finding.

Differential Diagnosis

- Bacterial pneumonia: gram-positive bacteria (*Streptococcus pneumoniae, Staphylococcus aureus*); gram-negative bacteria (*Haemophilus influenzae, Pseudomonas aeruginosa, Klebsiella pneumoniae, Moraxella catarrhalis*)
- Atypical pneumonias: *Mycoplasma pneumoniae, Chlamydia pneumoniae,* adenovirus, para-influenza virus, respiratory synctial virus, *Legionella pneumophila, Pneumocystis carinii*
- Anaerobic infection: aspiration pneumonia, lung abscess
- Influenza
- Bronchitis
- *M. tuberculosis*
- Congestive heart failure
- Pulmonary embolus

Diagnostics

- Oxygen saturation
- CBC/diff: may be normal
- Serum electrolytes, BUN, and creatinine: to determine fluid/electrolyte and renal status
- Chest radiograph: infiltrate may not be present if patient is dehydrated
- Sputum for Gram stain and culture and sensitivity: if drug resistance is suspected
- Consider blood cultures (aerobic and anaerobic) × 2: if fever and chills
- Consider sputum for acid-fast bacillus (AFB) if indicated.
- Consider two-step PPD if indicated.

Treatment Plan

There are often several factors to consider. The patient's wishes for treatment should be respected if advanced directives are in place. If there are no advanced directives, the family or significant other and the physician should be contacted and informed about the change in the patient's condition. If the patient wishes to prohibit antibiotic therapy, care and comfort measures should be initiated.

The second consideration is the ability of the facility to care for the patient. Hospitalization may be necessary if the patient is unable to take oral antibiotics and the facility does not provide intravenous therapy. Hospitalization is also essential for patients in acute respiratory distress.

Medications should be reviewed. Diuretics may need to be decreased or held, depending on the patient's hydration status. If the patient is lethargic, any medications potentially causing the change in mental status should be held.

- Give oxygen if indicated to maintain oxygen saturation > 90%.
- Antibiotic therapy should be started as soon as possible if pneumonia is clinically suspected. Nursing home patients are at increased risk for gram-negative pneumonia, *S. pneumoniae*, *H.influenzae*, and *S. aureus*, thus requiring specific antibiotic therapy. Oral hydration and oral antibiotic therapy are preferred.
    - If the patient is unable to take oral medications, IM, or IV Rocephin (ceftriaxone) 1 g every 24 hours or Claforan (cefotaxime) 500 mg every 12 hours is indicated (unless allergic). IV clindamycin, azithromycin, or fluoroquinolone therapy may be substituted for allergic patients.
    - If aspiration pneumonia is suspected, clindamycin (Cleocin) or amoxicillin-clavulanate (Augmentin) is recommended.
    - MRSA: occasionally, a sputum culture reveals the patient has MRSA. Sensitivities will reveal the appropriate antibiotic, although vancomycin (Vancocin) is often the medication of choice (see Chapter 16). Zyvox (linezolid), 600 mg PO or IV every 12 hours for 10 to 14 days may also be appropriate.
    - Oral antibiotics can usually be instituted after 3 to 5 days of IV therapy if the patient has been afebrile for 24 hours, is able to swallow, is well hydrated, and is clinically stable (i.e., no acute life-threatening or cardiac events).
        - Patients considered appropriate for oral antibiotic therapy should receive combination therapy with a β-lactam and an advanced-generation macrolide (doxycycline can be substituted for the macrolide) or monotherapy with levofloxacin (Levaquin, 250 to 500 mg PO every 24 hours) or other fluoroquinolone with anti-pneumococcal coverage. Antibiotic therapy should be continued for 10 to 14 days or longer if clinically indicated.
- Additional management recommendations:
    - Patients on antibiotics and warfarin (Coumadin) should have warfarin dose reduced and INR checked in 2 to 3 days to prevent excessive anticoagulation.
    - Diabetic patients require frequent Accuchecks and appropriate sliding-scale insulin coverage (see Chapter 9).
    - Patients with feeding tubes will require increased free water each shift while ill.

- Increased fluids to 2 L daily. (Intake should exceed output by 1 L.)
- At-risk patients should have renal status monitored. Antibiotic doses must be adjusted for patients with renal insufficiency.
- IV fluids, if indicated (poor oral intake, nausea, vomiting, or serum sodium > 155). Daily serum electrolytes, BUN, and creatinine are necessary for patients receiving IV fluid.
- Consider nebulizer with unit dose ipratropium bromide 0.017% and albuterol 0.083% (Duoneb), unit dose albuterol (0.083%), or unit dose ipratropium bromide (Atrovent 0.02%) QID and PRN × 2 during night especially if patient has dyspnea, dry cough, or wheezing. The patient's heart rate should be monitored on albuterol. If tachycardia occurs with albuterol or if patient has history of cardiac ischemia, Atrovent should be used.
- Encourage cough and deep breaths
- Chest percussion
- Acetaminophen (Tylenol) 650 mg PO/PR every 4 to 6 hours PRN for fever reduction (if fever > 100° F) and comfort
- Avoid cough suppressants.
- Consider Robitussin 2 tsp PO every 4 to 6 hours PRN.
- Cool-mist humidification for comfort
- Consider daily yogurt or lactobacillus tablets while patient is on antibiotic therapy to deter *C. difficile* colitis.

Consultation/Hospitalization

- Notify physician of change in patient status and if patient fails to respond to treatment within 48 to 72 hours, as antibiotic therapy may need to be changed.
- Most patients are now treated in the rehabilitation or long-term care facility, but some physicians, patients, and/or families choose hospitalization.
- Hospitalization may be indicated for patients who have new-onset unresponsiveness, have hypoxia (oxygen saturation < 90% on room air) and do not respond to oxygen therapy, are hypotensive, or have comorbid conditions such as CHF, COPD, or diabetes.
- Hospitalization is also recommended if the facility cannot provide laboratory access, IV therapy, or appropriate nursing care.
- Consider hospitalization if patient presentation warrants blood cultures to exclude bacteremia.
- Consult physician if sputum culture and sensitivities are positive for MRSA to discuss suitable antibiotic therapy.

Complications

- Dehydration
- Failure to respond to treatment

- Nausea, vomiting, or C. *difficile* colitis from antibiotic therapy
- Infection precipitating atrial fibrillation or CHF
- Respiratory arrest

Education for Nursing Home/Rehabilitation Staff

- Explain to nursing staff the importance of obtaining vital signs and oxygen saturation for patients with a change in status and reporting findings to the healthcare provider immediately.
- Discuss with nursing staff the importance of starting antibiotic therapy within 4 hours after the medication has been ordered.
- Use universal precautions. Wash hands after patient contact.
- Consider isolation in room for 48 to 72 hours to protect other patients.
- The importance of frequently changing the patient's positioning (every 1 to 2 hours) should be explained. Semi-recumbent positioning, if possible, may help prevent aspiration pneumonia.
- Discuss parameters for adequate fluid intake to prevent dehydration. Nursing staff should understand the importance of encouraging fluids and reporting poor oral intake to the healthcare provider.
- The importance of checking vital signs and oxygen saturation frequently every 4 hours for 48 hours or until patient improves; then each shift and prn should be stressed.
- The nursing staff should also understand that a drop in oxygen saturation to the low 90s (or lower), systolic blood pressure < 90, heart rate > 120, increasing dyspnea, or decreased intake or output (< 30 mL/hr) may be significant and requires that the healthcare provider be notified.
- If MRSA is positive, isolation is necessary.
  - Masks when entering room
  - Gloves and gowns for direct patient contact
  - Careful handwashing after removing gloves
  - Separate blood pressure cuff, thermometer, and stethoscope in patient's room
  - Patient to wear a mask if leaving the room
- If aspiration risk, institute aspiration precautions.
- Explain importance of oral hygiene for patients to help decrease the incidence of aspiration pneumonia.
- Discuss importance of feeding small amounts of food to patients at risk for aspiration, as well as avoiding sedative medications that can increase dysphagia.
- Discuss importance of monitoring patients for dysphagia (i.e., monitoring for drooling, pocketing food on one side of mouth, food remaining in mouth after swallowing, coughing when drinking or eating, gargly vocal changes after eating or drinking).
- Stress value of pneumococcal and influenza immunization.
- Explain importance of cleaning humidifiers daily.

Patient/Family Education

- The recommendation for hospitalization should be discussed with the patient and family. The importance of increased fluids, oxygen, and nebulizer treatment should be discussed.
- Explain need for isolation and careful handwashing.
- Explain the importance of coughing up mucus and avoiding cough suppressants.
- Explain importance of mobilization and not staying in bed.
- Discuss the reasons ill family members should not visit patient.
- For patients at risk for aspiration, family members should understand the importance of maintaining the head of the bed above 45°; feeding small amounts of food; and using appropriate, thickened liquids. If the patient has a neurologic impairment, education about food placement on unaffected side of the mouth is also important.
- Discuss importance of pneumonia immunization and yearly influenza vaccine.

Bibliography

American Thoracic Society. (2001). Guidelines for the management of adults with community-acquired pneumonia. *American Journal of Respiratory Critical Care Medicine*, 163, 1730-1754.

Drinka, P. (2002). The role of atypical pathogens in nursing home pneumonia. *Journal of the American Medical Directors Association*, 3(5), 345-346.

Gleason, P.P., et al. (1999). Association between initial antimicrobial treatment and medical outcomes for hospitalized elderly patients with pneumonia. Archivers of Internal Medicine, 159(21), 2562-2572.

Houck, P.M., et al. (2004). Timing of antibiotic administration and outcomes for Medicare patients hospitalized with community-acquired pneumonia. *Archives of Internal Medicine*, 164(6), 637-644.

Hutt, E., & Kramer, A.M. (2004). Evidenced-based guidelines for management of nursing home–acquired pneumonia. *Journal of Family Practice*, 51(8), 709-716.

Marrie, T.J. (2002). Pneumonia in long-term care facilities. *Infection Control and Hospital Epidemiology*, 23(3), 159-164.

Naughton, B.J., & Mylotte, J.M. (2000). Treatment guidelines for NH pneumonia based on community practice. *Journal of the American Geriatric Society*, 48(1), 82-88.

INFLUENZA

ICD 9: 487.1

An acute respiratory viral infection caused by influenza A or B, influenza causes significant morbidity and mortality in persons older than 65 years of age and is responsible for more than 110,000 hospitalizations each year. Spread by droplet infection and hand-to-hand contact, outbreaks occur between late December and early March in the United States. Annual outbreaks occur with variable severity from year to year. In this country, the 2002 to 2003 influenza season was not severe, but in the late 1990s, influenza-associated deaths were increasing. Up to 90% of deaths associated with influenza occur in elderly persons.

Risk Factors

- Age > 65
- Immunocompromised
- History of chronic cardiopulmonary disease
- Communal living (e.g., long-term care facility, group home)
- Exposure to school-aged children

History

- Symptoms differ from the common cold, as onset is abrupt and accompanied by fever (up to 104° F) and nonproductive cough within the first 48 hours.
- Chills
- Headache or chest discomfort
- Sneezing, rhinitis, or pharyngitis
- Myalgias or arthralgias
- Malaise, weakness, and fatigue
- Anorexia
- Change in mental status or functional decline (falls, diminished ability or inability to participate in rehabilitation facilities)

Physical Examination

- Physical findings may initially be unremarkable. High fever (in elders, temperature >100° F is significant for infectious process), mild pharyngeal injection with posterior pharyngeal cobblestoning, and cervical lymphadenopathy may be present.
- Dyspnea, cyanosis, hypoxia, and rales are indicative of pneumonia. Pulmonary examination is usually unremarkable in influenza.

Differential Diagnosis

- Acute viral respiratory illness
- Respiratory synctial virus, adenovirus, rhinovirus, coronavirus, or parainfluenza virus
- Pneumonia
- Acute bronchitis

Diagnostics

- Culture nasal, pharyngeal, sputum secretions for virus, if indicated. Viral cultures are most accurate test, but might take 48 hours or more and are more costly than rapid viral assays.
- Rapid viral tests (enzyme immunoassay or direct immunofluorescence) can rapidly (within 20 min) determine presence of influenza (BD Directigen Flu A & B can differentiate between influenza A and B).
- Chest radiograph if indicated
- CBC/diff: may be normal; leukocytosis > 15,000 suggests bacterial pneumonia
- Serum electrolytes, BUN, and creatinine if dehydration is a concern
- Sputum for Gram stain and culture and sensitivity if indicated

Treatment Plan

- Relenza (zanamivir) and Tamiflu (oseltamivir) are neuraminidase inhibitors indicated for treatment of both influenza A and B within 48 hours of symptom onset.
  - Zanamivir, contraindicated in asthma or COPD, is a dry powder that is inhaled (via a disk-haler) to treat influenza: two inhalations twice on day 1 (inhalations should be at least 2 hours apart); then two inhalations every 12 hours for 4 days. Discontinue if bronchospasms result with inhalation.
  - Oseltamivir is indicated for both chemoprophylaxis and treatment of influenza A and B.
    - Treatment: 75 mg PO every 12 hours with food for 5 days; if creatinine clearance is 10 to 30 mL/min, 75 mg PO daily with food for 5 days
    - Prophylactic treatment: 75 mg PO with food daily for 7 days or longer, depending on length of outbreak; if creatinine clearance is 10 to 30 mL/min, 75 mg PO with food every other day for 1 week or length of outbreak
    - Dosage should be decreased if creatinine clearance is < 30 mL/min.
- Symmetrel (amantidine) and Flumadine (rimantadine) inhibit viral replication and may be used to treat influenza A if given within 48 hours of symptom onset. These agents may also be used prophylactically and should be considered for all patients, but neither is efficacious against influenza B.
  - Amantidine dosage is based on serum creatinine (Cr < 1.0 = 100 mg daily; Cr > 1.0 < 2.0 = 100 mg every other day; Cr > 2.0 = 100 mg 2×/week; dialysis patient = 100 mg a week).
  - Rimantadine 100 mg PO daily is recommended for elders. Rimantadine also requires dose adjustment for patients with renal and hepatic insufficiency.

- Increase fluids as much as possible (e.g., soups, bouillon, popsicles). Fluid intake should exceed output by 1 L.
- Provide IV therapy if indicated.
- Rest.
- Use oxygen if indicated to maintain oxygen saturation > 90%.
- Provide acetaminophen, 650 mg PO/PR every 4 to 6 hours, for comfort.
- Antibiotic therapy is indicated for secondary bacterial pneumonia.
- Monitor carefully for deterioration in status.

Complications

- Primary influenza pneumonia: continued dyspnea, nonproductive cough, high fever, and hypoxia with diffuse rales
- Secondary bacterial pneumonia: fever, productive cough with purulent sputum production, usually occuring after brief period of recovery from influenza; consolidation on radiograph
- Mixed viral and bacterial pneumonia: fairly common, with steady progression of illness or minimal improvement followed by relapse
- Worsening cardiopulmonary or renal function
- Myositis: acute muscle tenderness
- Rhabdomyolosis
- Myoglobulinemia
- Dehydration
- Possible central nervous system association (e.g., encephalitis)
- Exacerbation of COPD or other lung disease (e.g., asthma)
- Acute bronchitis

Consultation/Hospitalization

- Notify the physician of a change in patient status and if the patient fails to respond to treatment within 48 to 72 hours.
- Hospitalization may be indicated for increasing respiratory compromise.

Education for Nursing Home/Rehabilitation Staff

- Unless contraindicated, yearly influenza vaccination is indicated for all patients from the beginning of October to mid-November.
    - Patients at high-risk for the complications associated with influenza may be immunized during September and October.
    - Caregivers (both personnel and household members) of high-risk patients may also be immunized during September and October.
- Persons with egg allergies should not receive the vaccine.
- Persons with acute illness and fever should not receive the vaccine until illness has resolved.

- Persons with previous anaphylactic reaction to vaccine should not be immunized.
- Persons with chronic illnesses (such as asthma) or those older than 49 years should not receive the intranasal influenza vaccine.
- Healthcare workers should be immunized.
- Influenza vaccine is an inactivated vaccine that targets influenza A and B.
- Notify the healthcare provider as soon as flu symptoms occur in any patient.
- Discuss possible isolation of infected patients for 72 hours to prevent further outbreak. Incubation period lasts 1 to 4 days, but the contagious stage may last for 5 days after symptom onset.
- If there is a serious facility outbreak, consider keeping all patients in their rooms for 72 hours.
- Use universal precautions and wash hands frequently **(between each patient).**
- Weekly updates are available at *www.cdc.gov/ncidod/diseases/flu/weekly.htm* and *www.PreventInfluenza.org.*

Patient/Family Education

- Annual vaccination from mid-October through mid-November is recommended for people older than 50 years of age, residents of long-term care or assisted living facilities, and for people who are immunosuppressed or with comorbid illness (e.g., COPD, CHF, diabetes).
- The vaccine does not provide permanent immunity or protect against colds or other illness. Additionally, the vaccine may not protect persons from acquiring influenza, because the virus can mutate.
- Coughing and sneezing spreads influenza. Careful, frequent handwashing helps prevent viral distribution.
- Friends and family with cold or influenza symptoms should not visit patients.
- Influenza, if uncomplicated, usually resolves within 5 days, but post-influenza weakness can last several weeks.

Bibliography

Antiviral agents for influenza: Background information for clinicians. *www.cdc.gov/flu/professionals/antiviralback.htm.* Accessed June 30, 2004.

CDC Prevention and Control of Influenza. (2003). Recommendations of the Advisory Committee on Immunization (ACIP). *Morbidity and Mortality Weekly Report (MMWR),* RR8, 1-34.

Kingston, B.J., & Wright, C.V. Jr. (2002). Influenza in the nursing home. *American Family Physician,* 65(1), 75-78.

Nichol, K.L., et al. (2003). Influenza vaccination and reduction in hospitalizations for cardiac disease and stroke among the elderly. *New England Journal of Medicine, 348,* 1322-1332.

Peters, P.H. Jr. (2000). The impact of influenza on the aging population. *Annals of Long-Term Care*, 8(supp), 16.

Thompson, W.W., et al. (2003). Mortality associated with influenza and respiratory synctial virus in the United States. *Journal of the American Medical Association, 289*, 179-186.

PULMONARY EMBOLISM

ICD-9: 415.19

Approximately 650,000 cases of pulmonary embolism (PE) occur in the United States each year, resulting in approximately 50,000 deaths. For elders and those living in nursing home facilities, the risk for PE is increased. PEs occur most often in patients with venous thrombosis but may also occur without deep vein thrombosis (DVT). Small thromboemboli might not cause symptoms, but a significant obstruction can be rapidly fatal with presenting signs and symptoms of complete circulatory collapse. Although clinical presentation can suggest PE, extensive diagnostic evaluation is necessary to confirm the presence of a PE.

Risk Factors

- Immobilization for 3 or more days in previous 4 to 12 weeks (relate to illness, pregnancy, surgery, or travel)
- Previous DVT or confirmed PE
- Family history of DVT, PE, or cerebrovascular accident
- Inadequate anticoagulation therapy
- Hormonal therapy (e.g., oral contraceptive, hormone replacement therapy, tamoxifen)
- Advanced age
- AIDS
- Bechet's disease
- Chemotherapy
- CHF
- COPD
- Hyperhomocysteinemia
- Inflammatory bowel disease
- Intimal vessel injury: burns, childbirth, fracture (fat emboli), IV access, cannulation, pregnancy (amniotic emboli), and trauma
- Lower-extremity paralysis
- Malignancy
- Obesity
- Polycythemia and sickle cell disease

- Smoking
- Hereditary clotting defects (e.g., protein S, protein C, antithrombin III deficiency, antiphospholipid antibody syndrome)

History

Symptoms are often vague and patients may be completely asymptomatic. Pain on inspiration, tachycardia, and an acute onset of dyspnea or an increase in chronic dyspnea should always prompt consideration of pulmonary embolism. The patient's personal and family history is important, although embolic events occur in patients without risk factors. Additional suggestive symptoms that require consideration include:

- Pleuritic chest pain, cough, and dyspnea present in a significant number, although not all, patients
- Chest-wall tenderness and back pain
- Hemoptysis
- Restlessness
- Anxiety
- New-onset wheezing
- Signs of right ventricular failure and myocardial ischemia: in massive PE
- Signs of pulmonary hypertension: substernal chest discomfort and lightheadedness
- Syncope, convulsions, and neurologic deficits

Physical Examination

Initially, there may be no abnormal physical findings. Some findings are indicative of a PE, but many PEs are missed because the symptoms and physical findings are nonspecific. Suggestive signs include:

- Constitutional: restless, anxious, diaphoretic, and feverish
- Vital signs
  - Temperature: some, but not all, patients will have fever.
  - Tachycardia: heart rate > 90
  - Tachypnea
  - Oxygen saturation < 92% on room air (initially oxygen saturation may be normal)
  - Hypotension: may be present with massive PE
- Skin: cyanosis
- Lungs: hypoxia, wheezes, rales, or pleural rub
- Cardiac: increased JVD; split S2, loud P2, S4, RV heave, murmur, arrhythmias may be present
- Extremities: edema may be present. Presence of DVT may indicate PE; absence of DVT does not exclude PE
- Musculoskeletal: chest-wall tenderness without history of trauma

Differential Diagnosis

The clinical presentation of PE may be similar to other disorders associated with chest discomfort and/or dyspnea. Frequently, the possibility of a PE is overlooked. Nevertheless, it may be helpful to also review Chest Pain (see Chapter 5) and consider the following conditions in the differential.

- Pericardial disease
- Pleural disease
- Pneumothorax
- CHF
- MI
- Pneumonia
- Malignancy
- COPD
- Septic shock
- Anxiety with hyperventilation

Diagnostics

- **If patient is in shock or hypoxic, hospitalization/emergency evaluation is required.** (Diagnostics should be deferred to the emergency department physician.)
- For patients who are stable, but for whom PE is a concern, urgent diagnostic evaluation is essential. Consultation with the physician is recommended to determine the most appropriate diagnostic and/or to discuss evaluation in the emergency department.
  - VQ scan: this is used most often as an initial diagnostic, but it may be misleading, especially in a patient with COPD or interstitial fibrosis. If lung is totally occluded with a clot, lungs can be ventilated but not perfused.
  - Spiral CT: increasingly reliable, but expensive and carries risk of reaction to dye
  - Pulmonary angiogram: considered the "gold standard;" invasive and expensive, but is the diagnostic of choice if ultrasound is negative and VQ scan results are unclear.
  - MRI: appropriate in some situations and indispensable for determining presence of DVT in an upper extremity
  - Duplex venous ultrasound: positive ultrasound is indirect evidence of PE.
  - Arterial blood gases: hypoxemia is present in many pulmonary conditions and is not specific for PE.
  - CBC: white blood count may be elevated but is not specific for PE.
  - D-dimer: not sensitive and not specific for PE
  - ECG: right-axis deviation; tall, peaked P wave; ST-T wave changes consistent with right ventricular failure
  - Chest radiograph: normal chest film does not rule out PE.

Treatment Plan

- Hospitalization may be indicated for anticoagulation (intravenous heparin or low molecular weight heparin), with possible fibrinolytic therapy (alteplase or retaplase).
- Oxygen is necessary for all patients with suspected PE (to maintain oxygen saturation > 90).
- IV access
- Consider heparin, 5000 units subcutaneously, or heparin infusion (bolus 80 mcg/kg, followed by 18 mcg/kg continuous infusion) before transfer to an acute care facility.
- Pain management
- Anxiety management
- Patient may need a Greenfield filter if PE develops despite anticoagulation.
- Patients will require long-term anticoagulant therapy with warfarin (Coumadin) after hospitalization (goal INR: usually 2 to 3).

Consultation/Hospitalization

- **Hospitalization/emergency department evaluation is indicated for suspected acute PE.** After starting oxygen, initiate pain medication, and, if possible, obtain IV access.
- Discuss with the physician appropriate pain medication.
- Discuss with the physician stat dose heparin, 5000 units SQ, for patients with suspected PE prior to hospitalization.
- Consultation with the physician is indicated for any patient with suspected PE.

Complications

- Cardiovascular collapse and death may occur quickly if a large clot occludes pulmonary system.
- Pulmonary hypertension
- Cor pulmonale
- Venous stasis syndrome (chronic peripheral edema and venous ulcers) may occur in patients with DVT.

Education for Nursing Home/Rehabilitation Staff

- Discuss with nurses the importance of monitoring the patient carefully for hemoptysis and other symptoms associated with PE. The nursing staff should also understand the importance of notifying the healthcare provider about the change in the patient's status.
- Educate the nursing staff to ensure that the anticoagulation protocol is carefully followed.

- Discuss with nursing staff the importance of exercise, mobilization, adequate fluid intake in preventing DVT and PE.
- See Chapter 16.

Patient/Family Education

- See Chapter 16.
- Explain to patient that anticoagulation is continued long-term after PE.
- Discuss with the patient and family the importance of compliance with medications and blood testing if on anticoagulation.
- If patient has had DVT, educate patient and family regarding signs and symptoms of PE.
- Prevention
  - Explain the relationship of immobilization to DVT and embolism, and encourage patients to exercise lower extremities frequently.
  - Explain to patients at risk for DVT that compression stockings (30 to 40 mm Hg might be beneficial in preventing DVT, but that thromboembolic disease stockings (TEDs) have not been proven valuable in preventing DVT.
  - Discuss the importance of adequate hydration to prevent DVT.

Bibliography

Gomes, J.P., et al. (2003). Incidence of venous thromboembolic events among nursing home residents. *Journal of General Internal Medicine, 18*(11), 936-938.

Horlander, K.T., et al. (2003). Pulmonary embolus mortality in the U.S., 1979-1998: An analysis using multiple cause mortality data. *Archives of Internal Medicine, 163*(14), 1711-1717.

Quinlan, D.J., et al. (2004). Low-molecular weight heparin compared with intravenous unfractionated heparin for treatment of pulmonary embolism: A meta-analysis of randomized controlled trials. *Annals of Internal Medicine, 140*(3), 175-183.

Thompson, B.T., & Hales, C.A. (2004). Clinical manifestations of and diagnostic strategies for acute pulmonary embolism. *www.uptodate.com*. Accessed March 5, 2004.

Writing Committee for the Galilei Investigators (2004). Subcutaneous adjdusted dose unfractionated heparin versus fixed-dose low-molecular weight heparin in the initial treatment of venous thromboembolism. *Archives of Internal Medicine, 164*(10), 1077-1083.

CHAPTER 5

Cardiovascular Disorders

ATRIAL FIBRILLATION

ICD-9: 427.31

Atrial fibrillation (AF) is one of the most common arrhythmias and may be paroxysmal or persistent in nature. Most often related to cardiac disease, hypertension, hyperthyroidism, rheumatic heart disease, heart failure, pericarditis, infection, hypoxia, pulmonary emboli, alcohol, or other stimulants, AF can also be idiopathic. If the ventricular rate is rapid, the patient's hemodynamic status may be significantly compromised. However, patients may be asymptomatic and AF can be an incidental finding. The characteristics associated with AF include an irregularly irregular rhythm with presence of fibrillatory waves on electrocardiogram (ECG). Other ECG changes include the absence of identifiable P waves or PR intervals and an atrial rate of 400 to 600 beats per minute (bpm) with a variable ventricular rate. The fibrillating atria cause inadequate atrial contractions, diminished cardiac output, and heart failure, and may allow emboli to develop within the atrial chambers. Elderly patients especially have an increased risk for developing AF and are also at greater risk for stroke secondary to this dysrhythmia.

History

Shortness of breath, palpitations, dizziness, chest pressure, lightheadedness, and weakness are symptoms that may be associated with AF. Angina or syncope is also a possible presenting symptom. A sudden neurologic deficit suggesting transient ischemic attack (TIA) or an embolic event may be related to AF. Medical history, medications, and allergies, as well as timing of symptoms and associated

75

events (e.g., chest discomfort), are important aspects to review with the patient, family, and staff.

Physical Examination

The aim of the physical examination is to identify the precipitating cause of the AF and determine the patient's hemodynamic status. Critical aspects of the physical evaluation include:
- Vital signs: determine blood pressure (BP; hypotension or hypertension is possible), heart rate, respiratory rate, oxygen saturation, and temperature. A recent weight gain may suggest fluid overload.
- Neurologic: assess mental status and presence of neurologic deficit (from possible embolus).
- Neck: palpate for thyroid enlargement or nodularity.
- Cardiac: auscultate for heart sounds, murmurs, rub. Evaluate presence of jugular vein distention, and hepatojugular reflex.
- Lungs: assess for signs of heart failure and pneumonia.
- Abdomen: evaluate for ascites.
- Extremities: assess for peripheral pulses, edema, and mottling.

Diagnostics

New-onset AF requires diagnostic evaluation to determine the underlying cause of the arrhythmia. The following diagnostics should be considered:
- ECG: indicated initially to determine cardiac rhythm and presence of AF
- Holter monitor or event monitor: if arrhythmia is suspected but not apparent on ECG
- Chest radiograph: to determine presence of heart failure, cardiomyopathy, and pneumonia (infection can precipitate AF)
- Complete blood count with differential (CBC/diff): to determine presence of anemia or infection
- Serum electrolytes: to evaluate potential electrolyte disturbances
- Thyroid-stimulating hormone (TSH) and free T_4: if hyperthyroidism is suspected
- Serum glucose
- Drug levels if indicated
- Echocardiogram if indicated: to assess for valvular disease or ventricular hypertrophy
- Transesophageal echocardiogram if indicated: to determine presence of atrial thrombi

Differential Diagnosis
- See Box 5-1.

BOX 5-1	Differential Diagnosis: Tachyarrhythmias

Narrow Complex
Atrial fibrillation
Atrial flutter
AV nodal reentry tachycardia
AV reciprocating tachycardia
Multifocal atrial tachycardia
Paroxysmal atrial tachycardia
Premature atrial contractions
Premature junctional contractions
Sinus tachycardia

Wide Complex
Supraventricular tachycardia with aberrancy
Ventricular fibrillation
Ventricular tachycardia

Treatment Plan

Treatment is based on patient presentation. The underlying cause of the arrhythmia should be determined and treated. Patients with acute new-onset AF are considered unstable if symptomatic or hypotensive. Airway, breathing, circulation, and responsiveness must be continually assessed. Oxygen should be administered and, if possible, intravenous (IV) access obtained. Rapid transport to the nearest emergency facility is recommended for treatment (synchronized cardioversion or IV amiodarone, β-blocker, calcium channel blocker, or other medication).

For patients who are stable and for whom hospitalization is not appropriate, the goals of treatment should include anticoagulation to prevent emboli, rate control, and, if possible, reinstatement of normal sinus rhythm. More recent studies suggest that heart rate control may be more advantageous for patients than restoration of normal sinus rhythm.

- Anticoagulation: warfarin (Coumadin) is the anticoagulant of choice as numerous trials suggest warfarin is more efficacious than aspirin (see Chapter 16). Dosage is adjusted as necessary to maintain international normalized ratio (INR) between 2 and 3 (goal INR is 2.5).
  - The INR range for patients with AF who are at increased risk for an embolic event may be 2.5 to 3.5.
  - A lower INR range (1.8 to 2.5) is sometimes suggested for patients older than age 75 with increased risk for bleeding, though the benefit of a lowered dose regimen is unproven.
  - Anticoagulation may not be necessary for patients with documented

onset AF < 48 hours in patients who are at low risk for thromboembolism.

- Warfarin is usually continued in older patients, even if the patient's rhythm converts to normal sinus rhythm (NSR) because there is a persistent risk of embolization. (Patients older than 65 years of age with a medical history of AF frequently have asymptomatic paroxysmal episodes.)
- If warfarin is contraindicated, daily aspirin may be appropriate, although the efficacy of aspirin is still unclear.
- Rate control: recommended medications for rate control include metoprolol, atenolol, diltiazem, and verapamil.
  - Digoxin (Lanoxin) may be considered for rapid atrial fibrillation in patients with congestive heart failure or hypotension.
  - Atrioventricular node ablation and pacemaker implantation may be beneficial for some patients if rate control is not achieved with medications.
- Rhythm reinstatement
  - The benefits of pharmacologic treatment and restoration of normal sinus rhythm continue to be studied as there are potential significant medication side effects, and often AF is recurrent. In theory, restoration of normal sinus rhythm should decrease the risk for stroke or other embolic events, but drug therapy can have considerable side effects. Drug therapy is also more beneficial if started within 1 week of the onset of AF.
    - Propafenone (Rythmol) and flecainide (Tambocor) are class IC antiarrhythmics used to reestablish sinus rhythm in some patients. These medications are not indicated for patients with a history of myocardial infarction (MI) or coronary heart disease (CAD) and may be proarrhythmic in some patients.
      - Propafenone is also associated with agranulocytosis, thrombocytopenia, leukopenia, and granulocytopenia.
      - Flecainide is associated with leukopenia and thrombocytopenia.
    - Amiodarone (Cordarone), a class III antiarrhythmic and sotalol HCL, a class II/III antiarrhythmic, may also be used to reestablish sinus rhythm in some patients. Amiodarone may be the most effective in reestablishing sinus rhythm, but is associated with more toxic side effects. Patients are often started on 400 mg PO three times a day, and the dose is tapered to 100 mg to 200 mg daily to prevent toxicity. Amiodarone may also cause prolongation of the QT interval. Because amiodarone is associated with pulmonary fibrosis, hepatotoxicity, and thyroid abnormalities, patients require an ECG, chest radiograph, TSH, and liver function tests (LFTs) every 6 months. Routine ophthalmic examinations are also indicated. Patients may also be transferred on a higher or lower

than expected dose of amiodarone, which also requires communication with the cardiologist. Amiodarone therapy requires careful monitoring (particularly in older patients) and is often tapered down to the lowest dose.

■ The efficacy of sotalol in converting AF to normal sinus rhythm is unclear, although sotalol may be helpful in maintaining NSR. Patients receiving warfarin and amiodarone require careful monitoring of PT/INR. Patients started on sotalol must be hospitalized and monitored, because sotalol may cause prolongation of the QT interval.

• Cardioversion may be recommended for some patients. Anticoagulation with warfarin is usually indicated for patients for 1 month both before and after cardioversion.

Some patients with a history of AF are admitted to rehabilitation or long-term care but are not on anticoagulation therapy. The AF may be long-standing, or it may be a complication of the hospitalizing illness. Because patients with AF are usually anticoagulated, if a patient is not on warfarin, it is necessary to determine if bleeding, overcoagulation, or some other complication contraindicates further warfarin therapy. It is also important to be certain that, if hospitalized, the patient has had the appropriate evaluation for AF.

Consultation/Hospitalization

• **Physician consultation/emergency department evaluation is indicated for patients with new-onset or rapid AF if a patient is symptomatic or unstable.**

• Hospitalization is indicated for elective cardioversion, AV node ablation, or pacemaker placement for rhythm and rate control. Hospitalization is also indicated for patients starting on sotalol, flecainide, or propafenone.

• Consultation with the physician is recommended for stable patients with new-onset AF who do not wish hospitalization, but require treatment to prevent complications associated with AF. Discussion should include anticoagulation choices, INR goal (if warfarin is anticoagulant of choice), and the appropriate medication (plus dosage) indicated for rate control. Necessary monitoring should be discussed.

• Physician consultation is recommended for patients not responding to treatment.

• Cardiology consultation may be indicated for patients not responding to therapy.

Complications

• Decreased cardiac output
• Embolism
• Cardiomyopathy

- Heart failure
- Hypotension
- Angina
- Side effects from medication therapy: bleeding with excessive anticoagulation, stroke if patient is not anticoagulated properly, and effects of antiarrythmic medications

Education for Nursing Home/Rehabilitation Staff

- Explain to nurses the importance of notifying healthcare provider for heart rate greater than 100 or for change in heart rhythm (from regular rhythm to irregularly irregular rhythm).
- Explain to nurses the potential drug interactions (especially with antibiotics) associated with warfarin and the importance of ensuring that drug monitoring (PT/INR) for patients on warfarin is scheduled on a regular basis (every 2 to 4 weeks).
  - Nursing should understand the importance of monitoring the patient for hematuria, bleeding gums, or other signs of excessive anticoagulation.
- Discuss with nursing staff the side effects of prescribed medications (particularly amiodarone) and the importance of notifying the healthcare provider if side effects occur.

Patient/Family Education

- Patient/family require careful explanation of the disease process, diagnostic, testing, and recommended treatments.
- Discussion with patient/family and subsequent documentation of the risks and benefits of anticoagulation therapy are essential (see Chapter 16). Patients and families need to understand that dietary changes and medications may affect the anticoagulation status.

Bibliography

ACC/AHA/ESC. (2001). Guidelines for the management of patients with atrial fibrillation. *Circulation, 104*(17), 2118-2150.

Atrial Fibrillation Follow-up Investigation of Rhythm Management (AFFIRM) investigators. (2002). A comparison of rate control and rhythm control in patients with atrial fibrillation. *New England Journal of Medicine, 347*(23), 1824-1833.

Crecelius, C.A., & Levenson, S. (2004). Atrial fibrillation: Assessment and treatment of the most common cardiac arrhythmia in the LTC setting. *Caring for the Ages, 5*(5), 22-25.

Israel, C.W., et al. (2004). Long-term risk of recurrent atrial fibrillation as documented by an implantable monitoring device: Implications for optimal patient care. *Journal of the American College of Cardiology, 43*(1), 47-52.

Skidmore-Roth, L. (2004). *Mosby's nursing drug reference.* St. Louis: Mosby.

Van Gelder, I.C., et al. (2002). Rate control versus electrical cardioversion for persistent atria fibrillation study group: A comparison of rate control and rhythm control in patients with persistent atrial fibrillation. *New England Journal of Medicine, 347*(23), 1834-1840.

STROKE

Stroke, the third-leading cause of death in the United States, is a sudden or rapid onset of neurologic deficits, related to vascular compromise and lasting longer than 24 hours. The two major types of stroke are ischemic and hemorrhagic. Ischemic stroke accounts for 80% to 85% of all cases of stroke and is caused by emboli, thrombi, or hypoperfusion. Hemorrhagic stroke accounts for 15% to 20% of all strokes and occurs with bleeding into the brain or meningeal spaces. Each of these subtypes has different causes, presentation of symptoms, and treatment. The degree of neurologic impairment is related to the type, location, and size of the stroke. If the neurologic signs and symptoms last for fewer than 24 hours, the event is called a TIA. About 90% of all TIAs resolve within 15 minutes.

Risk Factors

- Increased age
- Gender: strokes are more common in males
- Personal or family history of stroke
- History of TIA (especially within previous month)
- Hypertension
- History of AF, MI, valvular disease, carotid artery disease, or peripheral vascular disease
- Diabetes
- Hyperlipidemia/hyperhomocysteinemia
- Smoking
- Sickle cell disease
- Polycythemia
- Trauma
- Substance abuse: drug use (cocaine) or excessive alcohol use
- Physical inactivity and obesity
- Drugs: amphetamines, warfarin, phenylpropanolamine, oral contraceptives, and hormone replacement therapy

History

It is key to determine the temporal aspects of symptoms to establish when symptoms actually began. Patients who may be eligible for thrombolytic therapies have a therapeutic window of 3 hours from symptom onset in which to receive treatment. The history should focus on a review of the signs of stroke as described by the American Stroke Association and is obtained from the patient, staff, or family members. The history should also include a careful review of the patient's risk factors for stroke, allergies, current medications, past medical history, recent procedures or surgeries, and contraindications for thrombolytic therapy. Patients who have had recurrent TIAs remain at high risk for stroke. Because the differentiation between TIA and stroke is made at a later time, it is important to respond to the evaluation of symptoms as a potential stroke.

- Sudden numbness or weakness of the face, arm, or leg, especially on one side of the body
- Sudden confusion or trouble speaking or understanding speech (expressive receptive aphasia)
- Sudden trouble seeing in one or both eyes
- Sudden trouble walking, dizziness, or loss of balance or coordination
- Sudden, severe headache with no known cause
- Unexplained vertigo
- Nausea and vomiting
- Falls or recent trauma
- Difficulty swallowing

Physical Examination

Often, the signs of stroke are easily identifiable. However, in elders, stroke symptoms may be atypical or subtle and include mental status changes. The early course can range from mild or transient symptoms, to worsening or stepwise gradual deterioration, or to the immediate appearance of severe deficits. Deficits relate to the part of the brain that is compromised. The patient's level of consciousness, airway status, vital signs, and neurologic status need to be immediately assessed. The history and physical examination should be sufficient enough to obtain pertinent information, but should not delay immediate transport for emergency care.

Other important aspects of the physical examination include:
- Accucheck: to rule out hypoglycemia or hyperglycemia
- Vital signs: to determine presence of elevated BP, tachycardia, tachypnea, fever, or hypoxia
- Head, eyes, ears, nose, and throat (HEENT) examination should evaluate for evidence of:
  - Head trauma
  - Buccal or tongue lacerations: may be a sign of seizure
  - Meningeal irritation
- Cardiovascular: assess for murmur, arrhythmia, carotid bruits, and peripheral pulses.
- Neurologic evaluation: determine changes in mental status as well as slurred speech or swallowing dysfunction.
  - Facial droop, facial pain, or sensory or motor changes in the face
  - Diplopia, decreased visual acuity or visual fields, nystagmus, or pupillary changes

- Abnormal reflexes, ataxia, and altered level of consciousness
- Limb weakness or paralysis
- Skin: determine evidence of trauma, bruising, lacerations, cholesterol emboli, ecchymoses, or purpura.
- Extremities: assess for evidence of DVT.

Diagnostics

Symptoms of a stroke must be differentiated from other illnesses causing similar neurologic deficits. Oxygen saturation and Accucheck are immediately indicated to exclude hypoxia or hypoglycemia/hyperglycemia. Further diagnostic evaluation for suspected acute stroke is performed at the hospital/stroke center. A non-contrast enhanced cranial computed tomography (CT) scan to exclude hemorrhagic stroke is performed urgently. Other diagnostics include the following.

Laboratory Evaluation
- CBC/diff
- Serum electrolytes, glucose, and blood urea nitrogen/creatinine (BUN/Cr) ratio
- Coagulation studies: prothrombin time (PT), partial thromboplastin time (PTT), platelets, and INR
- Drug/alcohol levels
- Toxic screen
- Type and crossmatch
- Serum human chorionic gonadotropin (hCG)*: if patient is a female of childbearing age
- Isoenzyme of creatine kinase with muscle subunits (CK-MB) and troponin levels*: if a cardiac event is suspected

Other Diagnostics
- Carotid duplex ultrasound*
- ECG
- Chest radiograph
- Lateral cervical spine*: if fall or recent trauma
- Transesophageal echocardiogram: if embolization from the heart is suspected

Differential Diagnosis

- Acute confusional state
- Migraine
- Hypoglycemia/hyperglycemia
- Hyponatremia
- Tumor

*If indicated.

- Trauma
- Seizure
- Aneurysm
- Subdural hematoma/epidural hematoma
- Drug-, alcohol-, or toxin-induced
- Meningitis, encephalitis, or other central nervous system (CNS) infection
- Encephalopathy
- Post–cardiac arrest ischemia
- Syncope
- Temporal arteritis
- Vertebral disc disease

Treatment Plan

Acute Stroke

Acute stroke is considered a medical emergency, and patients with suspected stroke require immediate treatment at a stroke center for evaluation. The patient's and family's wishes for hospitalization must be determined expeditiously, and emergency rescuers should be called for transfer to the closest emergency facility. It is important to know what facilities in the area are designated as stroke centers and can offer comprehensive emergency treatment. While waiting for ambulance transport, it is necessary to begin appropriate treatment.

- Monitor and protect airway continuously.
- Oxygen should be started only if patient is hypoxic or in respiratory distress.
- Continuous vital signs should be obtained and documented.
- Elevated BPs usually should not be treated. Physician consultation is necessary for consistent systolic BP elevations higher than 220 mm Hg and diastolic elevations higher than 115 mm Hg.

The goals of evaluation of a patient with acute stroke symptoms at the stroke center are to:

- Confirm that the cause is actually a stroke.
- Determine the type of stroke.
- Provide information about the reversibility of the pathology.
- Give clues about the most likely etiology.
- Predict the likelihood of complications.

Management Plan for Acute Ischemic Stroke

For acute ischemic stroke, thrombolytic therapy with tissue–type plasma activator (tPA) is an option if patients meet criteria and fall within the 3-hour reperfusion window. It is important to document and provide any pertinent information to the hospital or stroke center.

Inclusion criteria

- Onset of symptoms within 3 hours
- Deficits measurable on the National Institutes of Health (NIH) stroke scale
- Baseline CT without evidence of bleeding

Exclusion criteria
- Previous stroke or head trauma within 3 months
- Major surgery within 14 days
- Any history of intracranial hemorrhage
- Systolic BP >185 mm Hg or diastolic > 110 mm Hg
- Gastrointestinal (GI) or genitourinary (GU) hemorrhage within 21 days
- Seizure at the onset of stroke
- Arterial puncture within 7 days
- Current use of warfarin (Coumadin) or elevated PT
- Platelet count less than 100,000
- Glucose below 50 mg/dL or above 400 mg/dL

Management for Hemorrhagic Stroke
- Supportive care.
- Craniotomy with surgical evacuation of hematoma
- Embolization for ruptured aneurysm
- Endovascular procedures with clips and coils

Rehabilitation management after acute stroke includes intensive rehabilitation to help restore functional and language ability. Recent research suggests that there is a definite benefit for continued rehabilitation. This ongoing rehabilitation should include some type of aerobic exercise (facilitating an increase in heart rate and peak oxygen uptake), weight training to improve flexibility and mobility in all the major muscle groups, and stretch training either in several 10 minute sessions or for 20 to 60 minutes 3 to 7 days a week. In addition, management must include careful monitoring of medications, hypertension, hyperlipidemia, and comorbid disorders.

Consultation/Hospitalization

- **Immediate transport to the nearest emergency department or stroke center is indicated for patients with a suspected stroke.**
- Immediate consultation with the physician is indicated for patients who have symptoms that resolve (TIA), as these patients should be aggressively evaluated for contributing factors and preventative measures.
- Post-stroke care requires a multidisciplinary approach and consultation with a rehabilitation specialist or physiatrist, as well as physical, occupational, and speech therapists.
- Patients with critical carotid stenosis should be evaluated for carotid endarterectomy.
- Patients with visual field defects after a stroke require consultation with a neuro-ophthalmologist.

Complications

- Complications of a delay in treatment include progressive cardiovascular or neurologic impairments, or cardiopulmonary arrest.

- Post-stroke complications include DVT, expressive and or receptive aphasia, dysarthria, dysphagia, decubiti, cognitive/perceptual deficits, contractures, nerve palsies, malnutrition, urinary retention or incontinence, visual field defects, shoulder subluxation, reflex sympathetic dystrophy, depression, sleep disturbances, sensory impairment, and recurrent stroke.

Education for Nursing Home/Rehabilitation Staff

- Educate nursing staff about the warning signs of stroke, the importance of notifying the healthcare provider as well as family, and the need to transfer the patient immediately to the emergency department/stroke center.
- It is important that nursing understands the importance of providing the emergency department physician with information about the patient's medications, allergies, comorbid conditions, and advanced directives.

Post-Stroke Care

- The focus of care includes a multidisciplinary approach to care, with physical therapy (PT), occupational therapy (OT), and speech therapy where appropriate.
- Emphasize the need for early mobilization and close monitoring of vital signs.
- Stress the importance of accurate intake and output (I&O) and weights to ensure adequate hydration.
- Meticulous skin care and positioning to prevent decubiti, nerve palsies, contractures, and subluxation of shoulders are essential.
  - Turn patient every 1 to 2 hours.
  - Frequently inspect sacrum, ischium, greater trochanter, and heels for erythema and signs of skin breakdown, applying protective cream as needed.
- Avoid urinary catheters, if possible, to prevent urinary tract infections. However, monitor patients closely for urinary retention.
- Bowel regimen
- Review with staff the risk of DVT in patients on bedrest. The importance of compression stockings, early mobilization, and leg exercises should be emphasized.
- Review with staff the importance of preventing contractures and foot drop.
  - When possible, patients should be seated with their feet on the floor to prevent foot drop.
  - Each joint should be carefully stretched and positioned during each shift.
- Teach and review aspiration precautions and individual feeding considerations with staff.
  - Patients should be seated in chair at a 90-degree angle while eating.

- Patients receiving tube feedings should have head of bed elevated 30° or more. Tube feedings must be turned off if patient is lying flat in bed.
- Good nutrition is essential.
- Discuss with the nursing staff the importance of reporting episodes of bleeding in gums, stool, urine, or bruising for patients on anticoagulation.
- Discuss with nursing staff the goals of anticoagulation.
- Educate staff concerning the increased incidence of recurrent stroke and depression for post-stroke patients.
- Explain the importance of reporting speech changes, pocketing of food, and/or swallowing problems to the healthcare provider.

Patient/Family Education

- Explain the need for control of risk factors, including smoking, excessive alcohol, sedentary lifestyle, and obesity.
- Explain the need for medical interventions, including pharmacologic therapies for optimal control of hypertension, diabetes, hyperlipidemia, and arrhythmias.
- Educate patient/family regarding the warning signs of stroke.
- Discuss with patient and family post-stroke care, the possibility of confusion and depression after a stroke, and the slow return of functional and language skills.
- Discuss with patient/family the psychosocial implications of stroke and refer for counseling if indicated.

Bibliography

Adams, R.J., et al. (2003). Coronary risk evaluation in patients with transient ischemic attack and ischemic stroke: A scientific statement for healthcare professionals from the Stroke Council and the Council on Clinical Cardiology of the American Heart Association/American Stroke Association. *Circulation, 108*(10), 1278-1290.

Albers, G.W., et al. (2001). Antithrombotic and thrombolytic therapy for ischemic stroke. *Chest, 119*(1 suppl), 300S-320S.

American Stroke Association. (2004). *www.strokeassociation.org*. Retrieved March 25, 2004.

Gordon, N.F., et al. (2004). Physical activity and exercise recommendations for stroke survivors. *Circulation, 109*(16), 2031-2041.

Kalra, L. (2001). Approaches to organization of stroke care: A review. *Clinical Geriatrics, 9*(12). www.hmpcommunications.com/CG/displayArticle.cfm?articleID=cgac215. Accessed March 28, 2004.

Solenski, N. (2004). Transient ischemic attacks: Part I. Diagnosis and evaluation. *American Family Physician, 69*(7), 1665-1674.

Wolf, G., et al. (1999). Preventing ischemic stroke in patients with prior stroke and transient ischemic attack: A statement for healthcare professionals from the Stroke Council of the American Heart Association. *Stroke, 30*(9), 1991-1994.

CHEST PAIN

ICD 9: 786.50

Chest pain is frequently only associated with acute myocardial infarction (AMI), but, in fact, is an indication of an array of illnesses and disorders. In fact, MI or unstable angina may account for only 1.5% of all chest pain, and more than 50% of all chest pain is not caused by cardiac, gastrointestinal, or pulmonary disease.

Clinically, it is necessary to always first exclude cardiac causes of chest pain as well as noncardiac causes that are life-threatening. Unfortunately, in women, in elders, and in patients with diabetes, the presentation for an AMI is often atypical, making diagnosis challenging. Symptoms can be vague, and aggravating factors absent. Careful observation for the constellation of clinical symptoms (shortness of breath, fatigue, heart failure, or epigastric symptoms) that may indicate cardiac ischemia or an AMI is essential. A detailed history and thorough physical examination will also help differentiate life-threatening noncardiac disorders.

Risk Factors

Cardiac (Including Risk Factors for Aortic Dissection and Pericarditis)

- Age: coronary artery disease is a common cause of chest pain in patients older than age 40 (aortic dissection more common after age 60)
- Gender: symptoms more vague in females
- Cigarette smoking
- Personal or family history of coronary disease: in patients younger than age 40, influence of family history is strong
- Hypertension
- Hyperlipidemia
- Diabetes mellitus: chest pain may present atypically
- Anemia
- Angina
- Left ventricular hypertrophy (LVH) and low ejection fraction
- History of cocaine use/abuse
- Recent history of infection, chest trauma, autoimmune disease, MI, or cardiac surgery, including coronary artery bypass graft (CABG) and stent placement
- Medications: use of drugs such as procainamide, hydralazine, and isoniazid (INH)
- AF: may suggest pulmonary embolus

Gastrointestinal

- History of gastroesophageal reflux disease (GERD) or peptic ulcer disease (PUD)
- History of recent heavy meal

- Alcohol use
- History of pancreatitis, esophageal spasm, gallstones, cancer, or hiatus hernia

Pulmonary
- Cigarette smoking
- Tuberculosis (TB)
- History of chest trauma
- Recent infection
- Cancer

Musculoskeletal
- Degenerative joint disease (DJD)
- Osteoporosis
- Cancer
- Recent strenuous activity
- Harsh cough
- Rib fracture
- Trauma

Neurologic
- History of herpes zoster

Psychogenic
- Personal or family history of anxiety, depression, or panic attacks

History

History is essential in determining the etiology of the chest pain and is best elicited from the patient when possible. Additional history from the nursing staff and/or family may be helpful. It is necessary to pay close attention to risk factors for coronary artery disease, such as family history, hypertension, diabetes mellitus, smoking, and hyperlipidemia, as well as medications (with attention to nonsteroidal antiinflammatory drugs (NSAIDs), aspirin, steroids, or illicit drug use). Further history consists of using the mnemonic "OPQRST" to assess the chest discomfort and of determining any accompanying symptoms.

"O"—Onset: Duration of Discomfort: When Did Pain Start? Was it Sudden or Gradual? What Was the Patient Doing when the Pain Started?
- Any chest pain that lasts longer than a few minutes and is not relieved by nitroglycerin requires medical attention.
- The pain associated with a pneumothorax, aortic dissection, or acute pulmonary embolism usually has an abrupt onset.
- The onset of ischemic pain is often more gradual but increases with time.
- Functional, psychogenic, or nontraumatic musculoskeletal chest pain may have a vague onset.

- Pain that is constant over a long period of time does not usually represent ischemia; fleeting pain less than 1 minute is rarely cardiac.
- Pain from a pulmonary embolism may occur after trauma, a DVT, or prolonged bedrest.
- Relate onset of pain to a recent stressful event, recent physical activity, recent illness, trauma, surgery, or fall.

"P"—Provoking and Palliative Factors: What Started the Pain or Discomfort? What Makes it Better or Worse?

- Many patients experiencing an AMI will have a specific precipitating factor (e.g., illness, stress, exercise).
- Pain related to eating suggests upper gastrointestinal or gallbladder disease.
- Postprandial chest pain may be cardiac or gastrointestinal.
- Anginal pain can occur with or without activity. Emotional stress can provoke anginal pain.
- Pain related to pericarditis or pleurisy often occurs in relation to a viral illness or malignancy.
- Costochondritis pain may occur after repetitive arm movements, may be a sudden or gradual "twinge," and may be evoked by a change in body position. The pleuritic pain of pulmonary embolism, pneumothorax, or pneumonia is often worse with inspirations.
- Cold, emotional stress, meals, or sexual intercourse may provoke ischemic pain.
- Pain relieved by antacids or food suggests gastrointestinal origin.
- Pain relieved by nitroglycerin may be either esophageal or cardiac.
- Pain aggravated by movement or deep breathing suggests a musculoskeletal origin.

"Q"—Quality of the Pain: How Is Pain Described (Pressure, Squeezing, Throbbing, Burning, Dull, Stabbing, Tearing, Crushing)?

- Myocardial ischemia
  - Pain can be described as pressure, squeezing, tightness, constricting, viselike, strangling, burning, fullness, or like a "lump" in the throat, or a "toothache." Pain has usually been present 20 minutes or more (but, not necessarily) and is without point tenderness.
  - Pain is usually gradual in onset.
  - Some patients will have no chest discomfort but may have an anginal equivalent (e.g., jaw pain, dyspnea, palpitations).
- Pain described as lasting less than a minute is noncardiac.
- Pain described as fleeting, stabbing, and localized is usually noncardiac (but may represent pleurisy or herpes zoster).

"R"—Region/Radiation/Referral of Pain

- Substernal, epigastric, or abdominal pain radiating to the jaw, neck, shoulders, arms, wrists, or back suggests cardiac ischemia.
- Localized, point tenderness suggests a musculoskeletal etiology.

- Pain in the area of T5-T6 dermatomes suggests a problem in the diaphragm, gallbladder, pancreas, duodenum or stomach, lungs, or ribs.
- Pain in the area of T1-T4 dermatomes suggests a problem in the myocardium, pericardium, aorta, esophagus, pulmonary artery, or mediastinum.
- Pain along any thoracic dermatome, not crossing the midline anteriorly or posteriorly, suggests herpes zoster, especially if accompanied by a rash.
- Interscapular, epigastric, and/or right shoulder pain suggests cholecystitis.

"S"—Severity of Pain
- Use a pain scale of 1 to 10, with 10 being the worst. (With elders or patients unable to communicate, it may be necessary to use a different pain scale.)
- Severity of pain may not indicate severity of illness.

"T"—Timing
- How long have you had the pain?
- Is the pain or discomfort fleeting, intermittent, constant?
- How long does the pain last?

Accompanying Symptoms
- Nausea, vomiting, indigestion, diaphoresis, dyspnea, weakness, fatigue, syncope, lightheadedness, and anxiety suggest cardiac origin but can be mistaken for gastric or other sources. In elders, especially, fatigue is a significant symptom often associated with cardiac disease.
- Respiratory symptoms, such as fever, cough, hemoptysis, wheezing, or dyspnea, suggest a pulmonary origin.
- Heartburn, odynophagia, hematemesis, or melena suggests gastrointestinal disorders.
- Diaphoresis occurs frequently with a MI.
- Cough, hoarseness, and wheezing may indicate GERD.

Physical Examination

A focused physical examination should support the diagnoses suggested by the history. The patient's appearance and vital signs are critical in determining the patient's stability.
- General appearance
  - Anxious presentation suggests cardiac origin.
  - An acute change in mental status may be related to hypoxia or infection.
- Vital signs
  - Normal vital signs suggest a noncardiac cause for the chest pain.
  - Hemodynamic instability is an ominous sign requiring immediate transfer to an acute care facility.
  - A difference in the BP in both arms may indicate aortic dissection. Unequal pulses in the extremities may also suggest aortic dissection.

- Fever suggests an infectious process.
- Tachycardia, tachypnea, fever, and hypotension may occur with pulmonary embolism and silent MI.
- Skin
  - Diaphoreses is more frequently associated with MI.
  - Contusions suggest trauma.
  - Unilateral rash suggests herpes zoster.
- Neck
  - Trachea deviation suggests pneumothorax.
  - Jugular vein distention suggests fluid overload.
  - Lymph nodes may suggest systemic illness or malignancy.
- Lungs/chest
  - Localized chest wall tenderness suggests costochondritis, rib fracture, trauma, or a musculoskeletal problem.
  - Unilateral absence of breath sounds suggests pneumothorax.
  - Tachypnea, shallow breathing, unilateral limited chest wall expansion, localized tenderness, and pleural friction rub suggest pleurisy (although a friction rub may not always be present in pleurisy).
  - Bronchial breath sounds, rales that do not clear with cough, egophony, and dullness to percussion suggest pneumonia.
  - Oxygen saturation may be decreased in pulmonary embolism, pneumonia, and heart failure.
- Cardiac: determine point of maximum impulse and presence of S3 (suggesting heart failure), S4, murmurs, or pericardial friction rub.
- Abdominal: determine presence of aortic bruit (aortic dissection), abdominal tenderness, guarding, and rebound.
- Musculoskeletal: pain is reproducible.
- Extremities: assess skin color, temperature, edema, and presence or absence of pulses (to confirm vascular compromise from aortic dissection); assess for DVT if PE is a consideration.

Differential Diagnosis

- Cardiac
  - Acute MI: poorly localized discomfort more than 20 minutes, often accompanied by nausea, vomiting, diaphoresis, shortness of breath, minimal relief with nitroglycerin. Pain/discomfort is retrosternal, may radiate to the arms, back, neck, or lower jaw and is often described as enduring, severe deep pressure. Patient may be hypotensive or diaphoretic. Pulmonary edema, the murmur of mitral regurgitation (MR), and ST changes (elevation or depression) are not uncommon. Non-ST segment elevation MI may be difficult to distinguish from unstable angina. New ST-segment deviation or T-wave inversion with symptoms is significant.
  - Unstable angina: may be increased angina in a patient with a previous

diagnosis of angina or can be new-onset angina, increased anginal severity, or angina that occurs at rest with little or no provocation. It generally lasts 20 minutes or longer.

- Stable angina: pressing, constricting, squeezing sensation, or heaviness in central anterior chest with radiation to neck, jaw, arms, and/or back; relieved with nitroglycerin. May be related to exertion, stress, or exposure to cold. Shortness of breath can be anginal equivalent. Discomfort may occur at rest or after a meal.
- Pericarditis: pain that increases with deep inspiration, cough, or change in position. Pain is often referred to the left shoulder and neck and relieved by sitting in a high Fowler's position and leaning forward. If the pain lasts for hours, it may be related to upper respiratory infection or malignancy. Pericardial friction rub may be present.
- Aortic dissection: acute onset of severe, stabbing pain in anterior chest, abdomen, or interscapular region. Pain radiates to both upper extremities and back. Other findings include unequal pulses and the murmur of aortic insufficiency (AI).
- Mitral valvular disease: pain is often fleeting, sharp, and not localized; may be associated with fatigue, syncope, palpitations, or dyspnea; associated with midsystolic click at apex, as well as tachycardia.
- Pulmonary
  - Pulmonary embolus: usually a sudden onset of deep chest pain with dyspnea or tachycardia; often accompanied by cough, hemoptysis, and/or hypoxia; hstory often positive for inactivity, trauma, AF, or DVT.
  - Pleurisy: chest pain increases with inspiration or cough; localized, stabbing pain associated with recent upper respiratory infection, cough, malignancy, or pneumothorax.
  - Pneumonia: often accompanied by mental status change, dyspnea, cough, fever, chills, sputum production, and decreased breath sounds; pain usually located in lower chest.
  - Pneumothorax: sudden acute, unilateral pleuritic chest pain accompanied by dyspnea, tracheal shift, reduced respiratory excursion, diminished breath sounds on affected side, and asymmetrical diaphragmatic excursion. Tachycardia and hypotension may be present.
  - Pulmonary hypertension: discomfort is poorly localized, accompanied by dyspnea.
- Gastrointestinal
  - Esophageal spasm/esophagitis: associated with eating and similar to anginal pain; pain is usually substernal and often radiates to the back; sometimes can be relieved with position change (to upright position) or antacids
  - Pancreatitis: sudden onset, usually acute (although can be mild), knifelike pain radiates to left shoulder, chest, flank, or lower abdomen; epigastric tenderness usually intense; possible Cullen's or Gray Turner's sign (see Chapter 6)

- Cholecystitis/cholelithiasis: intermittent or steady right upper quadrant and epigastric pain radiates to the right shoulder and scapula; sometimes accompanied by nausea and vomiting; often occurs after meals
  - GERD: radiates upward toward neck; can be associated with heartburn; often occurs after eating
- Musculoskeletal
  - Costochondritis: constant, stabbing, sustained pain. Pain is worse with coughing, deep respirations, or any movement. May be related to a viral illness or cancer. Pain may last for hours or days, and is often reproducible.
  - Trauma: fall or increased exercise of upper body
  - Rib fractures: related to metastatic disease, osteoporosis, and coughing; pain is sharp, sudden, aggravated by movement and respirations, and may worsen over time.
- Dermatologic
  - Herpes zoster: unilateral, sharp, localized, fleeting, burning discomfort along a dermatome; pain usually precedes eruption of vesicles by 48 hours; aggravated by clothes touching skin.
- Nonspecific pain
  - Psychogenic: vague, often diffuse pain; may be associated with hyperventilation

Diagnostics

Diagnostic testing should be based on presentation and clinical findings but any chest pain complaint, as well as "indigestion," persistent shortness of breath, loss of consciousness, or dizziness that suggests a cardiac etiology requires an immediate 12-lead ECG. Diagnosis of an AMI is based on the presence of two of the following three criteria: (1) clinical history consistent with ischemic chest pain, (2) ECG changes on serial ECGs, and (3) rise and subsequent fall in CK-MB and/or troponin. For this reason, patients with symptoms consistent with an MI require transfer to an acute care facility, unless the patient and/or family specifically requests no hospitalization (and understands the limitations of this decision). For patients wishing to remain in the facility, an ECG should be obtained as soon as possible. Pertinent ECG changes include ST segment elevation or depression (indicating ischemia) and/or new Q-wave development. Other ECG findings include:

- ECG can be normal, or ST segment elevation or depression may be evident.
- No ST segment elevation may suggest unstable angina or non–Q-wave MI.
- T waves may be inverted in MI.
- ST segment elevation indicates a need for reperfusion.
- ST segment elevation also occurs with pericarditis and some types of angina.

Other diagnostics necessary for further assessment of acute coronary syndrome include CBC/diff (including platelets), glucose, electrolytes, BUN, creatinine, lipid profile, PT/PTT, CK-MB, troponin T or I, myoglobin, and chest radiograph. CK-MB may not be elevated initially. Troponin I indicates myocardial necrosis but also takes time to elevate.

If cardiac emergency is excluded, appropriate laboratory and imagery diagnostics should be guided by patient history and physical examination findings. Further diagnostics to consider include:

- LFTs: if cholecystitis or pancreatitis is suspected
- TSH: hypermetabolic state may precipitate MI.
- Amylase: if pancreatitis suspected
- Doppler ultrasound/D-dimer: to evaluate for DVT if indicated
- Chest radiograph: to rule out rib fracture, pneumonia, and heart failure
- Spiral CT or ventilation/perfusion (VQ) scan: to rule out pulmonary embolus

Treatment Plan

The priority for every patient is to rule out a cardiac emergency or other life-threatening condition and, when indicated, transfer the patient expeditiously to an acute care facility. For cardiac-related chest pain, timing is important if thrombolytic therapy is a consideration. Any patient status-post a CABG or recent coronary artery stent needs to have chest pain evaluated in the emergency department for occlusion. Other matters of importance include clarifying code status and patient/family choices for hospitalization.

Treatment while awaiting transfer to an acute care facility is as follows:

Ischemic Cardiac Pain

While the emergency responders are en route, administer:
- Oxygen 2 to 4 L/minute
- Obtain IV access.
- Aspirin 160 to 325 mg chewed (if no aspirin allergy)

Nitroglycerin 1/150 sublingually (SL) may be given at 5-minute intervals as long as BP is not less than 90 mm Hg systolic and heart rate is more than 50 bpm in an effort to reduce preload and myocardial oxygen consumption. It is preferable to have IV access before administering nitroglycerin.

Morphine sulfate 2 to 4 mg IV or SL may be given if nitroglycerin does not stop the pain. Morphine also eases the respiratory effort, decreases afterload, and is indicated for anxiety, severe agitation, and pulmonary congestion. Morphine may be repeated every 5 minutes to control pain if systolic BP is > 90 mm Hg.

Pulmonary Disorders
- Pulmonary embolus
  - Oxygen to maintain saturation > 90%
  - Obtain IV access.
  - Transfer to an acute care facility.
  - Manage pain.

- Pneumothorax
  - Oxygen to maintain saturation > 90%
  - Obtain IV access.
  - Transfer to acute care facility.
- Pneumonia (see Chapter 4)
- Pleurisy
  - NSAIDs: should be used cautiously in patients with renal dysfunction, history of heart failure, or GI bleeding
  - Tylenol scheduled around the clock, but no more than 4 g in 24 hours (i.e., 1 g PO every 6 hours); dose must be decreased in patients on warfarin
  - Incentive spirometry 10 times an hour to prevent pneumonia
  - Warm packs 15 min/hr to affected area (use caution to avoid a burn)
  - Respiratory therapy evaluation for flutter valve therapy

Gastrointestinal Disorders (if Cardiac Workup Is Negative)

- Esophageal spasm
  - Antacids: Maalox 30 mL PO after meals and at the hour of sleep; use aluminum hydroxide (Amphojel) if there are renal concerns. There may be a need for further workup if there is no response to antacid.
- Pancreatitis
  - Transfer to acute care facility
- Cholecystitis/cholelithiasis
  - Transfer to acute care facility
- GERD
  - Antacids, H_2 blocker (ranitidine [Zantac] 150 mg PO every 12 hours), or proton-pump inhibitor (i.e., esomeprazole [Nexium] or pantoprazole [Protonix] 40 mg PO daily)
  - Elevate head of bed.
  - Avoid caffeine, chocolate, and spicy foods.
  - Avoid lying down until 2 hours after eating.

Musculoskeletal Disorders

- Usually a diagnosis of exclusion
- Pain management
- Local cool or warm packs 15 minutes per hour to the affected area, using caution to avoid burns (typically, cool packs are used for 48 hours after an injury and for any back discomfort)
- Arthritis-strength BenGay or other topical musculoskeletal cream as needed (if there is no alteration in skin integrity)
- Rest
- Physical therapy/occupational therapy consult

Dermatologic Disorders

- Herpes zoster
  - Acyclovir (dosage based on creatinine clearance)

- Contact precautions
- Pain management: Tylenol up to 4 gm/24 hr or Neurontin 100 mg PO three times a day (may increase dose)
- Cimetidine (Tagamet), 200 mg PO three times during the day and 400 mg PO at bedtime has been proven beneficial in other countries as an immunomodulator to decrease post-herpetic neuralgia.
- Dry dressing if necessary, with monitoring for superimposed infection

Nonspecific
- Psychogenic
  - Education
  - Relaxation techniques
  - Reassurance
  - Selective serotonin reuptake inhibitors (SSRIs) and anxiolytics

Consultation/Hospitalization

It is critical to identify and exclude life-threatening conditions that would dictate emergency hospitalization. **Physician consultation and/or immediate emergency department transfer is recommended for aortic dissection, myocardial ischemia, pneumothorax, pulmonary embolus, unstable vital signs, signs of bleeding, or unrelieved pain.**

Complications

- Aortic dissection, MI, pneumothorax, and pulmonary embolus are life-threatening emergencies requiring immediate transport to an acute care facility.

Education for Nursing Home/Rehabilitation Staff

- Nursing and rehabilitation staff should understand that chest discomfort may signify a serious disorder. Changes in patient behavior and complaints of chest discomfort should be reported quickly to the healthcare provider to prevent fatalities.
- Staff should also understand the importance of a complete pain evaluation and implementation of appropriate pain relief protocols.

Patient/Family Education

- Patient/family should have careful explanation about the importance of expeditiously notifying the nursing staff if chest discomfort of any kind occurs.
- Patients/family need careful explanation about the cause of the pain, appropriate diagnostic testing, and treatment.

Bibliography

American College of Cardiology/American Heart Association (ACC/AHA). (2003). Guideline update for the management of patients with chronic stable angina. *Circulation*, *107*(1), 149-158.

American College of Cardiology/American Heart Association (ACC/AHA). (2002). Guideline update for the management of patients with unstable angina and non-ST segment elevation myocardial infarction. *Circulation*, *106*(14), 1893-1900.

Aronow, W. (2003). Management of unstable angina non–ST segment elevation myocardial infarction. *Annals of Long-Term Care*, *11*(4), 19-23.

Birrer, R., et al. (2001). Cardiac emergencies in older adults. *Annals of Long-Term Care*, *9*(6), 54-60.

Glasser, S. (2003). Angina: Optimizing treatment and compliance. *Clinician Reviews*, supplement, 4-13.

Meisel, J.L. (2004). Diagnostic approach to the patient with chest pain 2004. *www.uptodate.com*. Accessed June 26, 2004.

Wasserman, A. (2000). Chest pain: Is it life threatening or benign? *Consultant*, *40*(7), 1205-1208.

HEART FAILURE

ICD9: 428.0

Heart failure is a common clinical syndrome associated with ventricular dysfunction, insufficient tissue perfusion, and fluid retention. Approximately 5 million Americans have heart failure, and 550,000 new cases are reported yearly. This disorder is the single largest expense for Medicare, and the 5-year mortality rate can be as high as 50%. Hemodynamic changes secondary to the neurohormonal activation contribute to most symptoms.

Physiologic classifications of heart failure include diastolic and systolic dysfunction. Systolic heart failure accounts for up to two thirds of all heart failure cases, is characterized by a reduced capacity to eject blood from the ventricle (ejection fraction < 40%), and is frequently related to coronary disease, hypertension, and valvular heart disease. In diastolic dysfunction, the ejection fraction is > 40% and the disorder is associated with impaired ventricular filling related to left ventricular stiffness and atypical left ventricular relaxation. Diastolic heart failure is more common in elders, but heart failure can be associated with both systolic and diastolic dysfunction. For elderly patients at risk for heart failure, ischemia, tachycardia, and anemia are specific stressors.

Risk Factors

- Increased age
- Hypertension
- Peripheral vascular disease
- Cardiac disorders

- Coronary artery disease
- Recent MI
- Valvular heart disease
- Congenital heart defects
- Cardiomyopathy
- Connective tissue diseases
- Endocrine disorders
  - Diabetes
  - Thyroid disorders
  - Hypercholesterolemia
- Chronic obstructive pulmonary disease (COPD)
- Pulmonary hypertension
- Recent blood transfusion
- Anemia
- Obesity
- NSAIDs
- Hemochromatosis
- Exposure to cardiotoxic agents (e.g., alcohol, radiation, antineoplastic agents, illicit drugs)
- Family history of cardiomyopathy, sudden death, or conduction defect
- Infection (e.g., bacterial, parasitic, HIV)

History

In elders, the symptoms of heart failure are often vague and attributed to aging. Eliciting a thorough symptom history and reviewing medical history, risk factors, and medications are helpful in identifying precipitants and reversible causes of heart failure.

Patients may be asymptomatic, but common symptoms associated with heart failure include:

- Fatigue, weakness, dizziness, and shortness of breath at rest or with exertion
  - In patients with low-grade chronic failure, complaints of worsening fatigue, increased shortness of breath, or cough, particularly at night, are significant.
- A decrease in the ability to perform activities of daily living (ADLs), or a change in mental status
- Anorexia, dysphagia, orthopnea, insomnia, paroxysmal nocturnal dyspnea, nocturia, nonproductive cough, hemoptysis (in advanced heart failure/pulmonary edema), wheezing, angina, weight gain, fluid retention or a sensation of extremity heaviness, restlessness, and/or palpitations

Physical Examination

The examination should focus on determining the presence of heart failure and any underlying precipitant (e.g., infection, arrhythmia), but physical findings may be variable. For example, in elderly patients, the rales classically associated with heart failure may be absent. Pertinent assessment includes the following:

- Weight and vital signs, including temperature, BP (narrowed pulse pressure indicates decreased cardiac output), heart rate, respiratory rate, and oxygen saturation, should be assessed.
  - Weight gain (especially if recent) may signify fluid retention.
  - Tachycardia, tachypnea, and low oxygen saturation may indicate fluid overload.
- A careful cardiac and pulmonary examination is necessary to determine signs of diastolic or systolic heart failure as well as document the presence of extra heart sounds or adventitious lung sounds.
  - The left ventricular apical impulse should be located. Extra heart sounds such as an S3 and S4 (gallops) may be heard (most clearly if the patient is placed in the left lateral position). The S3 suggests the possibility of left ventricular dysfunction (a new S3 may indicate impending cardiac decompensation and failure); a solo S4 implies diastolic dysfunction.
  - The presence of any murmurs may indicate valvular or structural heart disease, both frequent causes of heart failure.
  - Jugular vein distention (JVD) is an indicator of fluid overload (often present in systolic failure), but may not be present in mild heart failure. JVD may increase with compression of the right upper abdominal quadrant (a positive hepatojugular reflex).
  - Although commonly linked with heart failure, crackles may or may not be present. Many patients with chronic heart failure do not have inspiratory crackles. If present, crackles are more likely to be present at the bases. Wheezing is possible, especially in patients with cardiac asthma.
- Liver enlargement, ascites, scrotal edema, sacral edema, and symmetric pitting peripheral edema may also be present.
- Acute dyspnea, accompanied by anxiety, restlessness, rapid, shallow breathing, and occasionally pink, frothy sputum are signs of pulmonary edema, a severe form of heart failure. BP and heart rate may also be significantly elevated in acute pulmonary edema.

Diagnostics

Testing is dependent on history and presentation and is necessary to guide treatment and determine correctable pathology, as well as the presence of systolic or diastolic dysfunction. In acute heart failure, diagnostic studies are reserved until after treatment of volume overload and/or immediate hospitalization. Initial diagnostics should usually include an ECG initially (to rule out ischemia), then a chest radiograph, CBC, basic metabolic panel (e.g., serum glucose, electrolytes, BUN, creatinine), and LFTs to determine presence and etiology of the heart failure. Recent studies also suggest that brain natriuretic peptide (BNP)

> 100 pg/mL is an inexpensive test that is diagnostic for heart failure.

New-onset heart failure may require more extensive diagnostic evaluation (e.g., thyroid and liver function studies, two-dimensional echocardiogram, lipids).

Laboratory Evaluation

- CBC/diff: to eliminate anemia and infection as precipitant
- Serum electrolytes, BUN, and creatinine: monitored initially and routinely
- Magnesium
- Calcium
- LFTs*
- TSH*
- Serum ferritin and transferrin*: to exclude hemochromatosis
- HIV screening*: possible cause of cardiomyopathy
- Fasting lipid profile*
- Serum brain natriuretic peptide (BNP): a diagnostic and prognostic indicator; level < 100 pg/mL suggests another cause of dyspnea
- Urinalysis: to exclude infection as precipitant of congestive heart failure (CHF)
- Antinuclear antibody (ANA)*: for suspected lupus

Other Diagnostics

- Chest radiograph: cardiomegaly usually present in systolic dysfunction; may be absent in diastolic dysfunction; prominent pulmonary veins, perivascular edema, and hilar and pulmonary edema indicate heart failure.
- ECG: to exclude ischemia or arrhythmia
- Echocardiogram: indicated in new-onset heart failure; aids in determining left ventricular ejection fraction, systolic dysfunction, diastolic dysfunction, valvular abnormalities, and ventricular wall motion; may be deferred until patient is stabilized
- Stress test if indicated

Differential Diagnosis

The differential diagnosis includes acute heart failure versus exacerbation of chronic failure, as well as systolic versus diastolic dysfunction. Other causes of respiratory distress should also be considered, and include the following:

- Airway obstruction
- Pneumothorax
- Pulmonary embolus
- Exacerbation of COPD
- Asthma
- Pneumonia or upper respiratory infection

---

* If indicated.

- Pleural effusion
- Neuromuscular disorders: consider Guillain-Barré syndrome and myasthenia gravis
- Anxiety

Treatment Plan

Treatment for acute heart failure is based on patient presentation and includes the patient's and family's wishes for hospitalization. Initially, volume overload, whether related to systolic or diastolic dysfunction, should be addressed to relieve the pulmonary congestion and prevent myocardial injury and improve comfort.

- Oxygen to maintain oxygen saturation above 90%; 100% non-rebreather should be used, if necessary.
- Diuretic therapy: usually a loop diuretic, such as furosemide (Lasix), 40 mg IV/IM/PO (in acute failure, IV furosemide is indicated; IM furosemide may be used if patient does not have IV access). This dose may need to be repeated, if the heart failure is severe or if renal insufficiency is present. It is important to note that some patients may respond better to other loop diuretics and that all diuretic therapy necessitates careful monitoring of urinary output, BUN, creatinine, and electrolytes.
- Morphine sulfate, 2 to 4 mg IV, may aid in decreasing anxiety and promoting vasodilation.
- Sublingual nitroglycerin 0.4 mg or topical nitroglycerin paste, 1 to 2 inches, to the chest wall also can promote vasodilation in acute heart failure accompanied by hypertension. BP should be assessed before administration because BP can decrease precipitously, resulting in syncope. In addition, NTG should not be given to patients with heart rate < 50 because severe bradycardia is a possibility.
- Bedrest is recommended (although a high Fowler's position or sitting in a chair [allowing blood to pool in the extremities] may alleviate some of the patient's distress).
- A low sodium diet should be followed (2 g for severe heart failure; 3 g for mild heart failure).
- Additional treatment should prevent recurrence, and, when possible, the underlying pathology should be identified and treated. Surgical treatment may be helpful for coronary artery disease, valvular disease, and pericardial disease, although surgical revascularization or other intervention may not always be feasible for older patients. Systolic and diastolic function should be evaluated to determine appropriate long-term pharmacologic therapies. Pharmacologic therapy is based on American College of Cardiology/American Heart Association (ACC/AHA) guidelines and should also be aimed at alleviating patient discomfort, preventing a recurrence, and preserving cardiac function (Box 5-2).

BOX 5-2 Treatment of Systolic and Diastolic Heart Failure

Systolic Dysfunction (EF < 40%)
No Evidence of Fluid Overload
- ACE inhibitor initially (dose can be doubled weekly as tolerated to titrate to target dose)
  - Monitor patient for postural BP changes.
  - Monitor for electrolyte disturbances.
- In consultation with physician/cardiologist, β-blocker therapy should be considered if patient is stable and ACE inhibitor dose is stabilized (β-blockers are not recommended for patients with severe COPD, asthma, second- or third-degree heart block, bradycardia). β-blocker therapy must be started at a low dose and titrated slowly (every 2 weeks).* Monitor patient for bradycardia.
- In consultation with physician/cardiologist, consider diuretic or digoxin, 0.125 mg PO daily, if symptoms continue.‡ (An appropriate serum digoxin level ranges from 0.5 to 0.8 ng/mL; however, some patients may exhibit side effects even at this level.)

Fluid Overload as Evidenced by Jugular Vein Distention, Rales, and Edema
- Diuretic and ACE inhibitor* (dose titrated as above)
  - The loop diuretic should be given in morning rather than twice-daily dosing to promote patient comfort.
  - Patients with elevated creatinine may need increased diuretic dosages.
  - Consult with physician for cautious administration of metolazone (Zaroxolyn) 2.5 mg PO 1 hour before furosemide once or twice a week to augment diuresis in patients with severe fluid overload. These patients must be monitored carefully for postural hypotension and electrolyte abnormalities.
- When fluid overload is corrected, and patient is stable, consult with physician/cardiologist for consideration low-dose β-blocker (carvedilol, metoprolol, or bisoprolol), which can be slowly titrated to control symptoms. (β-blockers are not recommended for patients with severe COPD, asthma, second- or third-degree heart block, and bradycardia.) β-blocker therapy must be started at low dose and titrated slowly (every 2 weeks).*
- When stabilized, if patient is symptomatic, consult with physician/cardiologist concerning use of digoxin.†
- Discuss with physician/cardiologist benefit of ARBs in combination with ACE inhibitor and β-blockers in patients with class II to III systolic heart failure.
- For patients with severe heart failure who are on ACE inhibitors and diuretics, consult with physician/cardiologist concerning adding aldactone antagonist (contraindicated if patient is hyperkalemic or if creatinine > 2.5 mg/dL).

Continued

BOX 5-2 **Treatment of Systolic and Diastolic Heart Failure—cont'd**

Diastolic Dysfunction
- If possible, reverse underlying pathology.
- Control fluid volume with a diuretic.
- β-blocker, titrated slowly, to control heart rate and improve diastolic function.* (In consultation with physician, consider CCB, which can improve diastolic function, or ACE inhibitor or ARB).[‡]
- Control hypertension, myocardial ischemia, and AF.
- If patient does not tolerate ACE inhibitor, consider ARB or hydralazine combined with nitrate TID.[‡]

---

*β-blocker therapy should be initiated under guidance of an experienced physician or cardiologist. Patient must be carefully monitored for increased heart failure. β-blocker therapy should not be abruptly discontinued.
[†]Digoxin must be used cautiously in elderly patients and patients with renal disease to avoid digoxin toxicity.
[‡]ACE inhibitors, diuretics, nitrates, and dihydropyridine CCBs should be used cautiously to prevent decreased cardiac output and hypotension.

- NSAIDs should be avoided in patients with any history of heart failure.
- Thiazolidinediones and metformin generally should be avoided in patients with any history of heart failure.
- Smoking cessation should be encouraged.
- The cause of the acute episode (e.g., anemia, arrhythmias) should be determined and, if possible, corrected.
- Foley catheterization may be considered for patients with acute heart failure requiring careful monitoring of I&O, but if at all possible, it should be avoided.
- I&O and daily weights are helpful in managing acute and chronic heart failure.
- Monitor BP and heart rate.

Consultation/Hospitalization

- Patients willing to be hospitalized should be transferred to the hospital for new-onset heart failure, myocardial ischemia, severe respiratory distress, pulmonary edema, or if there is associated pneumonia, infection, or renal insufficiency.
- Consultation with the physician is indicated when the patient/family refuses hospitalization.
- Hospitalization should also be considered for patients requiring IV dobutamine or other therapies for decompensated fluid overload and heart failure.
- Cardiology consultation is indicated for improved management, medication review (i.e., some antiarrhythmics can precipitate heart failure), diag-

nostic evaluation (radionuclide angiography, cardiac catheterization, myocardial biopsy, cardiac magnetic resonance imaging [MRI], if indicated), as well as for control of arrhythmias and consideration for surgical therapy or automatic cardioverter defibrillator.
- Physical therapy consultation is indicated to assist patients with exercise recommendations.
- Consult a dietitian.

Complications

- Cardiac arrhythmias are common sequelae and require consultation with a cardiologist to determine appropriate therapy.
- Other complications include pulmonary edema, cardiac cachexia, electrolyte imbalances related to diuretic therapy, and death.
- Digoxin may cause toxicity in elderly patients, in patients with renal disease, and has been associated with increased mortality in women.

Education for Nursing Home/Rehabilitation Staff

- It is important that the nursing staff understand the importance of a low-salt diet, daily weights, appropriate exercise, and careful assessment of vital signs, oxygen saturation, and I&O in patients requiring careful medical management.
- Discuss with nursing staff the importance of monitoring medications and reporting side effects, enabling better titration of medications and improved patient care.
- Teach nursing staff the proper application of thromboembolic disease stockings (TEDs) for peripheral edema.

Patient/Family Education

- Patients and families should understand the importance of reporting any shortness of breath or other symptoms associated with heart failure, as well as recognize the untoward symptoms associated with medical therapy.
- When applicable, patients should be encouraged to lose weight, stop smoking, and exercise.
- Patients and families should also be educated about stress reduction and dietary and exercise recommendations, and they should understand that controlling hypertension and elevated blood sugars will be beneficial.
- The benefits of daily weights and the importance of calling the healthcare provider when weight increases more than 2 lb in 2 days should also be explained.
- Discuss with patient/family the benefit of avoiding alcohol (or limiting to a maximum of 2 oz/day) and limiting caffeine, which can increase heart rate and myocardial oxygen demands.
- Explain the importance of energy conservation.

Bibliography

American College of Cardiology/American Heart Association (ACC/AHA). (2001). Guidelines for the evaluation and management of chronic heart failure in the adult: Executive summary. *Circulation, 104*(24), 2996-3007.

American Heart Association. (2003). *Heart disease and stroke statistics: 2003 update.* Dallas: American Heart Association.

Apstein, C.S. (2004). Diagnosis, treatment, and prognosis of diastolic dysfunction. *www.uptodate.com.* Accessed January 7, 2004.

Colucci, W.S. (2004). Overview of treatment of heart failure due to systolic dysfunction. *www.uptodate.com.* Accessed January 7, 2004.

Ghosh, S., & Gupta, K. (2002). Congestive heart failure in the elderly population: Some common questions. *Annals of Long-Term Care, 10*(12), 29-39.

Rathmore, S.S., et al. (2002). Sex-based differences in the effect of digoxin for the treatment of heart failure. *New England Journal of Medicine, 347*(18), 1403-1411.

DEEP VEIN THROMBOSIS

ICD-9: 451.9

Deep vein thrombosis (DVT) occurs in approximately 2 million people in the United States. Early detection and treatment can significantly reduce the risk for complications, particularly life-threatening pulmonary embolus (PE). Because venous thrombosis is often clinically silent, it is important to reduce its incidence by identifying patients at risk. Those with more than three risk factors are at highest risk. Most DVTs occur in calf veins or in the femoral/popliteal area. Although the exact cause is unclear, the disorder is typically associated with stasis, hypercoagulability, and platelet aggregation in the wall of the deep vein (which may be related to trauma or inflammation). The resulting blood clot may cause partial or complete obstruction of venous circulation. Patients with documented DVT must be evaluated for the use of anticoagulation to prevent progression of the clot, formation of new clots, and pulmonary emboli.

Risk Factors

- Obesity
- Advanced age
- Smoking
- Spinal cord injury: high risk
- Immobilization secondary to surgery (especially gynecologic, hip, or knee), illness, fracture, injury, paralysis, or travel
  - Pelvic fracture: pelvic vein DVT has high risk for PE.
- Hypercoagulable state
  - Inherited or acquired deficiencies: antithrombin III, protein S, protein C, factor V Leiden, anticardiolipin antibodies, and hyperhomocysteinemia

- Polycythemia vera
- Liver disease
- Malignancy
- Trauma (7 to 10 days after injury)
- Estrogen use: oral contraceptives, hormone replacement therapy, and tamoxifen
- Family history
- Abrupt discontinuation of anticoagulants
- Indwelling central venous catheter in upper extremity
- Varicose veins
- Cardiac dysfunction: AF, ventricular aneurysm, and cardiomyopathy
- Prosthetic valves: highest risk with tricuspid valve defect
- Recent history of MI or heart failure
- History of cerebral vascular accident, PE, or DVT
- Inflammatory bowel disease
- Systemic lupus erythematosus
- Pregnancy and postpartum

History

Eliciting a good symptom analysis is essential. Asymmetric extremity pain (may only be noted in the lower extremities with ambulation) or discomfort and edema are the most common presenting complaints. Chest discomfort, shortness of breath, and/or dyspnea are also possible if a PE has occurred. It is helpful to determine symptom onset as well as anorexia, weight loss, hemoptysis, hematuria, rectal bleeding, or other symptoms associated with malignancy. Any history of cancer, recent illness, injury, surgery, or other personal or family risk factors associated with DVT should also be explored. Allergies, medical history, a review of the patient's prescribed and over-the-counter medications (some medications can induce antiphospholipid antibodies), and any contraindications (history of falls, bleeding, or bleeding tendencies) for anticoagulation should also be obtained.

Physical Examination

The examination is directed at determining evidence of DVT as well as possible causes. Physical findings can be negligible and nonspecific, although the patient may seem fatigued or have other constitutional signs, such as weight loss. Factors to consider include the following:

- Vital signs, temperature, and oxygen saturation are important and can aid in differential diagnosis. Fever and tachycardia may be possible and are related to the inflammation.
- A careful skin examination, and cardiac, pulmonary, abdominal, and rectal examinations (including occult blood testing) are necessary to determine the presence of any abnormalities (e.g., malignancy, Budd-Chiari syndrome) that may be associated with DVT or other disorders associated with edema.

- Both lower extremities should be examined and the circumferences measured 10 cm below the tibial tuberosity.
  - Often, the affected extremity will have a greater circumference
  - Determine the presence of erythema, edema, warmth, prominent or tender superficial veins, cordlike tenderness, pulses, Homan's sign (considered an unreliable sign; calf pain with dorsiflexion of the foot is a positive finding that has been associated with DVT), thigh tenderness, and/or cyanosis.
- Upper extremity evaluation includes determining presence of edema and prominent tender veins (particularly axillary vein).

Differential Diagnosis

- Cellulitis
- Superficial thrombophlebitis
- Chronic venous valvular insufficiency
- Lymphedema
- Baker cyst
- Strained muscle
- Venous stasis
- Knee-joint pathology
- Underlying malignancy
- Connective tissue disorder

Diagnostics

Suspicion for DVT (despite negative physical findings) mandates diagnostic evaluation. Duplex ultrasound of the affected extremity is the most appropriate test (99% accurate, 95% specific, 50% to 80% sensitivity). It is less sensitive for detecting clots occurring in the calves, thereby requiring a repeat test in 5 to 7 days if the suspicion for a DVT is high, but the initial test is negative. Other diagnostics include:

Laboratory Evaluation
- Indicated in work-up for anticoagulant therapy
  - CBC/diff, including platelets
  - PT, PTT, fibrinogen, and INR if indicated
  - LFTs
  - BUN and creatinine
  - Stool for occult blood
- Patients with a documented DVT, younger than age 60 and no risk factors for a DVT may have a blood coagulation disorder and should have antithrombin III, protein S, protein C, factor V Leiden, homocysteine, and antiphospholipid antibody before treatment is started.
- Prostate-specific antigen (PSA) if indicated (males older than 50 years, to evaluate for malignancy)

Other Diagnostics
- D-dimer assay: insensitive and nonspecific
- Consult medical director (MD) for venogram if findings are highly suggestive and ultrasound is negative (venogram dye is nephrotoxic, and the procedure expensive).
- CT or MRI for inferior vena cava or pelvic vein DVT

Treatment Plan

Patients at risk for DVT (particularly surgical patients) require prophylaxis with intermittent pneumatic compression stockings (not elastic stockings or TEDS), low-molecular weight heparin, unfractionated heparin, or warfarin for prevention. For patients with documented DVT, the goal is prevention of recurrence and the complications, particularly clot proliferation and PE (which usually occurs within 2 weeks of DVT). Low molecular weight heparin (LMWH), unfractionated heparin, or subcutaneous heparin are initial pharmacologic medications used for treatment. Warfarin (Coumadin) is started and titrated to the appropriate dose for optimal anticoagulation (INR 2.0 to 3.0) (see Chapter 16). For patients experiencing pain, pain management with acetaminophen (Tylenol), tramadol (Ultram), or narcotics is necessary, though caution is necessary to avoid drug interactions with warfarin.

Other important aspects of care include bedrest for 2 days, elevation of the affected extremity, and, when ambulating, graduated compression stockings. Careful monitoring for signs of a pulmonary embolism is essential.

Complications

Complications may be related to the DVT or to anticoagulation therapy.

Deep Vein Thrombosis
- Chronic venous insufficiency
- Chronic brawny edema
- Pulmonary embolus

Anticoagulation
- Bleeding
- Thrombocytopenia with heparin use

Consultation/Hospitalization

- Hospitalization and physician consultation are indicated for patients who:
  - Are medically unstable
  - Require IV heparin therapy
  - Have symptoms suggestive of PE
  - Have uncontrolled bleeding with hypotension/shock
  - Require inferior vena cava (IVC) filter placement

- If pharmacologic intervention with anticoagulants is contra-indicated
- If recent history of cerebral bleed, quadriplegia/paraplegia after spinal cord injury, complex pelvic fracture, or major eye surgery.
- Consider filter if patient has had recurrent DVT despite appropriate anticoagulation therapy.

- Physician consultation is indicated to discuss treatment options for patients with known hemorrhagic tendencies, blood dyscrasias, malignant hypertension, and recent or contemplated CNS surgery, spinal puncture, eye surgery, traumatic surgery with large open area, GI, GU, or respiratory tract bleeding.
- Consultation with the physician is recommended for initiation of LMWH.

Education for Nursing Home/Rehabilitation Staff

- Discuss the use of a Coumadin book and tracking mechanism for patients on anticoagulation.
- Discuss the goals of anticoagulation with staff and the INR goal for each patient on warfarin (Coumadin).
- Demonstrate how to apply compression stockings correctly.
- Explain the value of exercise.
- Educate staff about signs and symptoms of DVT and PE.
- Educate nurses about the importance of monitoring patients for bleeding (hematuria, bleeding gums, excessive bruising) and reporting the bleeding promptly.
- Discuss the importance of documenting in the care plan that patient is on anticoagulants. Nurses should also understand that antibiotics and other medications may significantly increase or decrease the PT/INR for patients receiving warfarin.
- Discuss importance of documenting in nursing notes that the patient understands the impact of dietary changes on PT/INR.

Patient/Family Education

- Explain the disorder, diagnostics, and treatment to the patient and family.
- Discuss the importance of taking Coumadin as prescribed and maintaining a routine diet without drastic changes.
- Explain the importance of exercise to prevent DVT and the need to avoid sitting or standing for long periods.
- Explain the need for caution when shaving and brushing teeth for patients on anticoagulation therapy. An electric razor is preferable for patients on anticoagulation.
- Explain the necessity of promptly reporting any bleeding, as well as avoiding alcohol and hazardous activities while on anticoagulation therapy.
- Discuss the importance of following the medication schedule and having PT/INR tests regularly.

- Explain the importance of not rubbing or massaging lower extremities.
- Discuss the avoidance of constrictive clothing.
- Teach the use of a home monitoring device for the patient who needs Coumadin but has poor access to a laboratory.
- Discuss and give patient/family written information concerning dietary and medication influences (including over-the-counter and herbal drugs) on anticoagulation. Patient/family teaching should be documented in the medical record.

Bibliography

American Geriatrics Society. (1998). Current guidelines for practice, oral anticoagulation for older adults. Modified from *Chest, 114*, 439s-769s.

Buttaro, T.M., et al. (2003). *Primary care: A collaborative practice.* St. Louis, Mosby.

Chamberlain, T., et al. (2001). The assessment, management and prophylaxis of deep vein thrombosis (DVT) and related conditions in the senior care setting. *Annals of Long-Term Care, Multimedia HealthCare/Freedom Publication.*

Deblinger, L. (2000). The challenges of oral anticoagulation. *Patient Care for the Nurse Practitioner.* December, 12-25.

Ferri, J. (2001). *Clinical advisor: Instant diagnosis and treatment.* St. Louis, Mosby.

Hyers, T., et al. (2001). Antithrombotic therapy for venous thromboembolic disease. *Chest, 119*(Suppl 1), 176S-193S.

Landaw, S.A. (2004). Approach to the diagnosis and treatment of suspected deep vein thrombosis. *www.uptodate.com.* Accessed February 7, 2004.

Logan, P. (1999). *Principles of practice for the acute care nurse practitioner.* Stamford, CT: Appleton and Lange.

Nutescu, E., et al. (2002). Anticoagulation in long-term care: State of the art. *Annals of Long-Term Care,* Oct(Suppl 1) 1-4.

Pulmonary embolism and deep vein thrombosis. (2002). *Consultant,* June, 929-930.

Rich, M.W. (2004). Venous thromboembolic disease in the older surgical patient: Part 1. *Annals of Long-Term Care, 12*(6), 46-51.

Riggs, S. (2003). Preventing thromboembolism in patients with prosthetic heart valves. *Clinical Advisor,* 30-36.

HYPERTENSION

ICD-9: 401.1

It is estimated that more than two thirds of persons older than 65 years of age have hypertension, and, for those older than age 50, systolic hypertension (> 140 mm Hg) may be a more significant threat than diastolic hypertension. The Seventh Report of the Joint National Committee on Prevention, Detection, Evaluation, and Treatment of High Blood Pressure (JNC 7) has redefined normal BP as < 120/80 mm Hg. The new guidelines are based on research that indicates an increased risk for renal disease, retinopathy, and cardiovascular disease and its associated sequelae at BP levels over 120/80 mm Hg. Sustained systolic BP

> 140 mm Hg or diastolic BP > 90 mm Hg are diagnostic for hypertension and usually indicate the need for treatment. In elders, treatment is usually indicated. However, the risk/benefit ratio should always be considered, and, if pharmacologic therapy is initiated, the BP should be gradually reduced.

Risk Factors

- Age: men > 55, women > 65
- Family history of hypertension or premature cardiovascular disease
- Obesity
- Increased dietary fat or sodium
- Decreased physical activity
- Medications (NSAIDs, oral decongestants, chronic steroid therapy)
- Obstructive sleep apnea
- Endocrine disease: thyroid or parathyroid disease
- Renal disease
- Vascular disease
- Excessive alcohol ingestion

History

When possible, a detailed personal and family history should be elicited to help determine the cause of the hypertension as well as symptoms suggesting target-organ disease. Allergies, medical history, and any risk factors, along with current medications (including non-prescriptives), are a necessary component of the assessment. Important factors to consider include:

- Weight gain
- History of hypertension and previous treatments
- History of diabetes, hyperlipidemia, cardiovascular (angina, MI, stroke, or heart failure), renal, or endocrine disease
- Family history of hypertension or premature cardiovascular disease
- Smoking, alcohol, caffeine, sleep (sleep apnea), and exercise history
- Most often, patients with hypertension are asymptomatic, but back pain, chest discomfort, dyspnea, focal weakness, headache, eye changes, or other symptoms suggestive of target-organ damage should be elicited, if possible.

Physical Examination

The physical examination assesses for target-organ damage as well as secondary causes of hypertension.

- Weight
- BP in both arms (after sitting for 5 minutes): assessed first sitting with arm supported at level of heart, then assessed standing. BP should be taken with correct size cuff with proper cuff positioning.

- Fundoscopic examination: assess for arteriovenous nicking, arteriolar narrowing, hemorrhages, exudates, and papilledema.
- Thyroid examination for enlargement, nodules, and masses
- Cardiovascular examination: assess presence of carotid bruits, S3, S4, or murmurs.
- Pulmonary examination: assess for inspiratory crackles or wheezes.
- Abdominal examination to determine aortic/renal/femoral bruits, abnormal aortic pulsations, enlarged kidneys, or masses
- Peripheral vascular examination: assess peripheral pulses, lower extremity edema, and/or skin/nail changes/loss of extremity hair.
- Neurologic assessment

Differential Diagnosis

- Primary hypertension
- Secondary hypertension
  - Acromegaly
  - Alcohol
  - Coarctation of the aorta
  - Cushing's syndrome
  - Hypercalcemia
  - Medications
  - Pheochromocytoma
  - Primary aldosteronism
  - Renal vascular disease
  - Sleep apnea

Diagnostics

A new diagnosis of hypertension should be based on BP assessment on three or more occasions and diagnostics ordered accordingly. In new-onset hypertension, the following tests should be ordered if recent results are not available.

Laboratory Evaluation

- Urinalysis and urine: for microalbumin
- CBC/diff: to determine hemoglobin/hematocrit
- Fasting serum glucose, electrolytes, BUN, creatinine, calcium and phosphorus*: to identify end-organ disease and treatment planning
- Fasting lipid profile: to assess cardiovascular risk

Other laboratory studies that may be indicated in some circumstances include:

- TSH*
- 24-hour urine cortisol: if Cushing's is suspected
- 24-hour urine creatinine, catecholamines, and metanephrines: if pheochromocytoma is suspected

Other Diagnostics
- ECG: assess for left ventricular hypertrophy or ischemic heart disease
- Chest radiograph*: assess for cardiomegaly
- Echocardiogram*
- Renal angiogram, spiral CT, magnetic resonance angiography, or ultrasound*: to establish diagnosis of renovascular hypertension
- Abdominal ultrasound: if aortic aneurysm suspected

Treatment Plan

In the past, lifestyle changes for elderly patients were recommended before pharmacologic therapy was started. Elders with stage 1 hypertension (systolic BP 140 to 159 mm Hg or diastolic BP 90 to 99 mm Hg) should, if possible, try lifestyle changes for 6 months before pharmacologic therapy is started. Weight reduction, smoking cessation, increased exercise, and sodium restriction are beneficial for all patients. The Dietary Approaches to Stop Hypertension (DASH) eating plan, a low-fat, low-salt diet with increased fruits and vegetables, has been proven very helpful in decreasing BP.

Pharmacologic treatment, usually with a low-dose thiazide diuretic, is recommended for elderly patients with stage 2 hypertension (systolic BP 160 mm Hg or higher, diastolic BP 100 mm Hg or higher). Drug therapy is individualized, taking into consideration the patient's race, heart rate, electrolytes, renal condition, allergies, current medications, and comorbid conditions before a new medication is prescribed. Developing a treatment plan that addresses the hypertension as well as comorbid risk factors will benefit the patient (e.g., choosing a medication that addresses the coronary artery disease as well as the high BP).
- Goal of treatment for most patients is < 140/90 mm Hg if the patient does not have diabetes or renal disease.
  - For patients with diabetes or renal disease the BP goal is < 130/80 mm Hg. However, a recent study found a decreased risk for stroke, MI, sudden death, renal failure, and other complications if the systolic BP for type 2 diabetics was < 120 mm Hg.
  - In elderly patients with isolated systolic hypertension and low diastolic BPs, the goal of treatment is unclear, as tissue perfusion may be compromised. Diastolic BP should not be lowered to < 65 mm Hg.
  - Different parameters may apply to post-stroke patients (the concern being adequate perfusion to the brain).
- Treatment is usually based on two or three serial BP measurements.
  - Elderly patients should be started on low doses of antihypertensives; the BP should not be lowered precipitously, and the medication should be increased judiciously to prevent orthostatic hypotension and

* If indicated.

ischemia. "Start low and go slow" continues to be the best recommendation for pharmacologic therapy in elders.

- For most elders, diuretics are considered first-line therapy, and thiazides are most often recommended either alone or in combination with other antihypertensives. Hydrochlorothiazide 12.5 mg PO daily (titrated to maximum 25 mg PO daily) or chlorthalidone 12.5 mg PO daily (titrated to a maximum of 25 mg PO daily can be used.
- Most patients will require multi-drug therapy. An angiotensin-converting enzyme (ACE) inhibitor or an angiotensin-receptor blocker (ARB) is usually recommended as a second agent, although a β-blocker or calcium channel blocker (CCB) can be added.
- Reevaluate the BP frequently every 3 months until within goal, then every 3 months and PRN.
- Monitor serum electrolytes, BUN, and creatinine within 1 week for patients on started diuretics, ACE inhibitors, or ARB therapy. Frequent monitoring is recommended initially to monitor electrolyte and renal status. For stable patients, periodic monitoring (every 3 months) is suggested.
- Special situations
  - An ACE inhibitor or ARB should be considered as first- or second-line therapy in type 2 diabetics, but most diabetic patients will probably require multi-drug therapy.
  - Typically, the goal of BP management for patients with diabetes is to maintain the systolic BP at lower than 110 to 120 mm Hg and the diastolic BP lower than 80 mm Hg, but treatment must always be individualized to each patient.
  - Both ACE inhibitor and β-blocker therapy are indicated and should be considered in post-MI patients. An aldosterone antagonist may be considered for those patients requiring multi-drug therapy, but the patient must be monitored carefully for hyperkalemia.
  - Patients with heart failure require rigorous BP control with an ACE inhibitor and β-blocker. A loop diuretic is indicated for fluid management, particularly in ventricular dysfunction. An aldosterone antagonist is also often suggested if the patient has ventricular dysfunction.
  - Patients with chronic renal disease require skillful BP management. The goal of management with these patients is usually to decrease the systolic blood pressure to less than 130 mm Hg and the diastolic BP to less than 80 mm Hg. An ACE inhibitor or ARB, often with a loop diuretic, is indicated, unless the patient develops hyperkalemia (the creatinine must also be carefully monitored). An ACE inhibitor, combined with a β-blocker, is also considered renoprotective.
  - ACE inhibitors are indicated for left ventricular dysfunction, heart failure, and history of MI.
  - A β-blocker should be considered for patients with a history of MI, angina, heart failure, or tachyarrhythmias.

- Elderly patients with angina and systolic hypertension may benefit from isosorbide dinitrate, sustained release (Dilatrate-SR), 40 mg PO daily.
- Patients with normal lipid levels and isolated systolic hypertension that has been unresponsive to multi-drug therapy may benefit from the addition of a cholesterol-lowering medication to reduce the stiffness of the large arteries.
- Treat cardiovascular risk factors. Consider low-dose aspirin (once BP is controlled), lipid-lowering therapy if appropriate.
- Treat abdominal aortic aneurysm (AAA).

Consultation/Hospitalization

- Patients with hypertension associated with encephalopathy, unstable angina, pulmonary edema, suspected MI or cerebrovascular accident, head trauma, aortic dissection, or bleeding should be hospitalized, unless advanced directives indicate otherwise.
- Physician consultation is recommended for patients on multi-drug antihypertensive therapy and continued hypertension.

Complications

- Dizziness or fainting with increased risk for falling in older patients associated with a decrease in systolic BP > 10 mm Hg may indicate postural hypotension and warrant a change in medication management.
- If untreated, long-term complications of high BP include heart failure, left ventricular dysfunction, cerebrovascular disease, renal insufficiency, proteinuria, retinopathy, MI, and aortic dissection.
- Severe, acute hypertension is associated with hypertensive crisis.
- In elderly patients especially, treatment of hypertension can be associated with adverse drug reactions.
  - Cough with ACE inhibitor
  - Fatigue
  - Peripheral edema with CCBs
  - Bradycardia with α- and β-blockers
  - Fluid and electrolyte abnormalities

Education for Nursing Home/Rehabilitation Staff

- Discuss the importance of nonpharmacologic therapies: sodium restriction, diet, exercise, and weight loss.
- Reinforce the importance of using the correct sized BP cuff.
- Discuss the importance of appropriately scheduling antihypertensives (multiple antihypertensives should not be given at the same time; diuretics should be given in the morning).

- Discuss the risks associated with orthostatic and postprandial hypotension and the need to closely monitor patients.
- Explain the risks associated with various antihypertensives.
- Review the signs and symptoms of the fluid and electrolyte disorders caused by some antihypertensive medications.
- Explain to nurses the importance of reporting abnormal laboratory values to the healthcare provider.

Patient/Family Education

- Explain the benefits of lifestyle changes.
- Discuss the potential adverse effects associated with each antihypertensive medication.

Bibliography

ALLHAT Collaborative Research Group. (2002). Major outcomes in high-risk hypertensive patients randomized to angiotensin-converting enzyme inhibitor or calcium-channel blocker vs diuretics. *Journal of the American Medical Association, 288*(23), 2981-2997.

Chobanian, A.V., et al. (2003). The 7th report of the Joint National Commission on Prevention, Evaluation, and Treatment of High Blood Pressure. The JNC Report. *Journal of the American Medical Association, 289*(19), 2560-2571.

Ferrier, K.E., et al. (2002). Intensive cholesterol reduction lowers blood pressure and large artery stiffness in isolated systolic hypertension. *Journal of the American College of Cardiology, 39*(6), 1020-1025.

Flockhart, D.A., & Tanus-Santos, J.E. (2002). Implications of cytochrome P450 interactions when prescribing medication for hypertension. *Archives of Internal Medicine, 162*(4), 405-412.

Kaplan, N.M., & Rose, B.D. (2004). Treatment of hypertension in the elderly. *www.uptodate.com.* Accessed July 29, 2004.

Ruilope, L.M., et al. (2001). Renal function: The Cinderella of cardiovascular risk profile. *Journal of the American College of Cardiology, 38*(7), 1782-1787.

Whelton, P.K., et al. (1998). Sodium reduction and weight loss in the treatment of hypertension in older persons: A randomized controlled trial of nonpharmacologic interventions in the elderly (TONE). *Journal of the American Medical Association, 279*(11), 839-846.

Gastrointestinal Disorders

ABDOMINAL PAIN

ICD-9: 789.0

Abdominal pain, defined as any discomfort that is localized or referred to the abdomen, is a frequent occurrence in elderly patients and a major cause of morbidity and mortality in this population. Unfortunately, atypical presentations can obscure critical illness and complicate diagnosis, particularly in older or immunocompromised persons, who may not complain of pain or not be able to accurately describe symptoms or events associated with the discomfort. Diagnosis may also be difficult because of coexisting illness or because abdominal pain may be a symptom of organ pathology (abdominal aortic aneurysm, pulmonary infarct, pneumonia, and inferior myocardial infarction [MI]). As a significant number of older patients with abdominal pain will require hospitalization and/or surgical intervention, it is imperative to determine the presence of abnormal findings in a timely way.

Risk Factors

- Age; previous abdominal surgery; history of peptic ulcer disease; history of colorectal or other gastrointestinal cancer or gastrointestinal bleed; history of abdominal trauma, kidney stones, chronic alcohol use, drug use, or coronary artery disease (CAD)
- History of recent endoscopy, colonoscopy, or endoscopic retrograde cholangiopancreatography (ERCP)

History

A comprehensive history reviewing allergies, medications, and surgical and medical history is very important. Determining the history of present illness is often challenging, as not every patient will have the classic symptoms associated with the varied disorders that can cause abdominal pain. Furthermore, in some patients, it may be difficult to elicit a precise history. However, establishing severity and whether the pain is acute or chronic, constant or intermittent, is valuable. Abdominal pain usually results from a gastrointestinal disorder, but it can be referred pain from disorders of the reproductive, genitourinary, musculoskeletal, or vascular systems. Establishing location (Box 6-1), description of the discomfort (Box 6-2), radiation, timing to meals or activity, accompanying symptoms, generalized symptoms, and exacerbating and remitting factors may suggest the etiology. Other factors to consider include the following:

- Dietary: recent dietary changes, appetite change, and lactose intolerance
- Bowel habits: date of last bowel movement, stool consistency, frequency, color, volume, and presence of blood
- Presence of nausea/vomiting
- Vomitus: timing, color, content, volume, and presence of blood
- Sexual history/last menstrual period, if applicable
- History of trauma (e.g., fall, abuse)
- Other residents ill in the facility
- Recent weight loss or gain

Physical Examination

The general appearance is important, but may be deceiving. Significant signs of an acute medical condition include mental status changes, fever or hypothermia, tachypnea, and/or hypotension. Important aspects of the examination include the following:

- The patient's general appearance is quite important, as it may suggest the cause of the discomfort.
  - The motionless patient who does not want to move suggests peritoneal irritation, whereas the patient with acute pancreatitis will usually sit up and lean forward to ease the pain.
  - Guarding is ominous; rigidity suggests perforation.
  - Restlessness may indicate an obstruction, whereas writhing, spasmodic pain is usually associated with renal or biliary colic.
  - Mental status changes may indicate dehydration or sepsis.
  - Asterixis or liver flap occurs in hepatic failure or uremia.

Vital Signs

- Temperature, pulse, respiratory rate, and oxygen saturation
- Blood pressure in each arm and, if possible, postural blood pressure readings

---

BOX 6-1   Abdominal Pain Locations and Associated Pathologies

RUQ Pain
- Associated with pneumonia, pulmonary infarction, gall bladder or liver disease, gastric or bowel disorders, right kidney or ureter disease, or chest cavity disease

LUQ Pain
- Commonly related to cardiac, pulmonary, pancreas, stomach, spleen, left kidney, or ureter

RLQ Pain
- Suggests appendicitis, disorders of the bowel, kidney, pelvis, or ovaries

LLQ Pain
- May be related to bowel, ovaries, or pelvic or kidney disease

Diffuse Abdominal Pain
- Associated with trauma, bowel disease or inflammation, such as peritonitis, along with metabolic or psychogenic origin

Periumbilical Pain
- Associated with diseases of the small intestine

Suprapubic Pain
- Associated with the bladder, uterus, or prostate

Epigastric Pain
- Common with diseases of the gall bladder, common bile duct, pancreas, heart, duodenum, and stomach

Radiation to the Shoulders
- Associated with perforation of the intestine, gall bladder disease, and ectopic pregnancy

Radiation to the Back
- Associated with an aneurysm or pancreatitis

LLQ, Left lower quadrant; *LUQ*, left upper quadrant; *RLQ*, right lower quadrant; *RUQ*, right upper quadrant.

Skin
Observe for the following:
- Skin color: particularly jaundice
- Skin temperature: moist or diaphoretic or dry with loss of skin turgor

---

BOX 6-2   Pain Description

Visceral pain: related to distention of an organ and often described as dull, achy, and not well localized

Parietal pain: associated with peritoneal irritation; described as sharp and localized

Referred pain: occurs in a site remote from the problem; described as an achy discomfort; not deep, but closer to the surface

Burning, gnawing pain: often associated with an ulcer

Dull, steady pain that increases with movement (such as coughing) or increases with palpation (particularly if accompanied by guarding): suggests peritoneal irritation

Intermittent, wavelike, or colicky discomfort: often associated with obstruction in the bowel, ureters, or biliary tract

Constant aching: common with distention of the liver, kidney, spleen, or ovary

Crampy midabdominal discomfort that occurs after eating: may represent abdominal ischemia

Cramps with local or generalized distribution: suggests metabolic illness or altered bowel motility

Deep, boring pain: associated with an abdominal aortic aneurysm

---

- Grey Turner's sign (discoloration/bruising in flank area) or Cullen's sign (umbilical bruising), which suggests intraabdominal bleeding

Eyes
- Note any scleral icterus.

Cardiac Examination
- Determine presence of murmurs and rubs.

Pulmonary
- Assess for signs of pneumonia.

Abdominal Examination/Gynecologic Examination (if Indicated)/Rectal Examination
- Inspect for contour, distention, hematoma, abdominal scars, peristalsis, and masses.
- Auscultate for bruits.
- Auscultate for bowel sounds.
  - Sounds are absent in ileus, mesenteric thrombosis, intestinal obstruction, or peritoneal irritation.
  - High-pitched, increased bowel sounds suggest obstruction, usually of the small bowel.

- Peritoneal friction rub suggests peritoneal inflammation or hepatic metastases; friction rub in the left upper quadrant (LUQ) may signify splenic infarction.
- Perform percussion.
  - Percuss for tenderness, ascites, distended bladder, and liver/spleen size.
  - Tympany suggests distended bowel; dullness suggests a mass.
- Perform palpation.
  - Palpate femoral arteries: absent femoral pulse may indicate dissecting aneurysm.
  - Palpate for abdominal/inguinal lymphadenopathy.
  - Palpate for tenderness/rigidity.
    - Abdominal rigidity accompanied by abdominal tenderness suggests perforation.
    - Abdominal tenderness along with involuntary guarding or rebound tenderness in an elderly patient is an ominous sign.
    - Positive Murphy's sign: pain elicited when palpating under right rib cage with patient inspiring is often indicative of gallbladder disease.
    - McBurney's point: right lower quadrant (RLQ) localized tenderness between umbilicus and anterosuperior iliac spine.
    - Palpate for costovertebral angle (CVA) tenderness, which suggests pyelonephritis.
- Positive psoas sign. Supine patient keeps knee extended. Examiner asks patient to flex thigh while examiner exerts resistance on thighs. Eliciting pain in the pelvis indicates irritation of the iliopsoas muscle, which becomes inflamed with any abdominal abscess, often appendicitis.
- Positive obturator sign: supine patient flexes right thigh to 90 degrees. Examiner internally and externally rotates the knee. Pelvic pain occurs from an inflamed muscle secondary to an abdominal abscess; often appendicitis.
- Perform rectal examination.
  - Evaluate patient for impaction.
  - Tenderness or mass may or may not be present.
  - Obtain stool sample for occult blood, culture (if indicated).

Differential Diagnosis

Vascular Emergencies

- Abdominal aortic aneurysm (AAA): more common in adults older than age 50; usually abrupt onset with severe, constant back, flank, or groin pain radiating to back or chest; patient may have pulsatile mass, shock (hypotension), nausea/vomiting (N/V), lower extremity ischemia.
- Acute mesenteric infarction/ischemia: usually a diagnosis of exclusion; patient may have subtle, transient symptoms. Discomfort may be moderate or suddenly acute. Abdominal distention and/or obvious shock are possible.
- Splenic infarction: acute LUQ pain related to trauma.

Bowel Obstruction/Ileus

- Small bowel obstruction: presents with high-pitched to absent bowel sounds, colicky, mid-abdominal pain that lasts 1 or more days, accompanied by vomiting, distention, fluid volume loss, dehydration, and no flatus. Can be paralytic or mechanical.
- Large bowel obstruction: more common in the elderly; presents with a change in caliber of stool or constipation and no flatus.
- Incarcerated hernia: common in the elderly.
- Volvulus: a closed-loop bowel obstruction; usually occurs in sigmoid or cecum. Presentation is history of chronic abdominal pain or nausea, vomiting, diarrhea or constipation, hemorrhage, or anorexia.
- Malignancy
- Adhesions

Peritonitis

Pain generally localized with specific conditions, such as appendicitis, cholecystitis, diverticulitis; more generalized pain with perforated viscus. Abdomen can be rigid with guarding and rebound tenderness. Accompanied by n/v, fever, tachycardia, and diminished bowel sounds.

Acute Appendicitis

The usual initial symptoms include anorexia, N/V, fever, and a colicky epigastric or periumbilical discomfort that may dissipate. Localized RLQ pain or generalized abdominal pain with rebound tenderness and positive psoas or obturator sign may be present. Appendicitis can occur in elders and may be related to a tumor.

Pancreatitis

Abrupt or gradual severe gnawing, epigastric pain radiating to flank and back, steadily increasing in severity. Patient will sit slouched forward in an effort to relieve pain. N/V, distended abdomen, and fever are usually present. Ileus, hypoactive or absent bowel sounds, and jaundice are possible, accompanied by hypotension, dehydration, and hypocalcemia. Associated with heavy chronic ethanol (ETOH) use, sulfa or thiazide therapy, or post-ERCP.

Cholecystitis/Cholelithiasis

Usually associated with epigastric or RUQ pain that radiates to shoulder or back. Often occurs after a high-fat meal. Flatulence, eructation, fever, local tenderness, positive Murphy's sign.

Diverticulitis

Periumbilical pain that localizes most frequently in left lower quadrant (LLQ). Left scrotal or testicular pain, anorexia, constipation, fever, malaise, leukocytosis, and rectal bleeding are also common findings.

Perforated Peptic Ulcer
Acute, abrupt onset of severe epigastric pain followed by generalized abdominal pain, guarding, rebound tenderness, hypotension, diaphoresis. Usually afebrile.

Other Causes of Abdominal Pain
Cardiac
- Myocardial ischemia, acute myocardial infarction, congestive heart failure, myocarditis, endocarditis, and pericarditis

Pulmonary
- Pneumonia: lower lobe pneumonias especially can cause upper abdominal pain.

Gastrointestinal
- *Clostridium difficile* colitis: associated with recent antibiotic therapy, leukocytosis, frequent watery or mucoid diarrhea, abdominal cramping, and generalized tenderness.
- Constipation: infrequent, inadequate bowel evacuation can be associated with anorexia and more generalized abdominal discomfort.
- Esophageal spasm, esophagitis, and esophageal rupture
- Gastritis, gastroesophageal reflux disease (GERD), and gastric/duodenal ulcer
  - Ulcers are associated with acute epigastric pain that can radiate to the back. Duodenal ulcer pain is usually relieved by food.
  - Gastritis pain is usually located in the epigastric or LUQ area and is less severe than ulcer pain.
  - GERD is associated with mild epigastric discomfort, chest pain, heartburn, and regurgitation.
- Gastroenteritis: accompanied by fever, vomiting, then diarrhea. Abdominal discomfort is usually crampy. This is a diagnosis of exclusion.
- Hepatitis: associated with fatigue, anorexia, nausea, RUQ pain, fever, arthralgia, myalgias. Can be related to medications or infection.
- Ileus: history of surgery, narcotic use, spinal cord injury, diabetes mellitus (DM), hypokalemia, inferior MI, and peritonitis. Often associated with constipation and decreased or absent bowel sounds.
- Inflammatory bowel disease (Crohn's disease, ulcerative colitis): more commonly associated with crampy abdominal pain, loose (bloody or not) stool, and RLQ localized or generalized pain.
- Irritable bowel syndrome (IBS): alternating constipation and diarrhea, with recurrent, crampy diffuse abdominal distress with distention.
- Lactose intolerance: associated with abdominal discomfort, cramping, and nausea after ingesting dairy products.
- Toxic megacolon may occur in a patient with C. *difficile* or recent clindamycin use.

- Biliary colic: abrupt severe epigastric pain often accompanied by vomiting. Laboratory tests are frequently normal.
- Adhesions from multiple surgeries
- Constipation/impaction

Genitourinary
- Pyelonephritis: fever, chills, and CVA tenderness
- Bladder: obstruction/urinary tract infection (UTI) with low pelvic or suprapubic pain
- Renal colic: abrupt, severe pain, usually from a stone can radiate from flank to testicle; often with N/V and urge to void
- Pregnancy, endometriosis, and pelvic inflammatory disease must be considered if female resident in long-term care (LTC) is of child-bearing age.

Hematologic
- Leukemia/lymphoma
- Hemolytic or sickle cell anemia

Metabolic/endocrine
- Diabetic ketoacidosis: generalized abdominal pain that may be acute; accompanied by vomiting, ketotic breath, lethargy, coma, tachycardia, tachypnea, dehydration, and leukocytosis
- Addisonian crisis: low sodium, high calcium, and high potassium
- Thyrotoxicosis
- Hypercalcemia

Immunocompromised
- HIV infection: constitutional symptoms with episodic non-peritoneal, diffuse, colicky, epigastric pain; recurrent pain without specific diagnosis
- Steroid-dependent patients with vasculitis: abdominal pain as part of multiple systemic complaints

Trauma
- Abdominal wall pain, contusion, and hematoma

Other
- Drug induced: antibiotics, nonsteroidal antiinflammatory drugs (NSAIDs), and narcotics
- Somatization: diagnosis of exclusion, suggested by discrepancy between history and physical examination findings
- Infectious: herpes zoster pain (sharp, stabbing pain with tingling) along dermatome; accompanied by rash
- Testicular torsion: more common in young adult males; associated with scrotal edema, erythema, and acute pain
- Malignancy
- Muscle strain

Diagnostics

Diagnostics are individualized and dependent on patient history and presentation. For some patients, diagnostics are unnecessary. For patients requiring urgent hospitalization (suspected bowel obstruction, ischemia, perforation, or abdominal aortic aneurysm), diagnostics should be deferred to prevent delayed emergency department evaluation. For patients stable enough to remain in the subacute or long-term facility, the following diagnostics should be considered.

Laboratory Evaluation
- Urinalysis (U/A) and culture and sensitivity (C&S): to rule out urinary infection
- Stat complete blood count with differential (CBC/diff): to determine infectious process or blood loss
- Stat serum glucose, electrolytes, calcium, blood urea nitrogen (BUN), and creatinine: to monitor for dehydration and ketoacidosis
- Liver function tests (LFTs) if there is a concern about cholecystitis
- Amylase and lipase: if pancreatitis is suspected
- Stool for occult blood
- Stool for culture & sensitivity (C&S)
- Blood cultures: if febrile
- Hepatitis profile*
- Prothrombin time/partial thromboplastin time (PT/PTT)*
- PT/international normalized rate (INR)*
- Arterial blood gases*
- Pregnancy test*
- Tumor markers: CA 125 and carcinoembryonic antigen (CEA)*: for patients with a history of cancer
- C-reactive protein or ESR*: may be elevated in appendicitis or other inflammatory process

Imaging
- Stat flat plate of abdomen: looking for air/fluid lines, distended bowels, or perforation.
- Stat chest radiograph: looking for pneumonia or air under the diaphragm.
- Computed tomography (CT) scan of abdomen/pelvis: most appropriate imaging study for acute abdominal pain; CT with contrast must have recent BUN and creatinine
- Magnetic resonance imaging (MRI): appropriate for angiography of celiac artery or mesenteric vessels; otherwise, not usually indicated
- Abdominal ultrasound: more appropriate if gall bladder disease, testicular disorder, or gynecologic disorder is suspected

*If indicated.

Other Diagnostics
- Electrocardiogram (ECG): to exclude myocardial ischemia or infarction

Treatment Plan

The priority for each person is to rule out surgical abdomen or acute blood loss and determine the need for surgical intervention, hospitalization, and/or consultation.

- Oxygen as needed (PRN) to maintain O_2 saturation > 90%.
- Nothing by mouth (NPO) for acute abdominal pain during work-up until acute disease is excluded
- Determine patient/family wishes concerning hospitalization.
- Maintain hydration with intravenous (IV) fluids; treat infections; manage symptoms, including pain.
- Consider ketorolac (Toradol) 15 to 60 mg intramuscularly (IM) or IV, depending on age, renal status, *or*
- Consult with a physician regarding judicious treatment with a narcotic (morphine sulfate 2 to 4 mg sublingually [SL] or subcutaneously [SC] every 2 to 4 hours PRN).
- Symptomatic treatment for N/V: prochlorperazine (Compazine) 10 mg PO every 6 hours or 25 mg per rectum (PR) or IM every 12 hours PRN for comfort
- Stop hepatotoxic drugs or other implicated medications.
- Nasogastric tube if indicated to prevent increased abdominal distention
- Consider well-lubricated small rectal tube to aid in bowel decompression if indicated.
- Consider Foley catheterization to monitor output or obtain critical urine specimen.
- Change diet as appropriate: clear liquids, BRAT diet (i.e., bananas, rice, apples, tea).
- Stop aspirin (ASA) and Coumadin if bleeding; consult a physician.
- Minimize narcotics and establish bowel regimen if indicated to treat constipation.
- For constipation: Dulcolax suppository 10 mg PR *or* Fleet enema and sorbitol/lactulose 30 mL PO *or* 1 tbsp every hour until bowel movement (BM); maximum 60 mL/day

Other Medications

- If diagnosis of pneumonia: antibiotic therapy (see Chapter 4)
- If diagnosis of C. *difficle* colitis: metronidazole (Flagyl) 500 mg PO every 8 hours for 7 days (see Diarrhea)
- If diagnosis of GERD: consider pantoprazole (Protonix) 40 mg PO daily, ranitidine (Zantac) 150 mg PO Q 12h, famotidine (Pepcid) 20 mg PO BID, or cimetidine (Tagamet) 300 mg PO every 12 hours

- If diagnosis of peptic ulcer disease: same medications as GERD
- If diagnosis is heartburn: follow GERD
- If diagnosis is UTI: appropriate antibiotics
- If diagnosis is related to hypercalcemia: stop vitamin A and D, thiazides, and calcium products; increase fluids; consider diuresis with furosemide (Lasix); consider alendronate (Fosamax) to inhibit bone resorption
- If diarrhea without infection (i.e., IBS): consider Imodium 2 mg PO after each loose stool; maximum 16 mg/day

Consultation/Hospitalization

- Immediate hospitalization is indicated for patients with acute abdominal pain, suspected AAA, acute pancreatitis, acute cholecystitis, appendicitis, perforated gastric/duodenal ulcer, peritonitis, bowel obstruction, and gross blood in vomitus or stool; serum sodium < 123, serum potassium < 3 mEq, serum potassium > 5.8, and corrected serum calcium < 7.5 corrected.
- Hospitalization should be discussed with the physician if vital signs are unstable, pain is uncontrolled, or patient has uncontrolled vomiting or stooling.
- Consult physician for concerns regarding pain management.

Complications

- Peritonitis: sepsis, shock, and death
- Delay in treatment: pain, perforation, sepsis, shock, and death

Education for Nursing Home/Rehabilitation Staff

- Use universal precautions.
- Staff should understand the importance of reporting an episode of acute abdominal pain, changes in temperature (fever/hypothermia), bowel habits, decreased oral intake (both liquids and food), weight loss, change in mental status, diarrhea, or lack of recent bowel movement. Patients should be monitored for vaginal or rectal discharge.
- Staff should know the importance of monitoring vital signs, intake and output (I&O).
- Stool guaiac kits should be kept up to date.

Patient/Family Education

- Education is dependent on pathology responsible for symptoms.
- Patients/families should have careful explanation that abdominal pain may be a sign of serious illness or represent a chronic disorder or condition. Expected diagnostics and treatment with the risk/benefit ratio should be discussed.

Bibliography

Beeson, M.S. (1996). Splenic infarction presenting as acute abdominal pain in an older adult. *Journal of Emergency Medicine* 14(3), 319-322.

Brown, J.R., & Hricko, J. (1999). *Gerontological protocols for nurse practitioners.* Philadelphia: Lippincott Williams & Wilkins.

Eddy, L., et al. (2001). Introduction to differential diagnosis in management of abdominal pain across the life span. *American Journal for Nurse Practitioners*, 5(3), 10-24.

Parker, L.J., & Hricko, J. (1997). Emergency department evaluation of geriatric patients with acute cholecystitis. *Academy of Emergency Medicine*, 40(1), 51-55.

Rodney, W.M., & Pean, C. (2000). Acute abdominal pain in the elderly: Guide to cost-effective work-up. *Consultant*, 40(1), 25-39.

Vissers, R.J., & Call, J.H. (2002). Systemic disease causes of abdominal pain. *Clinical Advisor*, 5(5), 55-74.

CONSTIPATION

ICD-9: 564.00

A frequent concern in older adults, constipation is not usually considered life-threatening, although it can be associated with impaction, ileus, and carcinoma. Frequently, the cause is multifactorial. Hundreds of medications can potentially cause constipation. The most common are listed in Box 6-3. Illness, inadequate fiber or fluid intake, hypothyroidism, hyperparathyroidism, diabetes, hypokalemia, hyperkalemia, neurologic or psychologic disturbances, colonic obstructions, ileus, anatomic disturbances, irritable bowel syndrome, decreased mobility, weakness, spinal cord compression, and ignoring the urge to defecate are secondary causes of constipation. Disordered colonic transit and pelvic floor or anorectal dysfunction (a failure to adequately empty the rectal contents) that do not respond well to laxative therapy are the two primary causes of constipation. Patients may describe constipation as a straining sensation, difficulty defecating, or infrequent defecation. However, to fulfill the Rome II criteria for constipation, two of the following symptoms must have been present for at least 12 weeks in the past year: fewer than three BMs per week, the passage of hard or lumpy stools, a sensation of straining, a feeling of incomplete evacuation and/or anorectal obstruction, and manual maneuvers to aid defecation straining in more than 25% of defecations. A true clinical diagnosis is the finding of a large amount of feces in the rectal ampulla on digital examination and/or excessive feces in the colon, rectum, or both on the abdominal radiograph.

History

- History is important to determine potential causes and can be obtained from the patient, family, or staff members. Any change in bowel pattern, frequency of BMs, last BM, feeling of incomplete evacuation, fecal incontinence, diarrhea, abdominal pain, straining or difficulty passing stools,

---

| BOX 6-3 | **Medications Associated with Constipation** |

Amantidine
Amitriptyline
Antacids (aluminum and calcium)
Anticholinergics
Anticonvulsants
Antidepressants
Antiemetics
Antihistamines
Anti-Parkinson's
Aspirin
Calcium channel blockers
Calcium supplements
Chemotherapeutics (Vinca derivatives)
Diuretics
Iron supplements
Memantine (Namenda)
Muscle relaxants
Narcotics
Non-steroidal antiinflammatory drugs (NSAIDs)
Resins

---

bloating, cramping, flatulence, anorexia, nausea, vomiting, presence of blood or pain with defecation, and aggravating or precipitating factors should be determined.

- A complete medication review (including laxative use), medical and abdominal surgical history, 24-hour dietary and fluid review, as well as determination of the patient's mobility and privacy issues related to bathroom use should also be elicited.

Physical Examination

- Physical examination may be normal.
- Weight and vital signs are necessary to determine the presence of fever, dehydration, or weight loss.
- Oral examination may suggest poor dentition, ill-fitting dentures, lesions, or dehydration.
- Abdominal examination: scars indicate a surgical history. Peristalsis and bowel sounds may be increased or decreased, suggesting an impending obstruction or ileus. There may be increased dullness over areas of stool, and masses may be palpated. Rebound tenderness suggests a peritoneal inflammation.
- A gynecologic examination may demonstrate a rectocele.

- A careful rectal examination and/or anoscopy should determine sphincter tone, pain, lesions, scars, fissures, rectal prolapse, anal stricture, impaction, rectal masses, hemorrhoids, fissures, and presence of occult blood.
- Perineum should be examined at rest with patient lying down in left lateral position, then bearing down to determine perineal descent (usually 1 to 4 cm during straining is normal).
- Anal sphincter tone may be diminished in patients with neurologic disorders or increased if a stricture is present.
- The neurologic examination may elicit autonomic dysfunction or neuropathy.

Diagnostics

- Acute episodic constipation may be managed without diagnostics. However, a change in bowel habits may suggest malignancy, intestinal obstruction, or an underlying metabolic disturbance. A stool sample for occult blood × 3 may reveal occult gastrointestinal bleeding, but there can be false-positive results if hemorrhoids or fissures are present. Because hypokalemia, hypercalcemia, and hypothyroidism are common causes of constipation, a thyroid-stimulating hormone (TSH) and chemistry profile (specifically calcium, potassium, and serum glucose) should be considered if constipation persists or is refractory. A CBC should be obtained if there is evidence of bleeding or concerns about anemia or malignancy.
- Abdominal radiograph studies are indicated in the presence of abdominal discomfort, nausea, and/or vomiting to exclude obstruction, ileus, or volvulus. Abdominal pain with guarding in elders mandates an abdominal CT scan.
- A recent change in bowel habits, weight loss, or rectal bleeding requires an evaluation for an obstructing neoplasm with colonoscopy or a barium enema.
- Physiologic testing for primary, refractory constipation can be considered.

Differential Diagnosis

Medications, metabolic abnormalities, comorbid conditions, and obstruction are common causes of constipation. Frequent, specific causes include but are not limited to the following:
- Dehydration
- Hypothyroidism
- Hypokalemia
- Hypercalcemia
- Ileus
- Obstruction
- Colorectal carcinoma

- Irritable bowel syndrome
- Idiopathic slow transit
- Autonomic dysfunction

Management

Management of constipation is dependent on the underlying cause and should be individualized for each patient. The goal of therapy is the patient's comfort and a regular bowel pattern. Ensuring privacy, establishing a regular elimination routine, and encouraging exercise are helpful nonpharmacologic measures. If the constipation is related to a medication, the medication, if possible, should be discontinued or the dose decreased. Although management modalities, such as increased fluid, fiber, and exercise, have long been recommended, studies evaluating their effectiveness have been small and inconclusive. Laxative studies are also limited, but suggest they improve bowel function, particularly for patients with decreased mobility. However, there is no evidence that suggests one laxative is better than another, nor are any laxatives actually approved for treatment of chronic constipation.

- **Pathologic and life-threatening conditions must be excluded. Constipation associated with fever, nausea, vomiting, abdominal discomfort, and/or guarding requires immediate surgical evaluation to exclude volvulus, obstruction, or other pathology.**
- Ileus and pseudo-obstruction can be medically managed with careful monitoring, no oral intake, nasogastric suction, and IV fluid. Hospitalization is indicated if the facility and nursing staff are not equipped to monitor the patient safely.
- For acute constipation, manual disimpaction may be the initial intervention. A Dulcolax suppository and/or oral lactulose (or other osmotic laxative) is appropriate. Enemas (Fleet, oil retention, or water) to clear the rectum may also be necessary. Once the acute episode has been resolved, a treatment plan to prevent constipation should be initiated.
- For mild, chronic constipation, the following management strategies are recommended:
  - Encourage fluids to 2 L/day.
  - Gradually increase dietary fiber (such as 1 kiwi fruit or 5 stewed prunes daily or 2 tbsp of bran with meals followed by 8 oz of liquid) to 20 to 40 g a day. To prevent abdominal cramping, the fiber should be taken with fluids and increased gradually over several weeks.
  - Foods high in fats, such as cheese, should be limited.
  - Increase exercise periodically throughout the day.
  - Encourage patient to sit on the toilet, with feet placed on a stool, at approximately the same time daily, preferably within 30 minutes of eating a large meal or ingesting a warm liquid (to stimulate the gastrocolic reflex).

- When possible, toileting should be private.
- If the patient is unable to consume adequate dietary fiber, oral fiber supplements such as psyllium, methylcellulose, or polycarbophil are appropriate. All, however, require adequate fluid intake.
- Although the efficacy of docusate is controversial, docusate sodium, 100 mg PO one to three times a day with 8 oz fluid, may be added if fiber supplements are inadequate.
- For constipation not managed with fiber, laxatives are indicated, but can be associated with side effects.*
  - Lactulose, a hyperosmotic disaccharide, 30 to 60 mL PO daily with 240 mL water or juice, although costly, is an effective laxative for chronic constipation. It should be used cautiously in patients with diabetes and is contraindicated for patients on a low-galactose diet or hypersensitivity to lactulose.
    - Potentially can cause electrolyte disturbances with long-term usage.
  - Osmotic laxatives
    - Milk of magnesia, 30 mL PO prn qhs (use carefully in patients with a history of heart failure or renal insufficiency)
    - Magnesium citrate, 30 ml PO prn qhs
    - MiraLax (PEG 3350), 17 g in 8 oz water prn each day
    - Fleet enema, one enema PR
  - Stimulant laxatives
    - Bisacodyl*, 5 mg PO qd prn
    - Senna,* 2 tablets PO prn qhs
    - Bisacodyl suppository (Dulcolax), 1 PR every 3 days prn: usually given in the early morning (before breakfast), followed by toileting
- To minimize patient anxiety and preoccupation on bowel evacuation and to promote time management strategies for nursing staff, consider a bowel regimen with fiber or a stool softener three times a day, a laxative at bedtime, and (if necessary) a suppository when patient first awakens in the morning to ensure a bowel movement. This regimen may be done daily or 3 to 4 days a week. The bedtime laxative should be given the night before the morning suppository.**

Consultation/Hospitalization

- Physician consultation and/or hospitalization are essential for constipation associated with fever, nausea, vomiting, or abdominal discomfort and/or guarding.

---

*The chronic use of senna, castor oil, or bisacodyl has been associated with fluid and electrolyte abnormalities as well as intestinal mucosa damage and should be avoided when possible.
**The use of mineral oil has been associated with vitamin deficiency and (in elders) aspiration, and, therefore, is not recommended.

- Constipation that does not respond to conservative or pharmacologic management requires physician consultation.
- Physician consultation is necessary and hospitalization should be considered for patients requiring intravenous therapy to treat ileus. In facilities not equipped to provide IV therapy, hospitalization is indicated.

Complications

- Nausea, vomiting, anorexia, and dehydration
- Obstruction
- Urinary retention or overflow incontinence
- Fecal impaction
- Perforation
- Bleeding
- Ileus
- Megacolon
- Hemorrhoids
- Rectal or uterine prolapse
- Tenesmus
- Pain and anxiety
- Laxative dependency

Education for Nursing Home/Rehabilitation Staff

- Explain the importance of adequate fluid and fiber intake daily.
- Discuss importance of scheduling medications 1 to 2 hours before giving laxatives to prevent absorption disturbances.
- Explain the importance of assisting the patient to the toilet promptly, the need for privacy during toileting, ensuring that the toilet is at the correct height, and the advantage of encouraging patients to toilet at a regular time each day or after eating (to make the most of the gastrocolic reflex).
- Discuss the risk of mechanical injury associated with enemas.
- Explain the importance of notifying the healthcare provider if the patient experiences constipation associated with nausea, vomiting, abdominal pain, fever, chills, or bleeding.

Patient/Family Education

- Explain causes and treatment of constipation.
- Encourage patient to exercise regularly within their ability, increase dietary fiber and fluids, and toilet at a regular time daily (preferably after meals).
- Discuss the benefit of sitting on the toilet with feet on floor or on a slightly raised footstool to relax the pelvic floor muscles and decrease straining.
- Discuss the side effects of medications prescribed to treat constipation.

Bibliography

DeLillo, A.R., & Rose, S. (2000). Functional bowel disorders in the geriatric patient: Constipation, fecal impaction, and fecal incontinence. *American Journal of Gastroenterology, 95*(4), 901-905.

Howard, L.V., et al. (2000). Chronic constipation management for institutionalized older adults. *Geriatric Nursing, 21*(2), 78-82.

Hurdon, V., et al. (2000). How useful is docusate in patients at risk for constipation? A systematic review of the evidence in the chronically ill. *Journal of Pain Symptom Management, 19*(2), 130-136.

Jones, M.P., et al. (2002). Lack of objective evidence of laxatives in chronic constipation. *Digestive Diseases and Sciences, 47*, 2000-2230.

Karch, A.M. (2004). *2004 Lippincott's nursing drug guide.* Philadelphia: Lippincott Williams & Wilkins.

Management of constipation in older adults. (1999). *Best Practice: Evidenced-Based Practice Information Sheets for Health Professionals, 3*(1), 1-6.

Muller-Lissner, S. (2002). General geriatrics and gastroenterology: constipation and fecal incontinence. *Best Practice Res Clin Gastroenterology, 16*(1), 115-133.

Robson, K., & Lembo, T. (2001). Management of constipation in geriatric patients. *Long-Term Care Interface, 2*(10).

Robson, K.M., et al. (2000). Development of constipation in nursing home residents. *Diseases of the Colon and Rectum, 43*(7), 940-943.

Rush, E.C., et al. (2002). Kiwifruit promotes laxation in the elderly. *Asia Pacific Journal of Clinical Nutrition, 11*(2), 164-168.

DIARRHEA

Acute diarrhea has an abrupt onset but may be part of a chronic or recurring disorder. Although diarrhea may be a symptom of a self-limiting ailment related to medications, a virus, feedings, or food, it may be a symptom of a serious problem related to a preexisting illness, a metabolic problem, infection, inflammation, previous surgery, or an acute emergency. Diarrhea must always be addressed seriously because it puts the patient at risk for fluid/electrolyte imbalance, dehydration, and even death.

With so many patients being treated with antibiotic therapy, particular attention must be given to *C. difficile* colitis and the risk of pseudomembranous colitis, and toxic megacolon. Caused by an alteration in intestinal flora from antibiotic therapy, *C. difficile* is a common diarrhea in hospitals and rehabilitation and long-term care facilities and can cause significant illness and even death in elderly persons. There is more than one form of *C. difficile* infection. There is a mild, antibiotic-associated diarrhea without colitis, which can be somewhat self-limiting. Some diarrhea (3 to 4 loose stools daily) is present, and there can be slight abdominal tenderness, but fever, leukocytosis, and dehydration are absent, and the patient's symptoms will resolve with cessation of the offending antibiotic therapy. A second form is associated with more diarrhea (as many as 15 liquid stools/day), increased abdominal cramping and pain, fever,

Bibliography

DeLillo, A.R., & Rose, S. (2000). Functional bowel disorders in the geriatric patient: Constipation, fecal impaction, and fecal incontinence. *American Journal of Gastroenterology, 95*(4), 901-905.

Howard, L.V., et al. (2000). Chronic constipation management for institutionalized older adults. *Geriatric Nursing, 21*(2), 78-82.

Hurdon, V., et al. (2000). How useful is docusate in patients at risk for constipation? A systematic review of the evidence in the chronically ill. *Journal of Pain Symptom Management, 19*(2), 130-136.

Jones, M.P., et al. (2002). Lack of objective evidence of laxatives in chronic constipation. *Digestive Diseases and Sciences, 47*, 2000-2230.

Karch, A.M. (2004). *2004 Lippincott's nursing drug guide*. Philadelphia: Lippincott Williams & Wilkins.

Management of constipation in older adults. (1999). *Best Practice: Evidenced-Based Practice Information Sheets for Health Professionals, 3*(1), 1-6.

Muller-Lissner, S. (2002). General geriatrics and gastroenterology: constipation and fecal incontinence. *Best Practice Res Clin Gastroenterology, 16*(1), 115-133.

Robson, K., & Lembo, T. (2001). Management of constipation in geriatric patients. *Long-Term Care Interface, 2*(10).

Robson, K.M., et al. (2000). Development of constipation in nursing home residents. *Diseases of the Colon and Rectum, 43*(7), 940-943.

Rush, E.C., et al. (2002). Kiwifruit promotes laxation in the elderly. *Asia Pacific Journal of Clinical Nutrition, 11*(2), 164-168.

DIARRHEA

Acute diarrhea has an abrupt onset but may be part of a chronic or recurring disorder. Although diarrhea may be a symptom of a self-limiting ailment related to medications, a virus, feedings, or food, it may be a symptom of a serious problem related to a preexisting illness, a metabolic problem, infection, inflammation, previous surgery, or an acute emergency. Diarrhea must always be addressed seriously because it puts the patient at risk for fluid/electrolyte imbalance, dehydration, and even death.

With so many patients being treated with antibiotic therapy, particular attention must be given to *C. difficile* colitis and the risk of pseudomembranous colitis, and toxic megacolon. Caused by an alteration in intestinal flora from antibiotic therapy, *C. difficile* is a common diarrhea in hospitals and rehabilitation and long-term care facilities and can cause significant illness and even death in elderly persons. There is more than one form of *C. difficile* infection. There is a mild, antibiotic-associated diarrhea without colitis, which can be somewhat self-limiting. Some diarrhea (3 to 4 loose stools daily) is present, and there can be slight abdominal tenderness, but fever, leukocytosis, and dehydration are absent, and the patient's symptoms will resolve with cessation of the offending antibiotic therapy. A second form is associated with more diarrhea (as many as 15 liquid stools/day), increased abdominal cramping and pain, fever, dehydration, and leukocytosis, but does not cause pseudomembranous colitis.

mentioned type, but there are pseudomembranous changes throughout the

disorder.

Although C. *difficile* is probably the most common diarrhea associated with

creatic or biliary disease or AIDS), a malabsorption disorder, fecal impaction, or infection. *Campylobacter*, *Salmonella*, *Shigella*, and enterohemorrhagic *Escherichia coli* should be considered if C. *difficile* or other pathology is unlikely. Viral infections are possible causes of diarrhea, though vomiting may be the main symptom.

Risk Factors

- Medications, particularly bowel medications and antibiotics
- Endocrine disorder: hyperthyroidism and diabetes
- Fecal impaction
- Infectious process
- Irritable bowel disease
- Previous history bowel surgery or radiation
- Malignancy
- Tube feedings

The history is particularly important, especially in determining how ill the patient is (is the patient eating, drinking, alert, in pain?). Does the patient have a past history of IBS, ulcerative colitis, Crohn's disease, radiation of the lower

vomiting, abdominal discomfort, cramping, and response to previous interventions.

Acute diarrhea present for fewer than 48 hours accompanied by mental status changes; fever; nausea; vomiting; frequent, watery (or bloody) stools; and/or

- CBC/diff: leukocytosis suggests infection
- Serum glucose, serum electrolytes, BUN, and creatinine: to assess for fluid volume and electrolyte status
- TSH: if hyperthyroidism is suspected
- Zinc level: if there is persistent diarrhea to assess need for zinc replacement
- 24- to 72-hour stool collection for fecal fat: if malabsorption syndrome is suspected (patient must be on high-fat diet)

Other Diagnostics

- Radiograph: kidney-ureter-bladder (KUB) if bowel obstruction or fecal impaction is suspected
- Upper gastrointestinal series with small bowel follow-through*: persistent diarrhea
- Barium enema*: persistent diarrhea
- Abdominal CT scan: if diverticulitis is suspected
- Endoscopy/colonoscopy: if diagnosis is elusive and diarrhea continues despite appropriate interventions

Differential Diagnosis

Non-Infectious Diarrhea

- Post-bowel resection or other abdominal surgery (ileostomy, Whipple's procedure)
- Diverticulitis
- Endocrine disorder: hyperthyroidism, gastroparesis in diabetes
- Enteral feedings
- Fecal impaction
- Inflammatory bowel disease (ulcerative colitis, Crohn's disease)
- IBS
- Lactose intolerance
- Malabsorption syndrome (Sprue, Whipple's disease)
- Malignancy
- Medications: bowel medications, antibiotics, or other drugs
- HIV infection
- Pancreatic or biliary disease
- Radiation colitis

Infectious Diarrhea

- *Campylobacter:* associated with fever, watery or bloody diarrhea; related to undercooked poultry
- *C. difficile:* associated with acute watery, malodorous diarrhea, fever, lower abdominal pain, and history of antibiotic or chemotherapeutic therapy

---

*If indicated.

- Enterohemorrhagic *E. coli:* associated with undercooked ground meat; unpasteurized apple cider
- *Salmonella:* foodborne illness associated with fever, honey, eggs, milk, and poultry
- *Shigella:* foodborne illness or person to person transmission; associated with fever
- *Staphylococcus aureus:* associated with diarrhea that starts within 6 to 24 hours after ingestion of infected food
- Viral illness: associated with fever and vomiting

Treatment Plan

If the patient is eating and drinking, without constitutional signs, evaluation, and treatment can be more systematic. If the patient is acutely ill, hydration must be initiated and specific treatment started empirically once the specimen has been obtained, unless hospitalization is warranted. Intravenous fluid (see Chapter 10) is necessary for patients who cannot take oral fluids or who have severe dehydration. Fluid intake and output must be carefully monitored and fluid and electrolytes replaced as indicated (see Fluid and Electrolyte Disorders).

The underlying cause of the diarrhea must also be determined to guide further therapy. Most cases of acute diarrhea in rehabilitation or long-term care settings are related to a viral infection or *C. difficile,* but there are innumerable causes of diarrhea. General considerations in the treatment of diarrhea can be found in Box 6-4. More specific recommendations are as follows:

- If the diarrhea is medication induced, the offending medication should be discontinued or changed.
- Diarrhea associated with enteral feedings may be related to contamination, concentration, fiber, or rate intolerance. The enteral feedings should be handled, hung, and stored properly. All open cans must be refrigerated. Feedings should be started at low rates and run continuously, at least initially, then advanced as tolerated.

BOX 6-4   General Considerations in Diarrhea Management

- Stop all laxatives and stool softeners.
- Consider discontinuing diuretics if patient is at risk for dehydration associated with diarrhea.
- Isolation is usually indicated for diarrhea until the etiology is proven noninfectious.
- Imodium or Lomotil are not indicated for treatment of *C. difficile,* infectious diarrhea, or other diarrhea associated with fever or bloody diarrhea.
- If patient is not vomiting and is able to drink fluids, oral rehydration is best.

- Diarrhea associated with fecal impaction requires fecal disimpaction and/or enemas, plus attention to bowel regimen
- Diarrhea related to inflammatory or irritable bowel disease, pancreatic/biliary disease, malignancy, or endocrine disorder requires treatment of the underlying disorder.
- Lactose intolerance is treated with a lactose-free diet or lactase (Lactaid) tablets with meals.
- Patients with suspected food-borne illness require rehydration and antibiotic treatment (usually a fluoroquinolone, such as ciprofloxacin, every 12 hours for 5 days). Although clear liquids should be encouraged (if the patient is not vomiting), food is not indicated initially. After 12 to 24 hours, crackers, dry toast, or rice can be gradually added to the patient's diet.
- Viral infections require supportive therapy and careful monitoring to prevent dehydration.
- Anti-diarrheal medications are appropriate if an infectious source has been excluded.
    - Loperamide (Imodium), 2 mg PO after a loose stool (maximum dose of 16 mg in 24 hours), may be used for chronic noninfectious diarrhea, but it should be used cautiously if dehydration is suspected.
    - Monitor all patients with diarrhea (both acute and chronic) carefully for weight loss as well as fluid, electrolyte, nutritional, and mineral abnormalities.
- C. *difficile* colitis
    - If C. *difficile* is suspected and the patient is on antibiotic therapy, it is important to first stop the antibiotic and send stool for C. *difficile* toxin assay. For patients only having 3 to 4 stools per day, cessation of antibiotic therapy may ease the symptoms. If the patient is having more frequent stooling and the presentation is highly suspicious for C. *difficile* colitis, the offending antibiotic should be, if possible, discontinued, and the patient started on metronidazole therapy (see later).
        - If it is imperative that the patient be continued on antibiotic therapy, but is positive for C. *difficile*, the antibiotic can be continued, and the patient may be started on metronidazole 500 mg PO TID (every 6 to 8 hours) throughout the course of the antibiotic therapy and for 7 days after the offending antibiotic is completed.
    - Metronidazole, 500 mg PO TID (every 6 to 8 hours) can also be started and continued for 10 to 14 days. The diarrhea usually abates within 7 days after metronidazole is started.
    - Repeat stool testing to be certain that the infection has been eradicated is not recommended.
    - If the diarrhea continues, and the patient is not improving, vancomycin 125 mg PO every 6 hours (IV vancomycin is not effective) should be started and the metronidazole discontinued. If the diarrhea

and symptoms continue, the vancomycin can be doubled every 48 hours (maximum dosage is 500 mg PO QID [every 6 hours]).
- For patients still symptomatic, even with this therapy, the vancomycin should be continued. The addition of IV metronidazole, 500 mg every 8 hours, or vancomycin enemas may be beneficial.
- Recurrent infection
  - Patients who seem asymptomatic after therapy are still at risk for recurrent infection, which may be related to spores in colon diverticula not eradicated by the prescribed treatment.
  - Initial relapse may be treated with a repeat course of metronidazole, 500 mg PO TID (at intervals of 6 to 8 hours) for 14 days.
  - Subsequent relapses require repeat stool for C. *difficile* toxin to ensure accurate diagnosis. If the assay is positive, vancomycin pulsed and tapered therapy has been shown to be effective (Box 6-5).

Consultation/Hospitalization

- Physician consultation is indicated for patients with diarrhea accompanied by high fever, nausea, vomiting, abdominal pain or tenderness, dehydration, or bloody stools.
- Physician consultation is recommended for patients not responding to therapy.
- Hospitalization is indicated for patients with fever, nausea, vomiting, rigors, abdominal tenderness, and guarding.
- Surgical consultation is necessary for patients with suspected toxic megacolon.
- Gastroenterology consult is indicated for patients with suspected irritable bowel, gastroparesis and for patients requiring endoscopy/colonoscopy.
- Consultation with a physician or HIV specialist is recommended for immunocompromised patients and patients with HIV infection.

BOX 6-5   **Treatment of Recurrent *Clostridium difficile* Infection**

First week: Vancomycin 125 mg PO QID
Second week: Vancomycin 125 mg PO BID
Third week: Vancomycin 125 mg PO daily
Fourth week: Vancomycin 125 mg PO QOD
Fifth/sixth week: Vancomycin 125 mg PO every third day
Additional recommendations:
- Colestipol 5 g PO every 12 hours (3 hours after vancomycin) or cholestyramine 4 g PO TID or QID (3 hours after vancomycin) for up to 2 weeks
- Lactobacillus, 1 tablet PO TID*

---

*Evidence of benefit is unconfirmed.

Complications

Dehydration, electrolyte imbalance, and mineral loss are the most common complications associated with diarrhea. Skin breakdown, poor wound healing, and sepsis are other diarrhea-associated complications. Complications associated with *C. difficile* include:

- Cellulitis
- Reactive arthritis
- Fulminant colitis
- Ileitis
- Toxic megacolon
- Hypoalbuminemia
- Dehydration
- Metabolic acidosis
- Chronic carrier state
- Recurrent, relapsing *C. difficile* infection
- Superimposed yeast infection

Education for Nursing Home/Rehabilitation Staff

- Discuss with nursing the importance of monitoring patients on antibiotic therapy for diarrhea.
- Explain why anti-diarrheal medications are usually not indicated.
- Explain importance of hand washing as well as isolation and universal precautions to prevent spread of infection.
- Explain the importance of monitoring I&O and daily weight.
- Discuss ways to increase the patient's fluid intake with small sips of flat cola, ginger ale, bouillon, tea, Pedialyte, or other clear liquids.
- Discuss the importance of notifying the healthcare provider immediately if the patient develops nausea, vomiting, abdominal pain, bloody or dark tarry stools, oliguria, fever, or weakness.
- Explain importance of proper timing of antibiotic and cholestyramine therapy.
- Discuss importance of monitoring/preventing skin breakdown related to diarrhea. Gentle skin cleansing and prophylactic use of skin protectant after each stooling is imperative.
- Discuss the potential benefit of daily yogurt while patients are on antibiotic therapy.

Patient/Family Education

- Explain etiology and treatment of diarrhea.
- Discuss importance of increased fluid intake.
- Explain importance of hand washing and precautions to prevent spread of infection.
- Discuss the potential benefit of daily yogurt while on antibiotic therapy.

Bibliography

Akhtar, A. (2003) Acute diarrhea in the frail elderly nursing home patients. *Journal of the American Medical Directors Association, 4*(1), 34-39.

American Gastroenterological Association. (1999). Medical position statement: Guidelines for the evaluation and management of chronic diarrhea. *Gastroenterology, 116*(6), 1461-1463.

Kelly, C.P., & LaMont, J.T. (2004). Treatment of recurrent *Clostridium difficile* infection. *www.uptodate.com*. Accessed January 24, 2004.

LaMont, J.T. (2004). Clinical manifestations and diagnosis of *Clostridium difficile* infection. *www.uptodate.com*. Accessed January 18, 2004.

Wanke, C.A. (2004). Approach to the patient with acute diarrhea. *www.uptodate.com*. Accessed January 24, 2004.

Zaleznik, D.F., & LaMont, J.T. (2004). Treatment of antibiotic-associated diarrhea caused by *Clostridium difficile*. *www.uptodate.com*. Accessed January 19, 2004.

CHAPTER 7

Genitourinary Disorders

RENAL INSUFFICIENCY

ICD-9: 584.9 (ACUTE RENAL FAILURE); 585 (CHRONIC RENAL FAILURE)

Patients in rehabilitation and long-term care facilities often have some degree of renal failure. The cause may be acute (the result of prerenal, intrarenal, or postrenal injury) or chronic, but frequently the end result is renal injury. Acute renal failure is characterized by a significant increase in blood urea nitrogen (BUN) and creatinine (in a relatively short period of time) and is not infrequent in patients who have a urinary obstruction or who have experienced trauma, hypotension, infection, surgery, heart failure, or rhabdomyolysis, or who have been exposed to nephrotoxic substances (aminoglycosides, intravenous (IV) contrast dye, toxins). Efforts should be made to prevent acute renal failure by carefully monitoring patients with risk factors for its development. Prompt recognition and treatment of acute renal failure may prevent long-term complications.

Chronic renal failure, the result of vasculitis, atherosclerotic disease, diabetes, hypertension, renal artery stenosis, obstructions, medications, or any condition that causes nephron destruction, is associated with a decrease in the glomerular filtration rate (GFR) and a creatinine level > 2.0 mg/dL. Usually, chronic renal failure occurs over a period of months to years. Prudent management is necessary to deter complications.

Whether acute or chronic, impaired renal function requires careful assessment to determine the cause. Urinary obstruction must be excluded and patients carefully monitored to prevent the metabolic, cardiovascular, hematologic, and acid-base problems associated with this disorder.

Risk Factors

- Age
- Diabetes
- Hypertension
- Hypovolemia
- Liver disease
- Vascular disease
- Nephrotoxic medications
  - Nonsteroidal antiinflammatory drugs (NSAIDs)
  - Aminoglycosides
  - Radiographic contrast dye
- Infections
- Postrenal obstructions: prostate enlargement, tumor, bladder dysfunction, and nephrolithiasis
- Collagen disease

History

The history is particularly important, as a recently hospitalized patient may have been exposed to a radiographic contrast dye or medication during the hospitalization or experienced surgery, hypotension, or an infection. A history of anuria or oliguria, dysuria, urinary frequency, hesitancy, nocturia, and/or overflow incontinence should be determined. Medical history (including a history of cancer, renal/kidney disease, and baseline renal function), allergies, and a medication review are essential.

Patients are usually asymptomatic in the early stages of chronic renal failure. Symptoms begin to be notable when the GFR drops below 35% and may include nausea, vomiting, anorexia, confusion, pruritus, non-healing sores, and lethargy.

Physical Examination

The physical examination must be a comprehensive evaluation and should determine the presence of any associated abnormalities. Patients with long-standing renal failure usually appear chronically ill, whereas other patients may not. Each system should be assessed, and the occurrence of any of the following abnormalities noted.

- Weight and vital signs (including temperature and blood pressure measurements in both arms [sitting and standing])
- Urine output
- Skin: may be dry; rashes, ecchymoses, jaundice, or uremic frost may be present
- Eyes: conjunctiva possibly pale; bulbar conjunctiva injection associated with calcium or phosphate deposits; fundoscopic examination to assess presence of papilledema, arteriovenous nicking, and diabetic retinopathy

- Cardiovascular: extra heart sounds, murmurs, rubs, jugular vein distension, carotid bruits, and hepatojugular reflux
- Pulmonary: rales, wheezes, hypoxia, or other signs of fluid overload
- Abdomen: distention, bruits, hepatomegaly, bladder distention, suprapubic tenderness, or hiccups may be present
- Rectal: prostate evaluation and stool for occult blood
- Extremities: pulses and edema
- Neurologic: lethargy, poor concentration, asterixis, irritability, myoclonic twitching, peripheral neuropathy, and/or depression possible; mental status evaluation necessary

Diagnostics

Laboratory Evaluation

- Urinalysis: red blood cell casts suggest glomerulonephritis; positive broad casts are a specific finding indicating chronic renal failure (CRF); proteinuria and hematuria are nonspecific findings.
- Serum electrolytes: patients with renal failure are at risk for hyperkalemia.
- BUN and creatinine
- Calcium/ionized calcium
- Albumin/total protein
- Phosphorus
- Magnesium
- Uric acid
- Parathyroid hormone (PTH)
- Complete blood count with differential (CBC/diff): assess for anemia.
- Liver function tests (LFTs)
- 24-hour urine for creatinine clearance and microalbumin
- Hemoglobin (Hgb) A1C*

Other Diagnostics

- Ultrasound*: to exclude obstruction and hydronephrosis
- Renal biopsy*

Differential Diagnosis

- Acute renal failure: prerenal, intrarenal, or postrenal
- Chronic renal failure
  - Stage 1: normal GFR > 90 mL/min per 1.73 m^2 and persistent albuminuria
  - Stage 2: GFR ranges between 60 to 89 mL/min per 1.73 m^2 and persistent albuminuria

---

*If indicated.

- Stage 3: GFR ranges between 30 to 59 mL/min per 1.73 m^2
- Stage 4: GFR ranges between 15 and 29 mL/min per 1.73 m^2
- Stage 5: GFR <15 mL/min per 1.73 m^2 (end-stage)

Treatment Plan

When possible, the underlying pathology should be identified and reversible pathology (e.g., hypotension, hypovolemia, infection, urinary tract obstruction, offending medications) treated expediently. Appropriate treatment (i.e., discontinuing nephrotoxic medications, correcting hypovolemia, or relieving urinary tract obstruction) will possibly improve renal function. Continuing management goals should include the prevention of further deterioration in renal function and treating the complications associated with renal failure.

- Avoid nephrotoxic medications: NSAIDs, aminoglycosides, and radiographic contrast dye if at all possible; adjust dose if use is absolutely necessary.
- Assess renal function by determining creatinine as well as GFR; monitor creatinine and GFR periodically. (In elderly patients and in patients with risk factors for CRF, small increases in serum creatinine may indicate renal insufficiency, even if the GFR range is within acceptable limits.)
- Adjust medication dosages appropriately for patients with renal failure.
  - Determine creatinine clearance before prescribing medications.
    Men = (140 – age) × weight [kg]/72 × serum creatinine (mg/dL)
    Women = (140 – age) × weight [kg]/72 × serum creatinine (mg/dL) × 0.85
- Cardiovascular management
  - Control hypertension: BP goal < 130/80; systolic blood pressure < 110 is not advised.
    - Angiotensin-converting enzyme (ACE) inhibitors are usually indicated for patients with type 1 diabetes or for patients with proteinuria. If the patient is on a diuretic, the diuretic should be stopped before adding the ACE inhibitor (if possible) to prevent hypoperfusion to kidneys. Monitor serum potassium, BUN, and creatinine within 5 days after starting medication, then monitor carefully.
    - Consider angiotensin-receptor blockers (ARBs) for type 2 diabetics or for patients intolerant to ACE inhibitor therapy. Monitor serum potassium, BUN, and creatinine within 5 days after starting medication, then monitor carefully.
    - If blood pressure goal is not met with an ACE inhibitor or ARB, add a diuretic (usually a loop diuretic).
    - For continued elevated blood pressure, consider diltiazem, verapamil, or a β-blocker.
- Control hyperlipidemia: Goal LDL < 100 mg/dL because cardiovascular complications are significant in patients with CRF
- Glycemic control for patients with diabetes
- Consider dietary protein restriction 0.8 g/kg/day.

- Monitor fluid status and serum BUN, creatinine, calcium, hemoglobin/hematocrit, lipids, magnesium, phosphorus, sodium, potassium, uric acid, and PTH every 3 months and as indicated.
    - Prevent hypotension/hypovolemia.
    - Adjust medications in older patients or in patients with impaired renal function to minimize renal injury.
    - Keep serum potassium levels < 6 mEq/L (preferably < 5.5 mEq/L). Daily low-dose loop diuretic in combination with ACE inhibitor may maintain acceptable serum potassium levels. A low potassium diet may also be helpful, but some patients, especially if serum creatinine > 3, may not be able to tolerate ACE inhibitor or ARB therapy because of associated hyperkalemia.
    - Decrease or discontinue ACE inhibitors, ARB, potassium supplements, spironolactone, or other medications causing hyperkalemia if necessary.
    - In consultation with physician, consider Kayexalate therapy, 15 g PO PRN with food, to control hyperkalemia if necessary. Follow serum potassium closely.
    - Elevated serum phosphorus requires treatment to bind phosphorus. Consider calcium carbonate tablets given at mealtime (1 to 2 g PO BID to QID; up to 20 g daily) to maintain serum phosphorus between 4.5 and 5.5 mg/dL. Careful monitoring of serum calcium is necessary as hypercalcemia is a frequent result of this therapy.
    - Consider allopurinol 100 mg/day for treatment of gout.
    - Discuss fluid restriction (1000 mL daily) for hyponatremia.
    - Consult with endocrinology for treatment recommendations for patients with secondary hyperparathyroidism (usual treatment: calcitriol [vitamin D], calcium, and phosphate binder to maintain serum calcium and phosphorus within acceptable limits).
    - Consult with a nephrologist.
- Monitor hematocrit monthly if patient is receiving erythropoietin.
    - Serum iron and ferritin should be monitored periodically during erythropoietin therapy. If indicated, ferrous sulfate 325 mg PO daily to TID should be added to the medical regimen.
- Monitor for metabolic acidosis (serum bicarbonate between 10 and 20 mEq/L).
- Maintain serum protein and albumin within normal limits.
- A lowered sodium diet is usually indicated. Discussion with the nephrologist is necessary to determine the benefits of a low protein, low potassium, and/or low phosphorus diet.
- Avoid medications containing aluminum or magnesium.
- Pruritus usually responds better to skin moisturizers than antihistamines.

Consultation/Hospitalization

- Consultation with a nephrologist is recommended for patients with creatinine > 1.5.

- Endocrinology referral is indicated for patients with elevated PTH (secondary hyperparathyroidism).
- Consult with a physician for treatment of metabolic acidosis.
- Consultation with the physician and consideration for RenaGel therapy are recommended for patients who develop hypercalcemia while taking calcium carbonate for hyperphosphatemia. (RenaGel is suggested for persistent hyperphosphatemia, as RenaGel does not cause hypercalcemia.)
- Consultation with a nutritionist is recommended to maintain adequate nutritional status.
- Hospitalization is indicated for patients with suspected acute renal failure, congestive heart failure, pulmonary edema, pericarditis, or acute electrolyte imbalance.

Complications

- Anemia
- Congestive heart failure
- Depression
- Dialysis: peritoneal or hemodialysis
- Erythropoietin deficiency
- End-stage renal disease
- Gastrointestinal disturbances: anorexia, nausea, and vomiting
- Electrolyte abnormalities: hyperkalemia, hyperphosphatemia, and hyponatremia
- Encephalopathy
- Hyperlipidemia
- Hyperparathyroidism (secondary)
- Hypertension
- Leukopenia
- Malnutrition
- Metabolic acidosis
- Metabolic complications related to calcium, phosphorus, and vitamin D absorption
- Neuromuscular complaints
- Pericarditis
- Renal osteodystrophies
- Restless leg syndrome (RLS)
- Sexual dysfunction
- Thyroid dysfunction

Education for Nursing Home/Rehabilitation Staff

- The importance of monitoring blood pressure, fluid status, and electrolyte abnormalities should be discussed with the nursing staff so that acute renal failure can be prevented and the complications of CRF reduced.

- The importance of daily weights (early morning, before breakfast) to monitor fluid status should be explained to the nursing staff.
- The nursing staff should be educated and able to monitor arteriovenous fistulas.

Patient/Family Education

- Patients and families require continuous education about renal failure and the complications associated with the disorder.
- Treatments as well as associated risks and benefits for renal-related disturbances should be carefully explained.
- Long-term care planning, including explanation of the types of dialysis and risks and benefits, should be discussed.

Bibliography

National Kidney Foundation. (2004). *Clinical practice guidelines for chronic kidney disease.* *www.kidney.org.* Accessed February 16, 2004.

Post, T.W. (2004). Overview of the management of chronic renal failure. *www.uptodate.com.* Accessed February 16, 2004.

Yu, H. (2003). Progression of chronic renal failure. *Archives of Internal Medicine, 163*(12), 1417-1429.

URINARY TRACT INFECTION

ICD-9: 599.0

In women, urinary tract infections (UTIs) occur fairly frequently and are attributed to periurethral fecal contamination, a short urethra, and sexual intercourse. Young men typically do not experience UTIs, as they are not as exposed to fecal contamination, have a longer urethra, and are somewhat protected by prostatic secretions. For that reason, urologic consultation is usually indicated if a male experiences an infection in the urinary tract. Risk factors for developing a UTI increase as we age, however, and, as a result, after age 50, UTIs are common in both men and women.

Symptomatic bacteriuria (Box 7-1) causes both complicated and uncomplicated UTIs and requires antibiotic therapy. *Enterococci, Escherichia coli*, and *Proteus mirabilis* are the most common pathogens in nursing home populations, although patients with spinal cord injury or other illnesses are susceptible to other pathogens.

Asymptomatic bacteriuria is quite prevalent in all institutionalized patients, particularly in patients with diabetes or an indwelling Foley catheter. Often, staff or family notice malodorous urine, increased confusion, lethargy, or other subtle changes in a patient and request a urinalysis to exclude a UTI. The urine may be positive for bacteria because bacteriuria is very prevalent in this population. The patient is subsequently started on antibiotic therapy. This approach has led to increased use of antibiotics and contributes to growing antibiotic resistance. Antibiotic therapy is not indicated for patients with asymptomatic bacteriuria unless the patient is pregnant or scheduled for cystoscopy or other traumatic genitourinary evaluation (e.g., transurethral resection of prostate).

Risk Factors

- Advanced age
- Fecal incontinence/impaction
- Incomplete bladder emptying or neurogenic bladder
- Vaginal atrophy/estrogen deficiency
- Pelvic prolapse/cystocele
- Insufficient fluid intake/dehydration
- Indwelling Foley catheter or urinary catheterization/instrumentation
- Diabetes or immunosuppression
- Benign prostatic hypertrophy or loss of prostatic antibacterial secretions
- Bladder cancer or cancer of the prostate
- Urinary tract obstruction
- Spinal cord injury

History

Immunocompromised and older patients may not complain of the classic symptoms associated with a UTI: frequency, burning, dysuria, urgency, or suprapubic discomfort. Usually, cystitis even in elderly patients, has an acute onset. Fever, frequency, incontinence, foul-smelling urine, and/or vomiting may be noted by the patient or nursing staff. Falls, mental or functional status changes, increased or new urinary incontinence, hematuria, and/or anorexia or vomiting, although not specific signs of a UTI, suggest the need for further investigation.

Additional history includes determining recent history of urinary catheterization or urologic procedure as well as medical history (comorbid disease, urinary tract abnormalities, current medications, and allergies).

Physical Examination

Physical findings may also be subtle. Usually, the change in functional or mental status mandates a comprehensive examination to determine the cause of the change in behavior or functioning. Important assessment considerations include:
- Weight: determine if there has been recent weight loss, which suggests dehydration.
- Vital signs: presence of fever (a temperature of 100° F or 2° F above baseline is significant in elderly or immunocompromised patients, although some patients will have bacterial infections without fever), chills, tachycardia, orthostatic changes, and/or hypotension should be determined.
- Neurologic: mental status

- Skin: to exclude herpes zoster, decubiti, cellulitis, abscess, or other infection
- Head, eyes, ears, nose, and throat (HEENT) examination: conjunctiva, oropharynx, and neck for evidence of infection, nuchal rigidity, or lymphadenopathy
- Cardiopulmonary: exclude pulmonary infection as well as heart failure or pericarditis, which may be associated with UTI or other causes for change in patient status.
- Abdominal examination: any abdominal tenderness, bladder distention, or costovertebral angle (CVA) tenderness is significant.
- Rectal examination: monitor for impaction, prostate tenderness, masses, or enlargement.
- Vaginal examination: determine presence of atrophy, vaginal bleeding or discharge, lesions (particularly herpetic lesions that may be associated with herpes zoster), tenderness, uterine prolapse.
- Penile evaluation: assess for discharge, lesions, and edema.

Diagnostics

A clean-catch, mid-stream urine specimen from patients suspected of having a UTI is the initial essential diagnostic. It is preferable not to catheterize patients to obtain the specimen. New, clean external catheters may be used for male patients. In patients with an indwelling Foley catheter and suspected urosepsis (fever, chills, hypotension, new-onset confusion), the urine specimen may be aspirated from the catheter port. Urine dipstick may suggest the presence of urinary white blood cells (WBCs), but in older or institutionalized adults at risk for UTI, the urinalysis is necessary.

Laboratory Evaluation
- If 10 or more WBCs per high-power field are present in the urine, a culture and sensitivity is essential.
- Upper UTI is suggested by the presence of WBC casts in urine.
- CBC/diff and basic metabolic panel are dependent on patient presentation, but they are often indicated to determine presence of leukocytosis or dehydration.
- A patient presenting with an acute onset of illness or with fever, chills, anuria, hypotension, or CVA tenderness requires a urinalysis, culture and sensitivity, chest radiograph, CBC/diff, basic metabolic panel, and blood cultures as part of the fever work-up.
  - Blood cultures are recommended for suspected bacteremia. Depending on patient/family wishes, hospitalization should be considered for patients living in long-term care facilities for whom blood cultures are considered.

Other Diagnostics
- If obstructive uropathy is a consideration, ultrasonography or CT scan is recommended.
- Further testing (e.g., intravenous pyelogram, cystoscopy) may not be

necessary but is dependent on history and physical findings, especially if symptoms continue after treatment for UTI.

Differential Diagnosis

- Other infectious processes: consider appendicitis, cholecystitis, cholangitis, diverticulitis, and pneumonia.
- Acute urethral syndrome: usually present in younger women who have dysuria, frequency, and < 10 WBCs per high-power field
- Urethral caruncle
- Interstitial cystitis
- Bladder cancer or bladder abnormalities
- Prostate enlargement

Treatment Plan

The prevalence of asymptomatic bacteruria in older patients makes diagnosis challenging. Current criteria for treatment in patients with or without an indwelling Foley catheter are listed in Box 7-1. Because asymptomatic bacteruria is common in elderly patients, treatment should not be predicated on the presence of urinary bacteria, even in numbers > 100,000 colonies per mL. Treatment is also not indicated for patients with low-grade fever and nonspecific symptoms, such as change in mental or functional status. Increasing fluid intake is beneficial, as mental and functional status changes in older patients are often due to a fluid volume deficit rather than an infectious process. For patients unable to take adequate oral fluids to replace fluid loss or prevent dehydration, IV fluid replacement may be indicated (see Chapter 10). Hold diuretics and laxatives for patients with suspected and documented dehydration.

Further considerations are as follows:
- Patients with positive urinalysis who are symptomatic or have fever, chills, and/or other signs associated with systemic illness (see Box 7-1) should be treated with antibiotic therapy. Patients may be treated in the nursing home or rehabilitation facility. Hospitalization is suggested if urosepsis is a consideration. Stable patients able to take oral medication can be started empirically on antibiotic therapy while awaiting urine culture results.
  - Antibiotic therapy is indicated for patients without indwelling Foley catheter and dysuria, fever > 100° F (or 2.4° F above baseline), hematuria, frequency, new or increased urgency or incontinence, suprapubic discomfort, or CVA tenderness.
  - For patients with an indwelling Foley catheter, antibiotic therapy is indicated for fever > 100° F (or 2.4° F above baseline) and new-onset CVA tenderness, chills, or delirium.
    - Choice of antibiotic is based on patient profile and must be individualized. Historically, trimethoprim-sulfamethoxazole (TMP-SMX) (Bactrim) was used for patients without sulfa allergies, but

---

BOX 7-1   Symptomatic Bacteruria: Diagnostic Criteria for Patients with and without an Indwelling Foley Catheter

Patients without Indwelling Foley Catheter
Three of the following symptoms or signs must be present:
- New or increased burning on urination
- Frequency
- Urgency
- Decreased mental or functional status (may be new or increased incontinence)
- Fever (> 38° C)
- Chills
- New-onset hematuria, foul smelling urine, or presence of sediment
- New suprapubic pain, flank pain, or tenderness

Patients with Indwelling Foley Catheter
Two of the following symptoms or signs must be present:
- Decreased mental or functional status
- Fever (> 38° C)
- Chills
- New suprapubic pain, flank pain, or tenderness
- New-onset hematuria, foul-smelling urine, or amount of sediment

---

Adapted from Kania, T. (2004). The A-B-Cs of urinary tract infection prevention in the incontinent patient. *Extended Care Product News, May/June,* 1, 6, 7.

sulfa resistance is increasing in some areas and in some patients may cause hyperkalemia. If not contraindicated, nitrofurantoin (Macrodantin), 100 mg BID or a fluoroquinolone (Ciprofloxacin 250 to 500 mg PO BID) therapy for 10 to 14 days is appropriate in female patients. β-lactam antibiotics and nitrofurantoin are not appropriate for elder male patients, because of concerns regarding associated prostatitis. Ciprofloxacin, 500 mg PO for 14 days (unless contraindicated), should be prescribed for these patients.

■ Many patients (particularly if UTI is associated with azotemia, obstruction, or indwelling Foley catheter) in rehabilitation and nursing home settings should be treated for complicated UTI and require IV antibiotic therapy with a third-generation cephalosporin (ceftriaxone [Rocephin], 1 g IV every 24 hours) or a fluoroquinolone (Levofloxacin [Levaquin] 500 mg IV every 24 hours). IV antibiotic therapy should be continued until patient is afebrile a minimum of 48 hours and able to take oral medication and fluids adequately. The recommended treatment course is 14 days.

- ■ Antibiotic dosage must be adjusted for patients with renal insufficiency.
- ■ Phenazopyridine (Pyridium) is not appropriate for elderly patients or for patients with renal insufficiency.
- Foley catheterization should be avoided if at all possible, although patients with urosepsis/dehydration may require urinary catheterization to monitor output. Recording intake and output and obtaining daily weights may help assess improvement in fluid status.
- Although controversial, patients with recurrent UTI may benefit from cranberry extract tablets, 1 PO BID, or daily vitamin C.
- Urinary symptoms related atrophy may respond to topical estrogen cream; however, there is disagreement about the efficacy of topical estrogen in preventing UTIs in older women.
- Male patients with recurrent UTI should be evaluated for functional obstruction or prostatitis.
- Prophylactic antibiotic therapy is also controversial. Studies have not demonstrated value for UTI prevention.
- A follow-up urinalysis/culture and sensitivity is not usually indicated after antibiotic treatment.
- UTI relapse is indicated by recurrent signs and symptoms within 2 weeks of treatment. The bacteria causing the relapse will be the same strain that caused the initial infection.
- Recurrent UTI is indicated by return of signs and symptoms 4 weeks after treatment is completed for the initial UTI. The bacteria causing the recurrent infection may be different from the bacterial strain that caused the first infection.

Consultation/Hospitalization

- Transfer to an acute care facility is indicated for patients with hypotension, suspected urosepsis, or suspected obstructive uropathy.
- Concerns about appropriate antibiotic and IV therapy should be discussed with the physician.
- Consider urology consultation for both male and female patients with recurrent UTI or suspected obstruction.

Complications

- Pyelonephritis
- Urosepsis and death
- Complications associated with antibiotic therapy
- Hyperkalemia and metabolic acidosis have been associated with TMP-SMX in higher dosages in elderly patients.

Education for Nursing Home/Rehabilitation Staff

- It is important that the nursing staff understands the importance of monitoring patients for signs and symptoms of infection and recognizes the necessity of reporting temperature elevations and mental status changes to the healthcare provider.
- Discuss symptomatic bacteruria diagnostic criteria with nursing staff.
- Discuss preventative strategies with staff to prevent UTIs.
  - Universal precautions
  - Meticulous hand hygiene
  - Foley catheter care and perineal care for incontinent patients (daily and as needed)
  - Bladder/bowel training; patients should be regularly toileted on commode or toilet to promote bladder emptying.
  - Prevention of constipation/impaction
  - Adequate fluid intake
  - Importance of avoiding indwelling Foley catheters whenever possible
  - Importance of checking/changing incontinent patients frequently
  - Avoidance of irritating powders or cleansing agents on perineum

Patient/Family Education

- Discuss with patients the importance of increased fluids as well as the benefit of avoiding caffeinated beverages, citrus juices, and alcohol, which may irritate bladder.
- See Chapter 12.

Bibliography

Bentley, D., et al. (2000). Practice guideline for evaluation of fever and infection in long-term care. *Clinical Infectious Diseases, 31*, 640-653.

Loeb, M., et al. (2001). Development of minimum criteria for the initiation of antibiotics in residents of long-term care facilities: Results of a consensus conference. *Infection Control and Hospital Epidemiology, 22*(2), 120-124.

Richards, C. (2002). Infections in residents of long-term care facilities: An agenda for research. Report of an expert panel. *Journal of the American Geriatric Society, 50*(3), 570-576.

Stothers, L. (2002). A randomized trial to evaluate effectiveness and cost effectiveness of naturopathic cranberry products as prophylaxis against urinary tract infections in women. *Canadian Journal of Urology, 9*(3), 1558-1562.

Neurologic Disorders

DELIRIUM

ICD-9: 293.0

Delirium is a reversible clinical state, associated with numerous underlying medical conditions. It is characterized by an acute, fluctuating change in mental status; a reduced ability to focus, sustain, or shift attention; altered levels of consciousness; or perceptual disturbances. There are three subtypes of delirium: hyperactive, hypoactive, and mixed variants. Nearly 30% of hospitalized patients older than 70 years of age develop delirium during hospitalization. Patients with underlying dementia and severe physical illnesses are at greater risk, although the pathophysiology is not well understood.

Several physiologic theories have been proposed and include:

- A disturbance in global function as demonstrated by diffuse slowing on electroencephalogram (EEG)
- Increased anticholinergic response due to decreased acetylcholine from endogenous factors or drug therapy
- Alterations in neurotransmitter synthesis
- Increased cytokines, which are activated in the presence of underlying illness

Risk Factors

The etiology is most likely multifactorial. However, there seems to be a relationship with the following:

- Metabolic, cardiovascular, or primary cerebral diseases, including dementia
- Infections
- Urinary retention, presence of bladder catheter, or constipation
- Previous history of delirium

- Altered nutritional status
- Trauma
- Sensory deprivation or sensory overload
- Polypharmacy
- Environmental change or stress
- Use of physical restraints
- Alcohol/substance abuse or withdrawal
- Advanced age
- Postoperative state
- Pain

History

A complete and thorough medication review, including over-the-counter (OTC) medications and herbal products, as well as any recent additions or changes in the medication regimen, is beneficial. In addition, reviewing the past medical history, including head trauma, and eliciting the history of the change in mental status is imperative. Identifying the timing and onset of symptoms and determining the change from the patient's baseline aid in diagnosis. The hyperactive state in delirium is characterized by restlessness and agitation; the hypoactive state by apathy, lethargy, and somnolence. Other symptoms include:

- Distractibility/disorganized speech
- Hypervigilance emotional lability (hyperactive), short-term memory loss, fever, cough, anorexia, decreased urine output, disorientation, constipation, anxiety, altered sleep/wake cycle, a recent fall, or functional changes
- Perceptual disturbance

Physical Examination

A thorough physical examination includes mood assessment and neurologic evaluation. Other aspects of the examination include:

- General appearance
  - What is patient's level of consciousness?
  - Is patient able to focus during conversation?
- Vital signs and oxygen saturation
- Skin, cardiovascular, pulmonary, abdominal, and rectal examination
- Mental status examination: patients may not be able to pay attention enough to answer questions.
- Confusion Assessment Method (CAM) (Table 8-1): the diagnosis of delirium requires the presence of features 1 and 2 along with either 3 or 4.

Differential Diagnosis

- Cerebrovascular accident (CVA), transient ischemic attack (TIA), subdural hematoma, seizure, head trauma, or temporal arteritis

TABLE 8-1   Confusion Assessment Method (CAM)

1. Acute onset and fluctuating course	Usually, obtained from a family member or nurse and shown by positive responses to the following questions: "Is there evidence of an acute change in mental status from the baseline?" and "Did the abnormal behavior fluctuate during the day, that is, tend to come and go, or increase and decrease in severity?"
2. Inattention	Shown by a positive response to the following: "Did the patient have difficulty focusing attention—for example, being easily distractible or having difficulty keeping track of what was being said?"
3. Disorganized thinking	Shown by a positive response to the following: "Was the patient's thinking disoriented or incoherent, such as rambling or irrelevant conversation, unclear or illogical flow of ideas, or unpredictable switching from subject to subject?"
4. Altered level of consciousness	Shown by any answer other than "alert" to the following: "Overall, how would you rate this patient's level of consciousness?" Normal = Alert Hyperalert = Vigilant Drowsy but easily aroused = Lethargic Difficult to arouse = Stupor Unarousable = Coma

From Inouye, S., et al. (1990). Clarifying confusion: The Confusion Assessment Method. *Annals of Internal Medicine, 13*(12), 941-948. Reprinted with permission.

- Cirrhosis
- Depression
- Dementia
- Psychotic illness
- Endocrine disorder (e.g., thyroid disorder, hypoglycemia)
- Infection, anemia, myocardial infarction, or congestive heart failure (CHF)
- Metabolic illness: dehydration, electrolyte disturbance, acid-base imbalance, hypoxia, renal insufficiency, or vitamin deficiency
- Intoxication from poisons or drugs
- Withdrawal from drugs or alcohol
- Pain

Diagnostics

Laboratory Evaluation
- Diagnostics should be individualized and based on physical examination and medication review.

- Complete blood count with differential (CBC/diff): to exclude infectious process or anemia.
- Serum glucose, electrolytes, calcium, magnesium, phosphorus, BUN, and creatinine: to determine fluid, electrolyte, and renal status
- Liver function tests (LFTs) and ammonia: to determine presence of hepatic dysfunction
- Thyroid-stimulating hormone (TSH): to assess for thyroid disorder
- Vitamin B_{12}, folate, and thiamine: to assess for reversible factors
- Drug levels when appropriate
- Urinalysis: to exclude urinary tract infection (UTI)

Other Diagnostics
- Chest radiograph: to evaluate for pneumonia
- ECG: to assess for ischemia or infarction

Treatment Plan

The goal of management is to determine the underlying precipitants, establish the diagnosis, manage symptoms, prevent complications, and promote a safe environment for the patient and staff. Management considerations include:

- Establish and implement plan for substitutive decision making (e.g., health care proxy).
- Interventions should depend on the patient's degree of confusion and agitation. Management of cognitive impairment, sleep deprivation, immobility, visual impairment, hearing impairment, and dehydration has been shown to reduce the number and duration of delirium episodes in hospitalized elders.
- Nonpharmacologic
    - Provide a supportive environment and environmental manipulation.
    - Assist with sensory impairment through eyeglasses and hearing aids.
    - Encourage family support.
- Pharmacologic
    - Taper or discontinue nonessential medications.
    - Neuroleptics: small doses of haloperidol may be useful in controlling agitation and psychosis. Dosing should be guided by the patient's initial response and by frequent reassessment (see p. 170).
    - Utilize short-acting benzodiazepines for behavior management (useful in the management of alcohol or sedative withdrawal).
    - Optimize pain management regimen (see Chapter 16).

Consultation/Hospitalization

- Discuss change in status and use of neuroleptics or short-acting benzodiazepines with physician and family. (The family may need to sign an authorization for treatment.)

- Consider psychiatric evaluation, especially for unfamiliar patients.
- Hospitalization is dependent on staff's ability to support patient in current setting, severity of underlying medical etiology, and patient/family's choice for "do not hospitalize."

Complications

- Falls
- Agitation
- Dehydration and malnutrition
- Lack of essential medications
- Injury to self and others
- Progressive cognitive impairment

Education for Nursing Home/Rehabilitation Staff

- Teach preventive measures, such as hygiene, adequate nutrition and hydration, and optimal skin care.
- Promote safety measures to avoid falls.
- Teach signs and symptoms of early presentation of functional, physical, or mental status changes (e.g., decreased appetite, unsteady gait, any change from normal baseline functioning).
- Educate staff concerning the stressor of institutionalization in the elderly patient, other potential causes of change in patient status, and course of the disorder.
- Explain the importance of promoting a normalized sleep/wake cycle (see Insomnia in Chapter 16).
- Review aspiration precautions with staff.
- Educate staff concerning need for 1:1 observation to avoid physical restraints.
- Educate staff concerning behavior and agitation management.
- Educate staff concerning signs and symptoms of extrapyramidal symptoms (EPS) related to neuroleptics.

Patient/Family Education

- Offer reassurance concerning clinical presentation.
- Explain to family the likely cause of the delirium, the fluctuating course, and length of time symptoms may last.
- Educate family concerning need for one-on-one observation to avoid physical restraints and medication use when necessary.

Bibliography

Dyer, C., et al. (1995). Post-operative delirium: A review of 80 primary data-collection studies. *Archives of Internal Medicine, 155*(5), 461-465.

Francis, J. (1992). Delirium in older patients. *Journal of the American Geriatrics Society,* 40(8), 829-838.

Inouye, S. (2004). A practical program for preventing delirium in hospitalized elderly patients. *Cleveland Clinic Journal of Medicine, 71*(11), 890-896.

Inouye, S., et al. (1999). A multicomponent intervention to prevent delirium in hospitalized older patients. *New England Journal of Medicine, 340*(9), 669-676.

Inouye, S., et al. (1990). Clarifying confusion: The Confusion Assessment Method. *Annals of Internal Medicine, 13*(12), 941-948.

Johnson, J. (1990). Delirium in the elderly. *Emergency Clinics of North America,* 8(2), 255-264.

Marcantonio, E., et al. (2003). Delirium symptoms in post-acute care: Prevalent, persistent, and associated with poor functional recovery. *Journal of the American Geriatrics Society, 51*(1), 4-9.

DEMENTIA

ICD-9: 331 (ALZHEIMER'S DISEASE); 290.0 (SENILE DEMENTIA); 290.40 (VASCULAR DEMENTIA)

Dementia is a progressive, permanent deterioration of intellectual function and cognitive skills that leads to a diminished ability to perform activities of daily living. It is characterized by the gradual onset and progressive decline of cognitive function, manifested by memory impairment and at least one of the following: aphasia (language disturbance), apraxia (impaired ability to carry out purposeful movements despite intact motor function), agnosia (failure to recognize or identify objects despite intact sensory function), or a disturbance in executive functioning. These deficits cannot be related to other psychiatric, neurologic, or systemic diseases. There are a number of dementia syndromes, including Alzheimer's disease (AD), vascular syndromes, Parkinson's disease (including Lewy body dementia), frontal lobe (Pick's disease), and potentially treatable causes (normal-pressure hydrocephalus, vitamin deficiencies). Clinical presentation, including onset, course, and symptoms, may vary according to the type of dementia; many individuals may have mixed features of more than one dementia syndrome. An evaluation for dementia is important to:

- Establish cause and type.
- Identify treatable concurrent medical disease.
- Guide appropriate treatment and long-term planning.
- Facilitate education and counseling of family members.
- Provide genetic advice when appropriate.
- Identify pertinent psychologic stressors and family concerns.
- Determine prognosis.

Agitation, aggression, and psychosis are some of the more common behaviors noted with dementia. *Sundowning* is a term used to describe the increased agitation and restlessness often observed during the late afternoon or evening hours. Delusions and hallucinations are the psychotic behavioral symptoms demented patients may experience. Antipsychotic medications are sometimes used to control these symptoms but are not necessarily indicated.

Sleep disorders are also prevalent in patients with dementia. The type of disorder can differ depending on the particular dementia. Initial management strategies should consist of nonpharmacologic interventions, but medication may be necessary.

Risk Factors

- Age
- Family history: in AD, a first-degree relative
- ApoE4 allele for AD
- For vascular dementias: a history of stroke, TIAs, hypertension (HTN), coronary artery disease (CAD), peripheral vascular disease (PVD), and/or hypercholesterolemia
- Diabetes
- History of head trauma
- Lack of educational opportunities

History

Dementia is frequently unrecognized or misdiagnosed in its early stages. Often delays in diagnosis are due to preconceptions regarding symptoms: family members or patients may attribute changes to normal aging. Patients may also present with a known neurologic disorder and appear to be cognitively declining. An acute change in mental status with or without a known predisposing disorder is also common. For example, patients with no previous history of cognitive impairment who develop delirium during hospitalization for illness or surgery may be demonstrating an unmasking of a previously unrecognized dementia. In general, a complete history is key to differentiating acute versus chronic cognitive conditions. Pertinent information includes:

- Time of onset of symptoms and pattern of progression. This information is usually obtained from family members or caregivers who can provide key details regarding changes in behavior, as well as deficits in the patient's judgment, ability to learn and retain information, handle complex tasks, and reason.
- Careful review of any history of neurologic or cardiovascular disease
- Family history of any type of dementia, particularly in first-degree relatives
- History of head injury or trauma
- History of seizures
- Alcohol and substance use: common in the elderly
- Medication review, including prescription drugs, herbals, and OTC medications
- History of depression, mood disorders, psychiatric conditions, or mental retardation (e.g., Down syndrome)

- Recent surgery or medical illness
- Social history, including recent events, losses, or transitions

Physical Examination

The goal of the physical examination is to identify acute disorders or exacerbations of chronic conditions that may be contributing and to exclude focal neurologic findings. The Mini Mental State Examination (MMSE) (see Diagnostics) is useful in determining cognitive impairment. Other possible findings include:

- General appearance: restlessness, agitation, passive demeanor, poor hygiene, or blunted affect
- Vital signs: presence of fever, hypertension, or hypoxia
- Cardiovascular: elevated blood pressure (BP), carotid bruits, or murmurs
- Neurologic examination: MMSE, cranial nerve deficits, impairment in speech, gait abnormality, limb weakness, motor or sensory impairments, tremor, deficits in vision or hearing, or abnormal deep tendon reflexes (DTRs)

Differential Diagnosis

Delirium
Refer to p. 159 in this chapter.

Depression
See Depression in Chapter 13 for more information.

Mild Cognitive Impairment
Mild cognitive impairment (MCI) is thought to be a transitional state between normal aging and AD. Patients primarily have memory impairment without significant deficits in other cognitive domains, intact activities of daily living (ADLs), and do not meet the criteria for dementia. Because it is believed that these patients may progress to AD at a rate of 10% to 15% a year, MCI is considered a risk factor for AD, and these patients need close follow-up with early intervention, including pharmacotherapy.

Dementia Syndromes
Dementia syndromes include Alzheimer's disease, vascular dementia (post-stroke dementia, vascular lesions [infarcts]), Parkinson's disease with dementia, Lewy body dementia, progressive supranuclear palsy, and front temporal dementia (temporal and frontal atrophy associated with Pick's disease and other non-Alzheimer's dementia). Potentially reversible dementias include normal pressure hydrocephalus, medication- or substance-induced dementia, metabolic disorders (electrolyte, thyroid, hepatic, or renal dysfunction; vitamin B_{12} deficiency), and central nervous system disorders (subdural hematoma, meningitis).

Diagnostics

There is no single diagnostic test that is specific for dementia. Rather, the diagnosis of dementia is one of exclusion. The following diagnostics, if indicated, are suggested to rule out reversible illness and aid in diagnosis.

Laboratory Evaluation
- CBC/diff: to determine presence of acute illness or infection
- Serum glucose, electrolytes, BUN, and creatinine: to evaluate for electrolyte imbalance, dehydration, and renal dysfunction
- LFTs: to assess for hepatic dysfunction
- TSH: to exclude hypothyroidism
- B_{12} and folate: to assess for reversible causes
- Rapid plasma reagin (RPR): to exclude syphilis
- Therapeutic drug levels: if indicated

Other Diagnostics
- Neuroimaging: a non-contrast head CT or MRI to rule out structural lesions or acute process
- Mood assessment: Geriatric Depression Scale (GDS) (available at *www.hartfordign.org*)
- Functional assessment: Katz ADL (available at *www.hartfordign.org*) or Get Up and Go Test (*www.fpnotebook.com/GER4.htm*)
- Neuropsychologic testing to differentiate between:
  - Mild cognitive impairment and dementia
  - Dementia and depression
  - Dementia and focal syndromes of cognitive impairment (amnesia, aphasia, agnosia)
- Hachinski Ischemic scale (Table 8-2) if vascular dementia suspected:
  - Points are given for each feature that is present
  - Total score < 4 is consistent with primary dementia
  - Score of 4 to 7 is indeterminate
  - Score > 7 is consistent with vascular dementia
- Mental status assessment: essential for developing a multidimensional clinical picture, provides a baseline for monitoring the patient's course over time, and documents the presence of multiple cognitive deficits; there are many instruments available, but the Folstein MMSE is the most commonly used; MMSE scores range on a scale of 0 to 30, with lower scores representing increased impairment and decreased ability to perform ADLs; in general, scores less than 24 indicate impairment, but age and education level can influence scoring.

Staging of Dementia
Early stage (MMSE 22-28)
- Memory loss
- Time and spatial disorientation

TABLE 8-2 Modified Hachinski Score

Feature	Score
Abrupt onset of symptoms	2
Stepwise deterioration	1
Fluctuating course	2
Nocturnal confusion	1
Preservation of personality	1
Depression	1
Somatic complaints	1
Emotional liability	1
History or presence of hypertension	1
History of stroke	2
Evidence of atherosclerosis	1
Focal neurologic symptoms	2
Focal neurologic signs	2

From Rosen, W., et al. (1980). Pathological verification of ischemic score in differentiation of dementias. *Annals of Neurology, 7*(5),486-488.

- Poor judgment
- Personality changes
- Withdrawal or depression
- Perceptual disturbances

Mid-stage (MMSE 10-21)
- Recent and remote memory worsens
- Increased aphasia
- Apraxia
- Disorientation to place and time
- Restlessness or pacing
- Loss of impulse control

Late stage (MMSE ≤9)
- Incontinence
- Loss of motor skills or rigidity
- Decreased appetite and dysphagia
- Agnosia or apraxia
- Impaired communication
- Inability to recognize self

Treatment Plan

It is important to correctly diagnose the type of dementia to appropriately guide management. General treatment principles should include:
- Treatment or elimination of all correctable factors that impair cognition to improve daily functioning and delay disability

- Optimal treatment of hypertension, diabetes, and hyperlipidemia
- Treatment of depression, even if patient does not meet criteria for major depression
- Encouraging regular exercise and continued mental activities
- Encouraging the patient to appoint a healthcare proxy and write advanced directives
- Supporting caregivers
- Targeting most problematic behavior to promote patient comfort and staff/caregiver safety.

Cognitive Symptoms

Nonpharmacologic interventions for cognitive symptoms includes visual cues to identify self and room, reminiscing, memory books, and photographs.

Pharmacologic interventions include the following:

- Vitamin E: although previous studies suggested doses up to 1200 IU BID may be helpful, a recent study showed no benefit in treating dementia.
- Cholinesterase inhibitors: for use in mild to moderate stages of dementia; may be used in Alzheimer's, vascular, and Lewy Body dementias; no clear guidelines as to the duration of therapy, but these medications are generally discontinued in advanced stages of disease; choice is primarily based on provider experience, costs, and side-effect profile; patients should be monitored on a regular basis to ascertain treatment response, behavior, mood, and illness progression
    - Aricept (donepezil): start with 5 mg and reevaluate after 6 weeks; may increase to therapeutic dose of 10 mg daily if tolerated; best if given at bedtime, *or*
    - Exelon (rivastigmine): start at 1.5 mg PO daily and increase every 2 weeks by 1.5 mg to a maximum of 6 to 12 mg/day; available in liquid form; gastrointestinal side effects may be lessened if given with meals, *or*
    - Reminyl (galantamine): start with 4 mg PO BID and increase by 4 mg BID every 4 weeks to 12 mg (if tolerated)
- N-methyl-D-aspartate (NMDA) receptor agonist: a disease modifier used in moderate to severe dementia
    - Namenda (Memantine HCl): start with 5 mg/day and increase by 5 mg every week to a maximum of 20 mg BID; there may be increased benefit when used in combination with donepezil

Behavioral Symptoms

Nonpharmacologic interventions for behavioral symptoms include the following:

- Evaluate for delirium.
- Identify and treat precipitants, and discontinue or change offending medications.
- Ensure patient has eyeglasses and functional hearing aids.
- Provide daytime stimulation or distraction when indicated.
- Monitor amount of sensory stimulation.
- Maximize routine, structure environment, and provide consistency in caregivers.

- Maintain adequate levels of daytime light and consider late afternoon bright light exposure.
- Discourage stimulants and smoking near bedtime.
- Improve sleep hygiene with a consistent bedtime routine and removal of environmental factors that keep the patient awake.
- Avoid restraints and provide one-on-one supervision when indicated.
- Establish a regular medication dosage regimen for disturbing behavior if indicated.
- Avoid prn hypnotics, benzodiazepines, and antihistamines.

Pharmacologic interventions are indicated when nonpharmacologic interventions fail to work. They should be used when the psychotic symptoms are disturbing for the patient or when the patient, family, or caregiver situation is unsafe.

For agitation/aggression

- Trazodone (Desyrel): start at 25 mg PO at the hour of sleep, titrating up to 50 to 100 mg BID
- If agitation is related to an unrecognized depression, selective serotonin reuptake inhibitors (SSRIs) are usually indicated. Tricyclics, fluoxetine (Prozac), and paroxetine (Paxil) should be avoided in patients with dementia. SSRIs to consider include:
  - Sertraline (Zoloft): start at 25 mg PO every morning, titrating up to 100 to 150 mg/day if tolerated, *or*
  - Citalopram (Celexa): start with 10 mg PO every morning, titrating up to 20 mg/day if tolerated, *or*
  - Escitalopram (Lexapro): Start with 5 mg PO every morning, titrating up to 10 mg/day, *or*
  - Venlafaxine (Effexor): a serotonin norepinephrine reuptake inhibitor indicated for apathetic depression in the elderly; start at 37.5 mg PO every morning, titrating up to 150 mg/day if tolerated
- Antiepileptic medications are also used for agitated dementias, but there has been limited research to prove efficacy.
- Lorazepam (Ativan) is indicated in some situations for acute management, but it must be used cautiously because benzodiazepines can cause increased agitation or altered mental status.

For psychotic behaviors

- Olanzapine (Zyprexa)*: start at 2.5 mg/day PO, up to a maximum of 5 mg BID, *or*
- Quetiapine (Seroquel)*: start at 25 mg PO at the hour of sleep, up to a maximum of 75 mg/day, *or*
- Risperidone (Risperdal)*: start at 0.25 mg at the hour of sleep, up to a maximum of 1 to 1.5 mg/day; available in oral solution, *or*

---

* For psychotic behaviors, olanzapine, quetiapine, and risperidone are used in the treatment of dementia, but they are approved only for the treatment of schizophrenia and may be associated with serious side effects.

- Haloperidol (Haldol): start at 0.25 mg PO daily or BID, titrating slowly to maximum 1 to 2 mg BID; available in IM form
- Routinely monitor patient for extrapyramidal symptoms and attempt dose reduction of neuroleptics when appropriate.

For sleep disorders
- Trazadone (Desyrel): start at 25 mg PO at the hour of sleep, up to a maximum daily dose of 150 mg in the elderly, *or*
- Mirtazipine (Remeron): start at 75 mg PO at the hour of sleep, up to a maximum daily dose of 45 mg

Consultation/Hospitalization

Psychiatric hospitalization is sometimes indicated for behavioral disturbances, particularly if the patient is a danger to self or staff and has not responded to the usual treatment modalities. Consultation with neurologist and/or psychiatric provider is indicated when:
- The patient has symptoms consistent with MCI.
- The dementia presentation is atypical or unclear.
- The neurologic symptoms need further evaluation.
- Behavioral disturbances do not respond to standard treatment.
- The patient is a danger to self or staff.
- The patient develops tardive dyskinesia, involuntary movements, tremors, rigidity, body restlessness (akathisia), or neuroleptic malignant syndrome (fever, rigidity, labile blood pressure, or autonomic disturbances).
- For patients with end-stage disease, consult hospice for evaluation.

Education for Nursing Home/Rehabilitation Staff

- Teach supportive measures and maintain good patient care.
- Promote safety measures to avoid falls.
- Encourage exercise and activity to maximize function and to promote sleep.
- Teach signs/symptoms of early presentation of functional, physical, or mental status changes.
- Educate staff concerning the stressor of institutionalization in the elderly patient.
- Educate staff concerning behavior and agitation management, and refer to staff education or psychiatric provider if additional training/resources are needed.
- Review aspiration precautions.
- Educate staff concerning the need for one-on-one observation to avoid physical restraints.
- Educate staff concerning signs of EPS (tremors, rigidity, involuntary movements, or restlessness associated with some neurologic disorders and antipsychotic medications), as well as medication oversedation.

- Utilize resources available at the University of Iowa Geriatric Nursing Intervention Research Center (*www.nursing.uiowa.edu/centers/gnirc/protocols.htm*) and through the John A. Hartford Foundation Institute for Geriatric Nursing (*http://www.hartfordign.org/*).

Patient/Family Education

- Maintain ongoing discussion as to treatment preferences.
- Refer to social worker or community resources for support.
- Refer to Alzheimer's Association (*http://www.alz.org/*).

Bibliography

American Psychiatric Association. (1997). Practice guideline for the treatment of Alzheimer's disease and other dementias of later life. *American Journal of Psychiatry*, *154*(5; suppl), 1-39.

Beers, M., & Berkow, R. (Eds.) (2000). *The Merck manual of geriatrics*. Whitehouse Station, NJ: Merck.

Folstein, M., et al. (1975). Mini-mental state—A practical method for grading cognitive state of patients for the clinician. *Journal of Psychiatric Research*, *12*, 189-198.

Grundman, M., et al. (2004). Mild cognitive impairment can be distinguished from Alzheimer disease and normal aging for clinical trials. *Archives of Neurology*, *61*(1), 59-66.

Katz, I. (1998). Diagnosis and treatment of depression in patients with Alzheimer's disease and other dementias. *Journal of Clinical Psychiatry*, *59*(9; suppl), 38-44.

Lanctot, K., et al. Diagnosis and treatment of depression in patients with Alzheimer's disease and other dementias. *Canadian Medical Association Journal*, *169*(6), 557-64, 2004.

Peterson, R.C., et al. (2005). Vitamin E and donepezil for the treatment of mild cognitive impairment. *www.nejm.org*. Accessed May 1, 2005.

Small, G., et al. (1997). Diagnosis and treatment of Alzheimer disease and related disorders: Consensus statement of the American Association for Geriatric Psychiatry, the Alzheimer's Association, and the American Geriatrics Society. *Journal of the American Medical Association*, *278*(16), 1363-1371.

Tariot, P., et al. (2004). Memantine treatment in patients with moderate to severe Alzheimer disease already receiving Donepezil: A randomized clinical trial. *Journal of the American Medical Association*, *291*(3), 317-324.

CHAPTER 9

Endocrine and Metabolic Disorders

HYPOGLYCEMIA

ICD-9: 251.2

Hypoglycemia is a clinical syndrome with diverse causes. The low glucose concentration associated with hypoglycemia leads to symptoms of sympathoadrenal activation and neuroglycopenia. The blood sugar is less than 50 (normal fasting glucose is 70 to 100); however, patients with diabetes may experience hypoglycemia at different ranges. Usually, as blood glucose declines, hormonal counter-regulatory responses occur, well before the person is symptomatic. When plasma glucose falls below 80, insulin secretion decreases in the normal person. This drop in glucose and in insulin results in the breakdown of fat and protein stores to assist the liver in gluconeogenesis. When the glucose concentrations fall below 65 to 70, glucoreceptors in the hypothalamus respond by causing the release of glucagons and epinephrine. Growth hormone secretion increases when plasma glucose concentration falls below 60 to 65; cortisol is increased when the plasma glucose concentration falls below 60.

Hypoglycemia can occur in those with or without diabetes. Hypoglycemia is increased in patients with type 1 diabetes mellitus because of impairment in the normal counter-regulatory response in addition to the emphasis on tight glycemic control. Hypoglycemia is less common in type 2 diabetes, but does occur in some patients, particularly those taking sulfonylureas. Disrupted sleep may be a symptom of nocturnal hypoglycemia.

It is important to identify patients at risk for hypoglycemia and correlate symptoms with the blood glucose to validate the diagnosis. Closer monitoring is required for those with communication and cognitive deficits because these patients do not or cannot report early signs of hypoglycemia.

Healthcare providers need to know how to manage both the alert patient with hypoglycemia and the unresponsive patient with hypoglycemia. Hypoglycemia should be avoided if at all possible, as even a few minutes of serious hypoglycemia can be harmful. Management of hypoglycemia is critical for those in long-term care facilities. Patients with hypoglycemia can quickly progress to unresponsiveness and death if not treated at the earliest sign.

Risk Factors

- Intensive insulin therapy in type I diabetes mellitus: counter-regulatory hormone response is impaired
- Unstable diabetes mellitus
- Neurologic deficits: inability to recognize symptoms associated with decreasing serum glucose
- Inconsistent caloric intake, delayed meal consumption, or prolonged fast
- Exercise without attention to glucose level
- Previous episodes of severe hypoglycemia: a predictor of future episodes
- Ethanol (ETOH): inhibits gluconeogenesis in the liver
- Prolonged nausea and vomiting
- Post-gastrectomy
- Pancreatic disease, if glucagons producing cells are affected
- Acute illness: alters the body's insulin needs
- Nonselective β-blockers: reduce the effectiveness of the counter-regulatory response of epinephrine; can mask the early warning symptoms of hypoglycemia and prolong the recovery from hypoglycemia
- Angiotensin-converting enzyme (ACE) inhibitors: increase insulin sensitivity and glucose disposal

History

It is important to obtain a complete history regarding previous episodes of hypoglycemia, treatment, and response. A complete symptom analysis will detect specific times of hypoglycemia and its relation to food and medications.

Sympathoadrenal activation occurs first as plasma glucose falls below 70, and the following symptoms are possible:

- Sweating
- Anxiety
- Palpitations
- Hunger
- Tremor
- Nausea

- Tachycardia
- Sensation of warmth

Neuroglycopenic symptoms (listed next) are noted as plasma glucose drops below 50:

- Fatigue
- Headache
- Visual disturbances
- Drowsiness
- Difficulty speaking
- Dizziness
- Inability to concentrate
- Abnormal behavior
- Memory loss
- Confusion
- Loss of consciousness
- Seizures

A complete medical history is important to elicit. Medical issues associated with hypoglycemia include:

- Renal disease: particularly if on dialysis with decreased insulin clearance
- Psychiatric problems: possible increased incidence of diabetes related to psychiatric conditions and medications
- Heart failure with liver engorgement
- Leukemia: large numbers of white blood cells will consume glucose
- Severe hemolytic disease: nucleated blood cells consume glucose
- Medications associated with hypoglycemia include:
  - Steroids
  - Tylenol
  - Quinine
  - Pentamidine
  - Propoxyphene
  - Salicylate
  - Monoamine oxidase (MAO) inhibitors
  - Sulfa
  - Insulin
  - Allopurinol
  - Hypoglycemics: insulin and some oral agents
  - ACE inhibitors
  - β-blockers

Physical Examination

Common positive physical findings include:

- Constitutional: pale, diaphoretic, irritable, or change in mental status
- Vital signs: tachycardia

- Neurologic: tremor, slurred speech, decreased coordination and level of consciousness, or seizures

Differential Diagnosis

The hypoglycemia may be mild, moderate, or severe (Box 9-1). Once the hypoglycemia has been identified and expeditiously treated, the underlying precipitant must be identified. Potential causes are as follows:

- Insulinoma: fasting hypoglycemia, occasional postprandial symptoms secondary to high insulin levels
- Over-exercise
- Adrenal insufficiency
- Alcohol
- Non–islet cell tumor of pancreas: some tumors produce insulin-like growth factor 2
- Liver disease: hepatitis, cirrhosis, metastatic cancer, primary liver failure, and liver cancer
- Renal failure
- Sepsis
- Chronic CHF with liver engorgement
- Prolonged fast; delayed or missed meals
- Error in insulin dose
- False reading: related to blood sampling processing problems
- Leukemia
- Hemolytic diseases
- Recurrent hypoglycemia: occurs within 24 hours of first episode and is related to impaired counter-regulatory response
- Medications associated with hypoglycemia

BOX 9-1   Classifications of Hypoglycemia

Mild hypoglycemia: hunger, weakness, tremulousness, diaphoresis, pallor, tachycardia, paresthesias, difficulty concentrating, and irritability without change in mental state; individual can self treat.

Moderate hypoglycemia: impaired central nervous system functioning evidenced by decreased thinking, increased emotion (e.g., anger, irritability), inability to complete tasks, and some mental status changes; individual may or may not be able to self treat.

Severe hypoglycemia: confusion, drowsiness, progression to unconsciousness, and impaired neurologic function; episode is undetected by individual or detected so late that someone else needs to inject glucagons or IV glucose.

Diagnostics

To diagnose hypoglycemia, an immediate finger-stick to confirm glucose level is necessary. Once the patient has responded to intramuscular (IM) glucagon or ingestion of glucose, the evaluation can proceed to determine the underlying precipitant. Appropriate diagnostics include:
- Complete blood count with differential (CBC/diff): to exclude blood dyscrasia or sepsis
- Serum electrolytes
- Hemoglobin (Hb)A1c*
- Drug toxicology*
- Liver function tests (LFTs)*
- Thyroid-stimulating hormone (TSH): assess for thyroid abnormality*
- If diagnosis is elusive, patient may need referral for further evaluation of insulin and hormone levels

Treatment Plan

Treatment is indicated regardless of the severity of the hypoglycemia. Caution should be exercised to avoid giving too much glucose, causing hyperglycemia.

Mild Hypoglycemia
- Consume 15 g of simple-acting carbohydrate (CHO) (e.g., glucose gel, 4 oz of orange juice) by mouth.
- Stop activity.
- Retest blood glucose in 10 to 15 minutes. If blood glucose is < 60mg/dL, give an additional 10 to 15 g (CHO) by mouth.
- In 30 minutes, patient should eat snack or meal consisting of protein and CHO.

Moderate Hypoglycemia
- Consume 15 to 30 g of simple-acting CHO.
- Follow the same protocol as for mild hypoglycemia.

Severe Hypoglycemia
- If the patient can swallow, give 30 to 45 g of simple-acting CHO. If patient is unresponsive, give 0.5 to 1 mg of glucagon subcutaneously (SC) or IM. Patient should improve/recover consciousness in 10 to 15 minutes, although he or she may have nausea 60 to 90 minutes later.
- Unresponsive patients may also be treated with 25 to 50 g 50% glucose intravenous (IV). If no improvement in 15 minutes, and blood glucose is still low, repeat dose of 50 mL 50% glucose IV.

*If indicated.

- Complete cognitive recovery may lag 30 to 45 minutes behind normoglycemia.
- Repeat blood glucose every 1 to 2 hours or more often if mental status changes continue.
- Once blood glucose is normal and eating is at baseline, patient may resume previous regimen. Consider short-term use of short-acting insulin before meals for 24 to 48 hours to prevent rebound hypoglycemia.
- If applicable, consider changing patient's regimen to newer insulin analog (i.e., Lantus).
- In patients who have had previous episodes of severe hypoglycemia, the HbA1c goal may need to be raised.
- During acute illness, if patient is nothing-by-mouth (NPO) for surgery or a diagnostic procedure, or when food intake is diminished or stopped, the dose of long-acting insulin should be adjusted to prevent hypoglycemia. An alternative plan is to change to a sliding scale with regular insulin regimen for the short term.

Consultation/Hospitalization

- Evaluation in the emergency department/hospital is indicated for patients with uncontrolled hypoglycemia.
- Consider endocrinology evaluation if episodes are frequent or diagnosis unclear.
- Referral to nutritionist/diabetes educator for teaching program
- Consider referral to social worker or psychiatrist if compliance with the regimen or abuse of drugs or alcohol is a concern.

Complications

- Transient cognitive deficits
- Falls
- Hospitalization
- Accidents
- Emotional trauma related to fear of hypoglycemia
- Stroke, myocardial infarction, arrhythmias, or other cardiac event
- Convulsions
- Death

Education for Nursing Home/Rehabilitation Staff

- Review signs and symptoms of hypoglycemia with staff.
- Explain the importance of routinely calibrating blood glucose device.
- Reiterate the value of routinely checking the expiration date on glucagon.
- Stress the importance of notifying healthcare provider if patient exhibits mental status changes.
- Discuss importance of correctly documenting/reporting meal consumption.

- Notify healthcare provider of loss of appetite or diminished appetite, especially in diabetic patients.
- Explain to nurses the importance of giving the patient specific glucose as directed, rather than 4 oz of orange juice with multiple sugar packets added.

Patient/Family Education

- Discuss the value of keeping a record of blood sugars.
- Educate patient and family members about the signs and symptoms of hypoglycemia.
- Support those patients who fear hypoglycemia and have a tendency to overeat to maintain normal serum glucose.
- Educate those patients who drink alcohol: alcohol consumption should be limited, consumed slowly, and taken with food. Blood glucose should be checked frequently when drinking alcohol.
- Educate patients and family about over-the-counter cough syrups that contain alcohol.
- Stress the importance of always carrying glucose tablets or gel, hard candy, and/or sweetened fruit juice. Explain that 15 to 30 gm CHO is usually sufficient to raise serum glucose to safe levels without inducing hyperglycemia.
- Explain the importance of consuming a long-acting CHO or protein after an episode of hypoglycemia to prevent recurrent episode.
- Review use of diabetic equipment with patient/family until they are comfortable with use.
- Review diabetic regimen with patient/family.

Bibliography

Buttaro, T.M., et al. (2003). *Primary care: A collaborative practice* (2nd ed). St. Louis: Mosby.

McCullogh, D.K. (2004). Management of hypoglycemia during treatment of diabetes mellitus. *www.uptodate.com*. Accessed April 28, 2004.

Service, J.J. (2004). Diagnostic approach to hypoglycemia. *www.uptodate.com*. Accessed March 31, 2004.

Service, J.J. (2004). Overview of hypoglycemia disorders. *www.uptodate.com*. Accessed April 28, 2004.

HYPERGLYCEMIA

ICD-9: 790.6

New-onset diabetes mellitus can occur in hospitalized patients as well as in rehabilitation or long-term care settings. The hyperglycemia may be precipitated by an infection, medication, myocardial infarction, or other stressor. Hyperglycemia develops because the beta cells of the pancreas are dysfunctional. The hyperglycemia related to type 1 diabetes mellitus is caused by beta-cell failure and the subsequent lack of insulin production. The hyperglycemia in type 2 diabetes mellitus is associated with the pancreas' inability to produce enough insulin and the body's inability to use insulin efficiently (insulin resistance).

Diabetic ketoacidosis, a profound hyperglycemia associated with osmotic diuresis, dehydration, and acidosis, usually occurs in patients with type 1 diabetes mellitus. It can also occur under certain circumstances in patients with type 2 diabetes mellitus. Nonketotic hyperglycemia hyperosmolar syndrome affects patients with type 2 diabetes mellitus and is often related to pneumonia or other infection, or a medication. In some patients, the two syndromes may overlap.

Whatever the cause, hyperglycemia may have immediate life-threatening as well as long-term complications. During marked hyperglycemia, immune and neutrophil functions are impaired. Serious hyperglycemia should be avoided. In a long-term care facility, the healthcare provider must be able to manage the acute emergency of hyperglycemia in addition to the day-to-day hyperglycemia in a newly diagnosed or longstanding diabetic patient.

Risk Factors

- Metabolic syndrome: obesity, high triglycerides (> 250), low high-density lipoprotein (HDL) (< 35), and hypertension (> 120/80) significant for type 2 diabetes mellitus
- Genetic predisposition: in type 2 diabetes mellitus, beta-cell dysfunction may be an inherited trait
- Older age: > 45 years old; beta-cell function diminishes
- Obesity: body mass index (BMI) > 25 (kg/m^2) is an insulin-resistant state
- High caloric, high-fat diet
- Enteric feedings
- Ethnicity: American Indians, blacks, Hispanic Americans, Asian Americans, and Pacific Islanders at increased risk for developing hyperglycemia or type 2 diabetes
- Tumors that secrete glucagons or somatostatin
- ETOH
- Pancreatic disease or tumor: usually requires insulin for management
- Endocrinopathies: Cushing's syndrome, acromegaly, pheochromocytoma (epinephrine, glucagons, cortisol, and growth hormone antagonize the action of insulin in a counter-regulatory response to low blood sugar), hyperthyroidism, polycystic ovary syndrome (abnormalities in insulin receptors)
- Stress, sepsis, trauma, and acute illness: increased secretion of counter-regulatory hormone; insulin absorption can be erratic secondary to changes in blood flow to subcutaneous tissue during acute illness.
- Gestational diabetes mellitus: 40% of women with a history of gestational diabetes mellitus will develop type 2 diabetes mellitus 10 to 20 years later.
- Birth of a child weighing more than 9 lbs
- Impaired renal function

- Physical inactivity
- Chronic hepatitis C
- Hereditary hemachromatosis: diabetes mellitus present in 50% of patients
- Noncompliance: secondary to a complicated regimen, finances, knowledge deficit, or self-care deficit for diabetic regimen

History

It is important to recognize the signs and symptoms of hyperglycemia in order to respond promptly. The history should establish the cause of the hyperglycemia as well as allergies, medications, remote history of diabetes, symptoms (including time of onset), and complications. Classic symptoms of hyperglycemia include polyuria (glucose spills into urine when serum glucose is approximately 180 mg/dl), polydipsia, and polyphagia. A sudden onset (usually within 24 hours) associated with history of infection, vomiting, change in mental status, and weakness may be related to diabetic ketoacidosis (DKA). A more prolonged 3-day to 3-week history of malaise, polydipsia, and polyuria is more likely to be indicative of nonketotic hyperglycemic hyperosmolar syndrome. Other pertinent considerations include:

- Nausea, vomiting, weakness, mental status changes, and/or symptoms of an infection or dehydration usually readily apparent in DKA or nonketotic hyperglycemic hyperosmolar syndrome
- Blurred vision: when blood glucose is higher than 180, water is drawn into the lens secondary to the hyperosmolar gradient
- Weight loss
- Fatigue
- Paresthesias

Important medical history includes:
- Wounds that do not heal
- Yeast infections
- Recent infection or surgery
- ETOH ingestion
- Medications associated with hyperglycemia
  - Protease inhibitors
  - Cyclosporin
  - Calcium channel blockers
  - Rifampin
  - Nicotinic acid
  - Opiates
  - Glucocorticoids
  - Indomethacin
  - Pentamidine
  - Phenytoin
  - Thyroxine
  - Estrogen
  - Hydrochlorothiazide

- β-blockers
- Furesemide
- Isoniazid (INH)
- Interferon
- Epinephrine
- Lithium

Physical Examination

Depending on the blood glucose level, the patient may present with varying levels of consciousness. If the patient is not in an emergent situation, a thorough physical examination should be completed, looking for signs of infection, myocardial infarction, or another precipitant. If the patient is less than alert, the examination may be brief: an Accucheck should be obtained, an appropriate dose of insulin should be given; and an acute-care facility evaluation should be considered.

Physical findings suggestive of hyperglycemia or its precipitants include:
- Fruity or acetone breath in DKA
- Vital signs
  - Temperature: may be elevated or below normal
  - Heart and respiratory rate: tachycardia and shallow respirations may indicate sepsis.
  - Blood pressure: hypotension and/or orthostatic changes suggest dehydration
- Skin: dry, if patient is dehydrated; observe for presence of skin infection.
- Head, eyes, ears, nose, and throat (HEENT): evaluate for dry membranes, signs of infection, and nuchal rigidity.
- Cardiovascular: tachycardia
- Lungs: deep, labored, panting breaths suggest Kussmaul breathing (associated with diabetic ketoacidosis or renal failure), and shallow respirations suggest nonketotic hyperglycemia hyperosmolar syndrome; cough, rales, bronchial breath sounds, egophony, and/or percussion dullness suggests pneumonia, a frequent precipitant of nonketotic hyperglycemic hyperosmolar syndrome.
- Abdomen/rectal: assess abdomen for distention, bowel sounds, or tenderness, and rectum for perirectal abscess.
- Neurologic: seizures or unresponsiveness possible; positive focal deficits usually present in DKA, but may also be present in nonketotic hyperglycemic hyperosmolar syndrome.

For stable patients with new-onset hyperglycemia, and annually for patients with type 1 and type 2 diabetes, a comprehensive evaluation is indicated. Typical findings when making a new diagnosis of hyperglycemia might include:
- Obesity: often associated with type 2 diabetes mellitus, whereas patients with type 1 diabetes mellitus are often leaner.

- Skin: inspect for altered skin integrity (irritation, ulcers) or infections, especially on feet, between toes, and in skin folds.
- HEENT
  - Eyes: assess fundoscopic changes associated with diabetes (e.g., retinopathy, vascular changes, nicking, bleeding).
  - Pharynx: inspect for dental and gum disease, infections, and lesions.
  - Neck: palpate for thyroid enlargement or nodularity, and auscultate for bruits.
- Cardiovascular/peripheral vascular: assess for extra heart sounds, murmurs, decreased pulses, bruits, and lower extremity edema.
- Abdomen/rectal: determine presence of aortic or renal bruits, hepatomegaly, tenderness, or rectal infection.
- Gynecology: inspect for vaginal discharge.
- Musculoskeletal: assess for structural deformities.
- Neurologic examination: decreased sensation, vibratory, proprioception, and two-point discrimination possible.

Differential Diagnosis

- Acute ketoacidosis: associated with elevated blood sugar > 200 mg/dL (may be as high as 800 mg/dL), high serum osmolality (usually > 330 mOsm), pH < 7.3, HCO_3 < 15 mEq/L, and elevated ketones
- Nonketotic hyperglycemia hyperosmolar syndrome: significant hyperglycemia (serum glucose > 600 mg/dL), serum osmolality > 320 mOsm, HCO_3 > 20 mEq/L, pH > 7.3, with minimal or no ketones or lipolysis; usually precipitated by dehydration
- Diabetes mellitus: fasting plasma glucose > 126 mg/dL, casual plasma glucose > 200 with symptoms
  - Type 1 diabetes mellitus: Although possibly an autoimmune disease, usually the cause is unknown. Patients with type 1 diabetes mellitus require insulin at all times, whether or not they are eating. Blood glucose levels tend to fluctuate more during the course of an acute illness or procedure. Insulin dose is usually lower than in type 2 diabetes mellitus because there is no insulin resistance. Patient is usually thin.
  - Type 2 diabetes mellitus: initially hypersecretion of insulin until beta cells burn out. Accelerated hepatic glucose production occurs secondary to insulin resistance in the liver.
    - Postprandial hyperglycemia: often seen in obese patients; associated with decreased insulin, stimulated glucose uptake in muscles, and overproduction of free fatty acids by fat cells.
- Impaired fasting glucose: glucose between 100 and 125 mg/dL
- Impaired glucose tolerance: after 2 hours, oral glucose tolerance sugar is 140 to 199 mg/dL

Diagnostics

Diagnostic testing is necessary to determine the extent of the hyperglycemia as well as evaluate for dehydration, ketones, acidosis, and infection. A urinalysis, urine for ketones, serum glucose, electrolytes, BUN, and creatinine are always indicated. Further diagnostic evaluation is dependent on the patient's history and physical findings.
- Immediate finger-stick glucose test
- If patient is acutely ill and/or unresponsive, hospitalization may be necessary. If the patient remains in the facility, consult physician, and obtain appropriate diagnostics.

Laboratory Evaluation
- Urine for ketones: present in DKA, but minimal or absent in nonketotic hyperglycemia hyperosmolar syndrome
- Serum glucose: may range from 300 to 800
- Serum electrolytes
    - A normal or lower-than-normal serum sodium may indicate pseudo-hyponatremia, particularly if hyperglycemia is present. The following formula may be used to determine the actual serum sodium level: serum Na + 1.6 (serum glucose) − 100 ÷ 100
    - Arterial blood gases, if indicated, to determine pH
    - Determine plasma osmolality and anion gap
        - Plasma osmolality: 2 (Na) + glucose/18 + blood urea nitrogen (BUN)/2.8
        - Anion gap: Na − (Cl + HCO_3)
    - Renal function: increased BUN and/or increased creatinine in dehydration
    - CBC: elevated white blood cells (WBCs) if there is infection
    - TSH: thyroid disorders may be associated with hyperglycemia
    - LFTs: increased with hepatitis
    - Amylase: high in acute pancreatitis
    - Consider urinalysis and culture.*
    - Consider blood cultures.*

Other Diagnostics
- Electrocardiogram (ECG): patients with a history of diabetes mellitus for more than 10 years duration or with type 2 diabetes have a high risk for silent myocardial infarction
- Consider chest radiograph.*
- If the patient is not acutely ill, assess for a precipitant or complications of diabetes mellitus.

*If indicated.

- HbA1c: determines glucose level during the previous 2 to 3 months
- Fasting lipid profile: high incidence of dyslipidemia with diabetes mellitus
- 24-hour urine for creatinine clearance, protein (normal urine protein 25 to 30 mg in 24 hours), and microalbumin (microalbuminuria 30 to 300 mg in 24 hours [normal < 30 mg/day])
- If indicated, serum insulin and C peptides to differentiate between type 1 and type 2 diabetes

Treatment Plan

Any patient with suspected hyperglycemia requires an immediate finger-stick blood glucose and assessment of fluid volume status.

- If the blood glucose is >300, immediately give regular insulin SC (10 units or 0.1 unit/kg of ideal body weight [IBW]).
- Consult physician regarding treatment and/or disposition. Many facilities have limited diagnostic capability and/or protocols regarding IV administration, which may limit the ability to manage the patient without an acute-care hospitalization.
- If the patient is able to take oral fluids, encourage fluid intake to prevent dehydration. It is sometimes possible to abort DKA by increasing fluid intake and treating the hyperglycemia.
- Intake and output (I&O) documentation.
- If the patient is unable to take oral fluids, estimate free-water deficits (see Chapter 10) and replace fluids. Fluid resuscitation must be individualized for each patient, as some patients require significant fluid resuscitation whereas others stabilize with 1 to 2 L of IV 0.9% normal saline (N/S). Patients with nonketotic hyperglycemia hyperosmolar syndrome may be critically dehydrated and may require even more aggressive fluid resuscitation. It is imperative to carefully monitor fluid resuscitation in elderly patients and in patients with a history of heart failure. A Foley catheter will aid in monitoring the patient's fluid status.
  - According to the Joslin Diabetes Center (Boston, MA), for hypotensive patients not in heart failure, infuse 1 L 0.9% N/S (15 to 20 mL/ kg/hour) over 30 to 60 minutes via a large-bore IV catheter. Then, depending on the patient's hemodynamic status, continue 0.9% N/S at 500 to 1000 mL/hour over the next 3 hours. Elderly patients or patients who are hemodynamically stable with adequate urinary output may require lowered IV fluid replacement (80 to 100 mL/hour). All patients must be carefully monitored for signs of fluid overload.
    - After 4 hours, consider changing the IV fluid to 0.45% N/S (depending on corrected serum sodium), continuing to monitor fluid status and serum glucose carefully. Some patients will continue to require 250 to 500 mL of IV fluid hourly. Total IV fluid requirements vary with each patient and can range from 1 to 2 L up to 6 L over 6 hours (Joslin Diabetes Center).

- Monitor blood glucose: when the blood glucose is < 250, change from IV 0.9% N/S or 0.45% N/S to D_5 ½ N/S
- If sodium is >150, use D_5 0.2%N/S
- Check serum electrolytes, magnesium, and calcium with initial diagnostics. Check serum electrolytes every 2 hours; check serum phosphate every 4 hours until patient is stable for a minimum of 4 hours.
- Replace potassium (K) when indicated, if patient is not anuric (Joslin Diabetes Center):
  - If serum K < 3.5, give 40 meq/L IV fluid
  - If serum K 3.5 to 4.5 give 20 meq/L IV fluid
  - If serum K 4.5 to 5.5 give 10 meq/L IV fluid
  - If serum K > 5.5, hold K, and recheck serum K every 2 hours
  - If phosphate is below normal, consider replacing serum K with potassium phosphate
- In DKA or nonketotic hyperglycemia hyperosmolar syndrome, an insulin drip may be required. The patient should first be rehydrated with 1 to 2 L 0.9% N/S, then, an IV insulin drip started with regular insulin at 0.1 units/kg/hour or 1 to 2 units/hour to provide basal level of insulin (Joslin Diabetes Center).
  - Check blood sugar hourly.
  - If blood sugar does not fall 10% or 50 mg/dL in the first hour, increase insulin drip by 1 unit/hour. May increase insulin drip 1 unit every 1 to 2 hours to maintain continued decrease in serum glucose of 50 mg/dL/hr.
  - When blood sugar reaches 250 to 300, the insulin drip should be decreased by 1 to 2 U/hr. Goal of serum glucose is 250 mg/dL until patient is hemodynamically stable; then 140 to 180 mg/dL.
  - Insulin drip can be discontinued when the patient is eating and stable. A dose of SC insulin can be given and the insulin drip discontinued an hour later (Joslin Diabetes Center).
- Consult with physician correcting serum bicarbonate if pH < 7. Bicarbonate therapy is not always recommended, as insulin therapy will usually increase the serum bicarbonate.
- Follow renal function and electrolytes closely.
- Antiemetic therapy is appropriate if necessary.
- Once the patient is stable hemodynamically, determine underlying precipitant. Stop any medications that could be implicated.
- Once the patient resumes eating well, the previous regimen should be reestablished. Evaluate diet, activity, signs of infection, and hypoglycemic agent.

For stable, asymptomatic patients with new diagnosis of type 2 diabetes mellitus or impaired glucose tolerance, recommendations include:
- Diet and exercise for 4 to 6 weeks to reach a glucose level of <100
  - Decrease caloric intake by 80 calories/day with low fat, high fiber diet.
  - If appropriate, increase activity by 1 km more per day. (Institutionalized elders also will benefit from increased exercise.)

- If HbA1c > 8.5 after 6 weeks of diet and exercise, start oral agent

Therapy for obese patients includes:

- Glucophage (metformin), 500 mg PO daily, may be an appropriate choice in patients < 80 years old with normal kidney and liver function. In elderly patients, the dose may be increased to 850 mg PO BID.
  - Creatinine must be < 1.4 in females and < 1.5 in males.
  - Contraindicated if history of CHF, alcohol abuse, or dehydration.
  - Monitor renal function.
  - Hold 48 hours before and after radiology studies with contrast dye (*www.guideline.gov*).
- Thiazolidines: Avandia (rosiglitazone), 2 mg PO once or twice daily or Actos (pioglitazone), 15 to 30 mg PO daily if used for monotherapy
  - Contraindicated if history CHF (class III, IV) or hepatic dysfunction (ALT > 2.5 times normal). Monitor ALT every 2 months and stop medication if ALT increases > 2.5 times normal.
  - Monitor renal function.

Therapy for non-obese patients includes:

- Sulfonylurea: Glucotrol XL (glipizide), 2.5 to 10 mg PO daily or BID or Diabeta (glyburide), 1.25 to 20 mg PO daily (usually in divided doses—AM and PM.
- Chlorpropamide and first-generation sulfonyureas should not be prescribed for elderly patients (*www.guidelines.gov*).

Therapy for postprandial hyperglycemia includes:

- Meglitinide: prandin (Repaglinide), 0.5 mg PO 30 minutes before meals. May slowly increase dose up to 2 mg PO 4 times a day (maximum dose 16 mg/day). Do not administer if a meal will be omitted. Use cautiously if there is renal or hepatic dysfunction.

Management long-term is based on the HbA1c. Combination multi-drug oral therapy and/or insulin therapy is indicated to manage continued hyperglycemia and prevent complications.

- Immunizations
  - Yearly influenza immunization unless contraindicated
  - Pneumovax immunization indicated for patients without previous history of immunization
  - Tetanus update every 5 to 10 years

Other considerations include:

- In type 1 diabetes mellitus, the total insulin daily dose should start at 0.4 to 0.8 units/kg/day based on ideal body weight.
- In type 2 diabetes mellitus, the total insulin daily dose should start at 0.5 units/kg/day based on ideal body weight.
- When ordering twice daily injections of insulin, order two thirds of the dose in the morning and one third of the dose in the evening. In the morning, the ratio of long-acting insulin to short-acting insulin is 2:1. In the evening it is 1:1.
- Consider new insulin analogues (glargine is long-acting, lispro is short-

acting) for fewer incidents of peaks in glucose level. Lispro dosing is equivalent to short-acting insulins but is absorbed more quickly, peaks within 30 to 90 minutes, and may be associated with improved glycemic control. Patients must eat within 15 minutes of administration to prevent hypoglycemia.

- Glargine, a new long-acting insulin analogue is usually given only at bedtime.
- Glargine cannot be mixed with short-acting insulin.

- When blood glucose levels are unstable in a patient with type 2 diabetes on an oral agent, try adding a single dose of long-acting insulin at bedtime to the oral agent. When insulin is used with an oral agent, consider 0.2 to 0.4 units/kg/day based on ideal body weight.
- Use sliding-scale regular insulin when a patient's dietary intake is unstable or the patient is acutely ill. Accuchecks are usually done before meals and at bedtime, with regular insulin given before meals to decrease postprandial hyperglycemia. Sliding scales should be individualized. However, a frequently used scale is:
  - Serum glucose (Accucheck) 0 to 200: no insulin is needed
  - 201 to 250: 2 units regular insulin subQ
  - 251 to 300: 4 units regular insulin subQ
  - 301 to 350: 6 units regular insulin subQ
  - 351 to 400: 8 units regular insulin subQ
  - > 401: 10 units regular insulin subQ
- Increase the frequency of blood glucose monitoring in acute illness.
- Schedule skin and foot examinations on a regular basis.
- Encourage regular exercise (walking if possible). If wheelchair bound, encourage patient to elevate legs periodically and to exercise toes, ankles, and feet.
- A patient with diabetes mellitus and hypertension, hyperlipidemia, or coronary artery disease is at risk for other cardiovascular risk factors and should be considered for a statin, ACE inhibitor (or angiotensin-receptor blocker [ARB] if ACE inhibitor is not tolerated), and aspirin, unless contraindicated.
  - Goal blood pressure for patients with diabetes is usually < 130/80. Patient must be routinely monitored for orthostatic changes associated with autonomic neuropathy. More than one antihypertensive is common practice for optimum blood-pressure control. Renal function should be monitored every 3 months, and patients on an ACE or ARB should have the serum potassium routinely monitored because hyperkalemia is a possible effect of therapy.
  - The LDL goal for patients with diabetes is < 100 mg/dL. For patients considered at very high risk (e.g., diabetes with other risk factors, such as cardiovascular disease, metabolic syndrome, and smoking), the LDL goal is < 70 mg/dL (*www.nih.gov*).

- Unless contraindicated, enteric-coated aspirin 81 mg PO daily is indicated for patients older than age 40 with diabetes (American Diabetes Association: *Standards of Care: Prevention and Management of Complications*). If the patient is aspirin allergic, discuss clopidrogrel therapy with physician.

Consultation/Hospitalization

- Hospitalization is indicated if the patient is unresponsive, hemodynamically unstable, unable to take or maintain adequate oral intake, or has comorbid medical or surgical problems, especially if blood glucose is > 400 or the facility is unable to provide IV therapy. If patient is not hospitalized, ongoing consultation with the physician is indicated. Hospitalization should be considered for patients with newly diagnosed type 1 diabetes.
- Patients with hyperglycemia are at risk for many complications. When the blood sugars are unstable, physician consultation is recommended.
- Consultation with a nutritionist is recommended to assist with dietary recommendations for a newly diagnosed diabetic, ongoing dietary education, and for patients on tube feedings with hyperglycemia.
- The diabetic educator, if available, may be helpful, especially when arranging discharge home.
- Consultation with vascular surgery (to assess vascular status), neurology, dermatology, ophthalmology (monitoring for diabetic retinopathy), podiatry (footcare), and nephrology may assist in managing the complicated needs of a diabetic patient.
- Consultation with the cardiologist is recommended for patients with diabetes and one cardiovascular risk factor.

Complications

- The complications of acute hyperglycemia are acute renal failure secondary to hypovolemia. In addition, a patient is at risk for dehydration, shock, and death.
- Potential treatment complications include fluid and electrolyte abnormalities, their associated sequelae, and the risk of hypoglycemia.
- There is an increased risk for postoperative infections in patients with higher blood glucose concentrations.
- The complications of diabetes mellitus include hypertension; cardiovascular, cerebrovascular, and peripheral vascular disease; retinopathy; nephropathy; neuropathy (sensory, motor, and autonomic); poor wound healing; amputations; and immune system problems.
- Patients with diabetes mellitus are at risk for a silent myocardial infarction.

Education for Nursing Home/Rehabilitation Staff

- Explain the importance of notifying the healthcare provider if the patient has signs or symptoms of acute illness, hypoglycemia or hyperglycemia, cognitive decline, blood glucose < 60 mg/dL, reduced oral intake for 2 or more days (or two consecutive meals with oral intake < 50%), or additional symptoms such as fever, hypotension, lethargy, confusion, abdominal pain, respiratory distress.
- The nursing staff should understand the necessity of reporting elevated serum glucose levels (2 or more blood glucose levels of > 250 mg/dL if new or accompanied by a change in condition or a blood glucose level > 300 during all or part of 3 consecutive days).
- Explain to the nursing staff the importance of regular blood pressure monitoring as well as the necessity of reporting sustained blood pressure measurements > 135/80.
- Discuss with nursing staff that weight loss, frequent infections, urinary frequency, nocturia or incontinence, skin ulcers, delayed wound healing, dental caries, or periodontal disease may signify undiagnosed diabetes mellitus.
- Explain to nursing staff the differences between lispro insulin (e.g., Humalog, Novolog) and regular Humulin insulin. Stress the importance of administering lispro insulin immediately before meals to prevent hypoglycemia (which may occur within 15 minutes of administration). Discuss the importance of preprandial and postprandial Accuchecks in patients receiving lispro insulin.
- Stress the importance of good oral care, good foot care with daily observation for skin breakdown, good skin and pressure area care, and the importance of hydration and daily exercise for all patients, but particularly for patients with diabetes mellitus.

Patient/Family Education

Diabetes education is individualized for each patient. For most patients and families, a basic understanding of the disease process, awareness of the signs of hypoglycemia and hyperglycemia, and the side effects of medications are indicated. Although not indicated for every patient, other educational considerations include:

- The value of daily exercise (at least 5 days per week) should be stressed, as even wheelchair-bound elders can benefit.
- Dietary recommendations are not advised for frail elderly patients (*www.guideline.gov*). However, usual dietary recommendations include the following:
  - Restrict fats to 35% or less of daily total calories.
  - Protein should be 10% to 20% of total calories.
  - Consume 20 to 30 g of fiber daily.

- Keep sodium intake to 2000 mg/day or less.
- Artificial sweeteners should be used.
- Cholesterol should not exceed more than 300 mg/day.
- The importance of adequate hydration with low sugar, nonalcoholic beverages should be stressed.
- Explain the appropriate medication regimen, including the importance of taking medications in relation to meals.
- Daily foot care and daily skin inspection for open areas.
- When appropriate, patients and families should be taught blood glucose monitoring, calibration of Accucheck machine, and glucose parameters (for notifying healthcare provider).
- Discuss the importance of personal hygiene, yearly eye examinations, and regular dental and podiatry care.
- Discuss importance of mouth care. Sustained hyperglycemia leads to prolonged oral infections, accelerated periodontal disease, and dry mouth.
- When indicated, discuss weight management measures.
- Encourage smoking cessation and alcohol avoidance.
- Discuss preventative safety measures (e.g., avoiding crossing legs, not using electric blankets or heating pads, not putting abrasive products on skin, no prolonged foot soaks).
- Educate both patients and families about the early signs of DKA as well as symptoms of hypoglycemia.
- Patients with diabetes should carry sugar or hard candy at all times to abort hypoglycemia.
- Explain the importance of wearing a medical alert bracelet.
- Explain the importance of avoiding foot soaks; wearing white, cotton socks without seams; and wearing appropriate (i.e., smooth linings, no foreign objects in shoes) footwear at all times. Patients should never go barefoot.
- Before discharge, patients and families should understand how to use a glucagon emergency kit and have one available at all times.

Bibliography

American Diabetes Association. (2002). Standards of medical care for patients with diabetes mellitus. *Diabetes Care, 25*(suppl 1), S33-S49.

American Medical Directors Association. (2004). Managing diabetes in long-term care settings. *http://amda.com/info/cpg/diabetes.htm*. Accessed June 5, 2004.

Joslin Diabetes Center. (2002). Guideline for management of hyperglycemia emergencies for adults. *http://joslin.org/education/library/guidelines*. Retrieved June 5, 2004.

McCullock, D.K. (2003). Definition and classification of diabetes mellitus. *www.uptodate.com*. Accessed June 1, 2004.

McCullock, D.K., & Sawin, C.T. (2004). Management of diabetes mellitus in the acute care setting. *www.uptodate.com*. Accessed June 1, 2004.

McDonald, K. (2003). Insulin therapy today: Focusing on the basal-bolus balance. *Advance for Nurse Practitioners, 11*(7), 40-44.

Mltzner, L. (2003). Selecting the best medication for type 2 diabetes. *The Clinical Advisor*, 6(7), 23-26.

Pandya, N. (2003). Diabetes management in long-term care. *Caring for the Ages*, 4(2), 21-24.

HYPOTHYROIDISM

ICD-9: 244.9

Hypothyroidism affects more women than men and is the most common thyroid disorder. Primary hypothyroidism is usually related to thyroid gland disease or destruction; secondary hypothyroidism is associated with a disorder of the pituitary gland that results in decreased thyroid stimulating hormone (thyrotropin) production. Regardless of the cause, the effects of hypothyroidism include fatigue, confusion, constipation, depression, paresthesias, impaired lipid metabolism, hypertension, musculoskeletal effects, and myxedema coma (advanced, untreated hypothyroidism). Unfortunately, in elderly patients, the symptoms associated with hypothyroidism can be misunderstood and attributed to aging. And, in this population, untreated hypothyroidism may have deleterious cardiac, neurologic, and psychiatric effects.

History

In elders, symptoms are frequently subtle or nonspecific, but even younger patients may be asymptomatic. Rarely, patients may complain of inability to concentrate or exhibit signs of depression or, in severe cases, slowed mentation, a sign of myxedema. More commonly, patients have concerns about fatigue; weight gain; constipation; cold sensitivity; dry skin; brittle hair; facial puffiness; muscle stiffness or aches; burning, tingling paresthesias in hands and fingers (carpal tunnel syndrome); or (in premenopausal women) irregular or heavy menses. Secondary hypothyroidism is suggested by complaints of headaches or visual disturbances. Past medical history, including recent upper respiratory infection, surgery, history of thyroid disease, or history of irradiation to the head and neck area, is significant and may explain the thyroid hormone deficiency. A through review of medications is also indicated because several drugs are also associated with hypothyroidism.

Physical Examination

A full physical examination is indicated, and should include weight (which may be increased), vital signs (including postural vital signs, as postural hypotension could suggest associated endocrine disorders, such as autoimmune adrenal insufficiency), and a general overview of the patient's appearance, noting mental alertness and comprehension. Myxedema coma should be suspected if the patient is unresponsive, appears to have facial puffiness, and a thickened nose and lips accompanied by hypothermia, hypotension, bradycardia, and hypoventilation. Key aspects of the examination include the following:

- Skin and hair: dry skin with possible facial, hand, and lower-extremity puffiness; dry, brittle hair
- Neck: check thyroid for goiter, nodules, and tenderness.
- Cardiovascular: blood pressure may be elevated, heart rate may be slowed; possible cardiomegaly
- Pulmonary: respiratory rate may be slowed or shallow.
- Abdominal: bowel sounds may be hypoactive.
- Musculoskeletal: possible entrapment neuropathies (i.e., carpal tunnel syndrome) or myopathic disorders
- Neurologic: lethargy, mentation, and deep-tendon reflexes slowed
- Psychiatric: depression

Diagnostics

- Initially the thyroid-stimulating hormone (TSH) should be checked to determine if the value is elevated. Normal TSH ranges from 0.5 mU/L to 5 mU/L.
  - If the TSH is above 5 mU/L, the free T_4 should be measured and the TSH rechecked. Often the repeat TSH will be normal. The previously elevated TSH may have represented a transient hypothyroidism, or possibly a laboratory error.
  - If the TSH is still elevated and the thyroxine (free T_4) is low, primary hypothyroidism is suggested.
  - When the TSH is elevated and free T_4 is normal, the patient may have subclinical hypothyroidism.
  - A low T_4 in combination with a TSH that is not elevated in proportion to the lowered T_4 suggests secondary hypothyroidism.
- Other diagnostics that should be considered include:
  - Fasting lipid profile*: to determine lipid abnormalities (hypercholesterolemia and hypertriglyceridemia)
  - CBC/differential*: to determine presence of anemia (often associated with hypothyroidism)
  - Antimicrosomal antibodies: antithyroid Abs, antimicrobial Abs, anti-TPO Abs (elevated in chronic autoimmune thyroiditis), and anti-Tg Abs*
  - Thyrotropin-releasing hormone (TRH)*
  - Thyroid ultrasound*
  - Fine-needle aspiration biopsy*
  - ECG*: to determine associated cardiac abnormalities

---

*If indicated.

Differential Diagnosis

- Chronic autoimmune thyroiditis
- Idiopathic hypothyroidism
- Infiltrative diseases: leukemia, hemachromatosis, scleroderma
- Iodine deficit or excess
- Hypothalamic dysfunction
- Medication-induced hypothyroidism: amiodarone, iodine, lithium, radiographic dyes, interferon alpha, and medications used to treat hyperthyroidism (e.g., methimazole, propylthiouracil [PTU])
- Pituitary tumor
- Post-infection thyroiditis
- Post-surgical subtotal or total thyroidectomy
- Radiation-induced thyroid dysfunction
- Subclinical hypothyroidism

Treatment Plan

The etiology of the thyroid deficiency should be established, because hypothyroidism can be transient or related to medication, infection, or a dysfunction in the hypothalamic-pituitary-thyroid axis. Hypothyroidism is most often treated with the synthetic thyroid hormone, levothyroxine. Elderly patients can be started on 12.5 to 25 mcg of oral levothyroxine daily; patients with coronary artery disease should be started on 12.5 mcg daily to prevent cardiac ischemia or arrhythmias. In elders, the TSH should be repeated every 8 weeks and the daily dose increased by 25 mcg (patients with cardiac ischemia or arrhythmias should have the daily dose increased by only 12.5 mcg) if the TSH remains above normal. This gradual titration should continue until the TSH is within normal limits. Once the patient is on the correct dose, the levothyroxine should be continued daily, and the serum TSH level checked once or twice yearly (or more often if the patient is symptomatic). Particular care should be taken to not overcorrect the hypothyroidism and cause subclinical hyperthyroidism, characterized by a low TSH and normal T3 and T4. For at risk patients, the over correction could precipitate atrial fibrillation.

Younger patients without a history of cardiac disease may be started on 50 mcg of oral levothyroxine each day. The TSH should be checked every 4 to 6 weeks, and the levothyroxine increased by 25 mcg daily if the TSH is still greater than normal. Drug titration should continue in this manner until the TSH is within normal limits.

If the hypothyroidism is transient or related to a medication that can be discontinued, no treatment is recommended. In patients with subclinical hypothyroidism (asymptomatic, but elevated TSH), treatment is suggested if the patient has symptoms suggestive of hypothyroidism, antithyroid Abs, elevated LDL cholesterol, a previous history of hypothyroidism, goiter, or if the TSH is > 10 mU/L.

In some patients, hypothyroidism may be difficult to correct. This may be related to the timing of the medication and interaction with foods or other medications. Usually, thyroid replacement medication should be given on an empty stomach without other medications in the early morning, before breakfast, or at bedtime. Crushing the medication may also enhance absorption in some patients.

Consultation/Hospitalization

- Consultation with the physician is recommended for levothyroxine dose adjustments for patients with a history of thyroid cancer (patients with thyroid cancer or thyroidectomy require life-long levothyroxine therapy).
- Physician consultation is recommended for patients with elevated TSH prior to elective or urgent surgical procedures.
- Consult with physician if patient is unable to take oral medications for more than 5 days to discuss IM/IV therapy (IM/IV dose is reduced).
- Physician consultation is indicated for suspected secondary or central hypothyroidism for patients who do not seem to be responding to the prescribed treatment.
- Hospitalization is recommended for patients with suspected myxedema as these patients require extensive supportive therapy in addition to IV levothyroxine.

Complications

- Myxedema coma
- Overtreatment of hypothyroidism can cause hyperthyroidism, cardiac arrhythmias, and increased bone loss.
- Untreated hypothyroidism is associated with anemia, bradycardia, cardiomegaly, hyperlipidemia, hypertension, hyponatremia, depression, psychiatric disturbances, entrapment neuropathies, myopathic disorders, paresthesias, cold intolerance, weight gain, fatigue, constipation, altered kidney function, obstructive sleep apnea, and decreased auditory acuity.

Education for Nursing Home/Rehabilitation Staff

- Explain to nursing staff the importance of scheduling medications so that drugs that may interfere with thyroid absorption are given several hours after thyroid medication.
- Discuss with nursing staff importance of notifying healthcare provider if patient is unable to take thyroid replacement for more than 5 days.
- Explain to nurses the importance of reporting patient complaints (e.g., palpitations).

Patient/Family Education

- Explain to patients and families the cause of the hypothyroidism, the need for daily medication, and regular drug monitoring.

- Explain that symptoms associated with the disorder may take several months to abate.
- Ask patients to report any palpitations or chest discomfort.

HYPERTHYROIDISM

ICD-9: 242.90

Hyperthyroidism is caused by a variety of disorders, including Grave's disease (the most common cause of hyperthyroidism), multinodular goiter, and thyroiditis. Younger patients are frequently symptomatic, complaining of weight loss despite increased appetite, palpitations, hyperdefecation, heat intolerance, insomnia, gynecomastia, menstrual irregularities, and other symptoms associated with a variety of organ systems. The disorder is more difficult to identify in elders, as older patients may not notice physical changes, or the expected symptoms may be absent. Apathetic hyperthyroidism occurs primarily in elders and is associated with lethargy, weight loss, muscle weakness, and constipation. Whatever the cause, hyperthyroidism places patients at risk for atrial fibrillation, arrhythmias, and increased bone loss.

History

A personal and family history of thyroid disease should be elicited, and a list of all current medications should be obtained. Many medications interfere with laboratory test results, and some medications can induce hyperthyroidism. Typical symptoms include failure to thrive, weight loss, angina, palpitations, shortness of breath, muscle weakness, tremor, pruritus, anxiety, and sleeplessness. Some older adults may present with anorexia, decreased appetite, muscle weakness, increased shortness of breath; others present with apathy, heat intolerance, angina, heart failure, confusion, lethargy, tachycardia, arrhythmias, dyspepsia, abdominal discomfort, diarrhea, or even constipation. It is important to note that elders may have minimal symptoms and still be hyperthyroid; thus, even subtle signs or symptoms in this population should be concerning.

Physical Examination

A thorough physical examination is indicated. Weight and vital signs should be assessed to determine weight loss, systolic hypertension, tachycardia, or other changes. Other possible findings include:

- Hair: thin; fine
- Skin: hyperhidrosis, brittle nails, or possible palmar erythema
- Eyes: lid lag, staring, soft-tissue edema, exophthalmos, proptosis, extraocular muscle paresis, or decreased visual acuity
- Mouth: possible tongue tremor

- Neck: thyroid bruit, asymmetric thyroid, goiter, nodules, or tenderness
- Cardiac: tachycardia; possible atrial fibrillation or evidence of heart failure
- Respiratory: dyspnea on exertion
- Extremities: tremors; possible edema localized over tibial areas
- Neurologic: muscle weakness, hyperreflexia, or tremor
- Mental status: confusion, lethargy
- Psychiatric: hyperactive, anxious, or irritable

Diagnostics

- Patients with suspected hyperthyroidism should first have the serum TSH evaluated. Low or undetectable TSH indicates primary hyperthyroidism.
- If the TSH is below normal, a T_3 (triiodothyronine) and free T_4 or free T_4 index must be assessed to aid in determining the type of hyperthyroidism.
  - A low TSH combined with an elevated free T_4 or free T_4 index indicates overt hyperthyroidism.
  - A low TSH combined with a high T_3, but normal T_4 or free T_4 index indicates T_3-thyrotoxicosis or T_3-hyperthyroidism.
  - A low TSH combined with a high free T_4 and normal T_3 indicates T_4-thyrotoxicosis.
  - A low TSH combined with normal T_4 and T_3 indicates subclinical hyperthyroidism.
  - An elevated TSH combined with increased T_4 indicates secondary hyperthyroidism.
- Other tests that may be indicated include:
  - ESR*: elevated in thyroiditis
  - LFTs*: abnormal in many patients with hyperthyroidism
  - Radioactive iodine uptake: to differentiate Grave's disease (high radio-iodine uptake) from thyroiditis (low radioiodine uptake)
  - Thyroid scan: to distinguish nodules, thyroid lesions, and metastases
  - Fine-needle aspiration biopsy*: to evaluate thyroid nodules
  - MRI*: to establish presence of pituitary adenoma

Differential Diagnosis

- Exogenous hyperthyroidism: overtreatment of hypothyroidism
- Graves' disease: an autoimmune disorder associated with symmetric diffuse goiter (possible thyroid bruit)
- Transient hyperthyroidism
- Thyroiditis

---

*If indicated.

- Trophoblastic disease and germ cell tumors: women with choriocarcinoma or a hydatidiform mole can develop hyperthyroidism
- Subacute thyroiditis
  - Chronic immune thyroiditis (Hashimoto's): nontender goiter
  - Subacute thyroiditis: viral, subacute lymphocytic thyroiditis (painless; amiodarone induced or induced by other medications; radiation induced; postpartum)
- TSH-secreting pituitary adenoma
- Toxic nodule: suggests toxic adenoma
- Toxic multinodular goiter
- Iodine-induced hyperthyroidism: related to amiodarone or iodine from CT scan
- TSH-secreting adenoma of pituitary gland
- Hypothalamic disorder causing overproduction of TRH
- Thyroid cancer
- Subclinical hyperthyroidism: tender thyroid

Nonthyroid disorders include:
- Anxiety
- Pheochromocytoma
- Metastatic cancer
- Sprue
- Cirrhosis
- Hyperparathyroidism
- Myasthenia gravis
- Muscular dystrophy

Treatment Plan

Therapeutics are based on the etiology of the disorder. Endocrinology referral is usually indicated for older patients. Symptomatic patients require treatment with a β-blocker such as propranolol or atenolol to alleviate the tremors or palpitations contributing to their discomfort.

- Thyroid malignancy usually requires a thyroidectomy and subsequent lifelong levothyroxine replacement to maintain the TSH level below normal levels.
- Graves' disease is treated in several ways. The symptoms are first managed with a β-blocker, then a thionamide, such as methimazole, 10 mg PO daily, or propylthiouracil (PTU), is used to induce a euthyroid state. The TSH is tested every 4 to 6 weeks and the medication adjusted accordingly. Other therapies for Graves' hyperthyroidism include radioiodine ablation (usually after pretreatment with methimazole or PTU), surgery for the goiter (if obstructive), a glucocorticoid, cholestyramine in combination with methimazole, carnitine, or, rarely, because of the associated toxicity, lithium.
- Subacute thyroiditis is treated with β-blockers to control symptoms. Prednisone, nonsteroidal antiinflammatory drugs (NSAIDs), or aspirin are used to manage the pain associated with the inflammation.

- Toxic adenomas and toxic multinodular goiter: methimazole or PTU is used for elderly patients, for patients with cardiovascular disease, or to induce a euthyroid state before surgery or radioiodine treatment. Radioiodine treatment, surgery, and inorganic iodine are other therapies. Ethanol injection therapy is also used for toxic adenomas. β-blocker therapy with propranolol or atenolol may also be used to relieve the symptoms associated with the hyperthyroidism.

Consultation/Hospitalization

- Hospitalization is necessary for patients with thyrotoxic crisis, an endocrine emergency.
  - Thyrotoxic crisis may occur in untreated patients and is precipitated by a serious illness or surgical emergency. Signs and symptoms include agitation, restlessness, fever, tachycardia, hypotension, vomiting, diarrhea, delirium, and possibly coma.
- Consultation with the physician or endocrinologist is necessary for treatment recommendations after diagnostic evaluation is complete.
- Methimazole and PTU can cause agranulocytosis. CBC/diff should be obtained on a regularly scheduled basis and if patient develops pharyngitis or fever.
- Consult with physician/endocrinologist if patient develops rash or pruritus on methimazole and PTU. (Antihistamine can be prescribed and medication is often continued.)
- Consultation with the cardiologist and endocrinologist is necessary for patients with suspected amiodarone-induced hyperthyroidism.

Complications

- Untreated hyperthyroidism can result in osteoporosis, angina, CHF, atrial fibrillation, or thyrotoxic crisis.
- Athralgia, rashes, pruritus, agranulocytosis, and fever are associated with both methimazole and PTU.

Education for Nursing Home/Rehabilitation Staff

- Discuss with nurses the disorder, treatment, expected outcomes, and potential side effects of medications.
- Explain to nurses the importance of calling the healthcare provider if a patient treated with methimazole or PTU develops rash, myalgias, arthralgias, fever > 101, or signs and symptoms of infection.
- Explain to nurses the importance of monitoring patients on β-blocker therapy and notifying healthcare provider, if the patient develops light-headedness, dizziness, falls, or pulse rate less than 50.
- Discuss signs and symptoms of hypothyroidism, hyperthyroidism, and thyrotoxic crisis.

Patient/Family Education

- Patients and families need to understand the risks associated with hyperthyroidism and the need for careful monitoring and treatment.
- Treatment options, as well as risks and benefits, should be carefully explained.

Bibliography

Braimon, J.C., et al. (2003). Thyroid disorders. In Buttaro, T.M., et al. (eds): *Primary care: A collaborative practice* (2nd ed; pp. 1050-1063). St. Louis: Mosby.

Burman, K.D. (2004). Subacute granulomatous thyroiditis. *www.uptodate.com*. Accessed January 11, 2004.

LoBuono, C. (2001). Keeping older patients healthy: Managing geriatric endocrine disorders. *Patient Care for the Nurse Practitioner, 4*(11), 23-36.

Ross, D.S. (2004). Diagnosis of hyperthyroidism. *www.uptodate.com*. Accessed January 8, 2004.

Ross, D.S. (2004). Treatment of Graves' hyperthyroidism. *www.uptodate.com*. Accessed January 11, 2004.

Ross, D.S. (2004). Treatment of hypothyroidism. *www.uptodate.com*. Accessed January 5, 2004.

Ross, D.S. (2004). Treatment of toxic adenoma and toxic multinodular goiter. *www.uptodate.com*. Accessed January 11, 2004.

CHAPTER 10

Fluid and Electrolyte Disorders

HYPERNATREMIA

ICD-9: 276.0

In older adults, sodium disorders are particularly prevalent. A serum sodium > 145 mEq is indicative of hypernatremia. Most times, the hypernatremia is related to a water deficit and associated with renal or extrarenal water loss. Sodium retention may also cause hypernatremia. Whatever the cause, the increase in serum sodium causes an increase in serum osmolality, resulting in cellular dehydration.

Risk Factors

- Inadequate thirst response
- Poor oral intake
- Increased insensible water loss
- Diarrheal conditions
- Osmotic diuresis
- Excessive use of diuretics, lactulose, or other laxatives
- Fluid restrictions
- Impaired level of consciousness
- Immobility/inability to obtain fluids
- Deficiency of antidiuretic hormone (ADH)
- Central diabetes insipidus (decreased production of ADH by hypothalamus or decreased release of ADH by pituitary)
- Nephrogenic diabetes insipidus (decreased kidney responsiveness to ADH)
- High-solute tube feedings

- Poor kidney excretion
- Intravenous (IV) hypertonic saline or excessive IV isotonic saline
- Primary aldosteronism

History

Determining the sources of the water loss or increased sodium intake is fundamental. Fever, vomiting, diarrhea, diuretic therapy, polyuria, high solute tube feedings, or IV normal saline (N/S) are possible causes of hypernatremia. The past medical history and all current medications should be determined. Presentation varies; patients may be completely asymptomatic, but the elevated serum sodium usually results in a change in cognitive and functional ability. Other possible symptoms include:
- Thirst
- Polyuria
- Lightheadedness
- Other symptoms/signs usually occur when serum Na is > 150 mEq/L and are nonspecific.
  - Confusion, change in personality, irritability, and agitation are some of the early changes that may be noted.
  - Lethargy, delirium, muscle twitching, seizures, and coma may develop as the serum sodium increases.

Physical Examination

The patient's appearance, weight, and vital signs (including temperature and oxygen saturation) should be evaluated. Careful examination of the cardiac, pulmonary, gastrointestinal (GI), and neurologic systems is indicated to determine subtle changes. Possible changes include:
- Change in mental status: agitation, confusion, irritability, or lethargy
- Weight loss
- Hypotension; postural blood pressure and/or heart rate changes
- Flattened neck veins: related to dehydration
- Diminished urine output, except in patients with diabetes insipidus or osmotic diuresis
- Dried mucous membranes and poor skin turgor (unreliable signs)
- Muscle twitching, spasticity, hyperreflexia, or seizures

Diagnostics

A serum sodium > 145 mEq/L is diagnostic for hypernatremia. If the cause of the hypernatremia is readily apparent, evaluation may be limited to serum glucose, electrolytes, blood urea nitrogen (BUN), and creatinine in order to calculate the serum osmolality. Other diagnostics are dependent on the history and physical findings and may include the following:

- Serum glucose, electrolytes, BUN, and creatinine
  - Calculate serum osmolality: 2(Na) + serum glucose/18 + BUN/2.8
- CBC/differential (CBC/diff): to determine presence of infection
- Urine*
  - Urine volume
  - Urinalysis/culture sensitivity: if infection is suspected
  - Urine sodium: < 25 mEq/L if volume depletion associated with water loss; > 100 mEq/L if related to excess sodium intake (IV or oral)
  - Urine osmolality: if less than serum osmolality, suggests diabetes insipidus; urine osmolality > 200 mOsm/kg suggests hypovolemic hypernatremia
  - Specific gravity: increased in dehydration; < 1.005 suggests diabetes insipidus

Differential Diagnosis

Usually, the clinical presentation and the physical examination establish the underlying cause of the hypernatremia and guide treatment. Water loss with inadequate water intake, increased renal water loss with insufficient fluid intake, excessive sodium intake with indequate water intake, and hyperactivity of the adrenal cortex should be considered. If the cause of the hypernatremia is unclear, consultation and further diagnostic evaluation are necessary.

Treatment Plan

Treatment consists of restoring fluid balance and correcting the underlying cause of the disorder.
- Attempt to determine underlying pathology.
- Calculate fluid deficit; plan to replace fluid deficit plus maintenance (insensible losses, urine and GI losses) fluids over 48 to 72 hours
  - Calculated water deficit for elders: 0.45 × (current weight in kg) × (serum Na/140 − 1)
- If the patient is not hypovolemic and can take oral fluids, oral rehydration is the safest.
- Hold laxatives and diuretics.
- Patients who are hypovolemic (as evidenced by hypotension) in addition to being hypernatremic (i.e., hypovolemic hypernatremia) will need IV fluid resuscitation with 0.9% N/S. Once the hypovolemia is corrected (normalized vital signs), the serum sodium should slowly be corrected (0.5 mmol/L or 0.5 mEq/hour) with free water via nasogastric tube or with IV D_5W or hypotonic saline solution (0.45% N/S). Only half of the fluid deficit should be replaced within the first 24 hours. Serum sodium and electrolytes must be monitored closely to prevent too rapid of a decrease in serum sodium and prevent cerebral edema.

---

*If indicated.

- Dietary sodium restriction
- Patients with central diabetes insipidus require intranasal or subcutaneous desmopressin acetate (DDAVP) or, in certain circumstances, chlorpropamide, clofibrate, or carbamazepine.
- Patients with nephrogenic diabetes insipidus are treated with a low-salt, low-protein diet and/or thiazide diuretics or nonsteroidal antiinflammatory drugs (NSAIDs).

Consultation/Hospitalization

- **Physician consultation is needed for serum sodium > 155 mEq/L and for treatment of central or nephrogenic diabetes insipidus.**
- Hospitalization should be considered for patients with critical hypovolemia or requiring IV therapy.

Complications

- Hypovolemic shock, if fluid volume not replaced
- Neurologic deficits
- Seizures
- Cerebral vascular damage
- Subarachnoid or intracerebral hemorrhage
- Coma
- Death

Education for Nursing Home/Rehabilitation Staff

- Adequate fluid intake should be incorporated into each patient's plan of care.
  - Fluids are needed between meals as most nursing home patients receive approximately 1200 mL of fluid with meals, but require 2000 mL/day. The nursing staff should understand that small, frequent drinks might be preferable and more easily tolerated by patients. Nursing assistants require education and supervision to ensure that patients receive adequate fluid and nutrition.
  - It is important to consider individual and cultural patient preferences when offering fluids.
- The importance of carefully monitoring each patient's fluid intake and output (I&O), as well as monitoring patients for changes in mental status and other symptoms of electrolyte disorders should be explained and stressed.
- Nursing should understand that correcting hypernatremia too rapidly with hypotonic fluids (D$_5$W or 0.45% N/S) might cause cerebral edema.
- Explain the importance of mouth care for patients with dehydration.

Patient/Family Education

Patients and families should understand the nature of the disorder, the treatment plan, and strategies to prevent further occurrences.

HYPONATREMIA

ICD-9: 276.1

Hyponatremia is associated with congestive heart failure (CHF), cirrhosis, nephrotic syndrome, infections, malignancies, medications, endocrine disorders, the syndrome of inappropriate antidiuretic hormone (SIADH), psychogenic polydipsia, AIDS, and other illnesses. When chronic, hyponatremia may be asymptomatic; acute hyponatremia can result in seizures, neurologic compromise, coma, and death. Whether acute or chronic, hyponatremia is classified into four different categories: hyponatremia with hypervolemia (increased extracellular volume); hyponatremia with hypovolemia (decreased extracellular volume); hyponatremia with euvolemia (normal extracellular volume); and pseudohyponatremia. The first three are considered hypotonic hyponatremias, whereas pseudohyponatremia is associated with hypertonic or isotonic hyponatremia.

History

The patient's history is very important. Symptoms may be vague or associated with other disorders. However, the following symptoms should prompt consideration for hyponatremia:
- Altered mental status: combativeness, confusion, disorientation, irritability, lethargy, restlessness, seizures, stupor
- Blurred vision
- Dizziness
- Dysgeusia
- Extrapyramidal signs
- Falls
- Fatigue
- Flulike symptoms
- GI complaints
- Headache
- Muscle cramps
- Polydipsia
- Polyuria
- Weakness
- Weight change

Physical Examination

Patients with mild hyponatremia may be asymptomatic, and physical signs of hyponatremia may be difficult to discern. The patient's weight and vital signs should be determined, and a focused physical examination, including neurologic assessment, is necessary.

Diagnostics

Diagnostics are indicated to classify the type of hyponatremia and determine the underlying precipitant.

Laboratory Evaluation
- Serum glucose, electrolytes, BUN, and creatinine: to determine serum osmolality and categorize hyponatremia into a hypertonic, hypotonic, or isotonic state
  - Serum osmolality = 2(Na) + serum glucose/18 + BUN/2.8
- CBC/differential: if infection is suspected
- Urine for sodium, specific gravity (may be decreased), and osmolality: to aid in discerning volume status and type of hyponatremia
- Calcium, magnesium, and phosphorus*
- Uric acid*: decreased in SIADH
- Thyroid-stimulating hormone (TSH)*: to exclude hypothyroidism
- Fasting lipid profile: if hyperlipidemia is suspected
- Liver function tests (LFTs)*: if cirrhosis is a consideration

Other Diagnostics
- Chest x-ray*: to evaluate for malignancy

Differential Diagnosis

The hyponatremia should first be categorized appropriately. Hyponatremia with hypervolemia is associated with CHF, cirrhosis, nephrotic syndrome, or advanced renal failure. Characterized by serum Na < 135 mEq/L and serum osmolality < 280 mOsm/L, increased urine osmolality, and usually urine Na < 20 mEq/L (if renal failure is present, urine Na will be > 20 mEq/L), hyponatremia with hypervolemia is a condition associated with edema.

Hypovolemic hyponatremia can be related to renal causes or nonrenal causes. Renal causes include chronic renal disease, osmotic diuresis, mineralocorticoid and glucocorticoid deficiency, NSAIDs, thiazides, and angiotensin-converting enzyme (ACE) inhibitors, whereas diarrhea, vomiting, and dehydration are nonrenal causes. If renal causes are the basis of the hypovolemic hyponatremia, the serum osmolality will be < 275 mOsm/L; urine Na > 20 mEq/L; and the BUN and creatinine elevated. If nonrenal causes are the source of the disorder, the

---

*If indicated.

serum osmolality will be < 275 mOsm/L; urine Na < 20 mEq/L; the urine osmolality increased; and the BUN and creatinine increased.

Euvolemic hyponatremia can be related to SIADH, psychogenic polydipsia, beer potamia, postoperative conditions associated with pain or stress, and the reset osmostat. SIADH, the most common of the euvolemic hyponatremias, is associated with many conditions.

Pseudohyponatremia with normal serum osmolality is associated with hyperproteinemia or hyperlipidemia, and pseudohyponatremia with elevated plasma osmolality is related to hyperglycemia, mannitol excess, or glycerol therapy. The absorption of isotonic genitourinary irrigant solutions containing glycine or sorbitol may also cause lowered serum sodium. This type of hyponatremia is also considered a pseudohyponatremia and is associated with both normal and elevated serum osmolality.

After determining the serum osmolality and fluid status, the underlying reason for the hyponatremia should be considered. Possible causes of hyponatremia include:

- Asthma
- Cerebrovascular accident (CVA)
- CNS infection or head trauma
- Depression
- Endocrine abnormalities: adrenal insufficiency, hypothyroidism
- GI illness with vomiting and diarrhea
- Illness or infection
- Malignancy: head and neck cancers; small and non-small cell lung cancer
- Medications: diuretics (particularly thiazides), selective serotonin reuptake inhibitors (SSRIs), chemotherapeutic agents, carbamazepine, and narcotics
- Metabolic illness such as diabetes
- Positive pressure ventilations
- Pregnancy
- Pseudohyponatremia related to hyperglycemia, hyperproteinemia, or hyperlipidemia
- Pulmonary disorders/infections

Treatment Plan

Treatment of the underlying cause of the hyponatremia is necessary, is aimed at increasing the patient's serum sodium, and is guided by the history, physical findings, and determination of the patient's volume status.

- Hyponatremia with hypervolemia
  - Characterized by serum Na < 135 mEq/L, serum osmolality < 280 mOsm/L, and increased urine osmolality and urine Na < 20 mEq/L; in renal failure, urine Na will be > 20 mEq/L
  - Management: correct underlying condition
    - If patient is asymptomatic and serum Na is 125 to 135 mEq/L, maintain dietary Na at 2 to 5 g/day, institute fluid restriction 1000 to 1500 mL/day.

- ▪ If serum Na is < 125 mEq/L, consult with physician (MD) concerning cautious use of loop diuretics.
- • Hyponatremia with hypovolemia
  - • Renal causes: chronic renal disease, osmotic diuresis, mineralocorticoid and glucocorticoid deficiency, NSAIDs, thiazides, or ACE inhibitors
    - ▪ Characterized by serum osmolality < 275 mOsm/L, urine Na > 20 mEq/L, and increased BUN and creatinine
    - ▪ Management: review medications. Discuss with MD discontinuing offending medication, if possible. Treat underlying pathology; consult with MD concerning isotonic fluid replacement. If serum Na <125 mEq/L, discuss hospitalization with MD.
  - • Nonrenal causes: diarrhea, vomiting, or dehydration
    - ▪ Characterized by serum osmolality < 275 mOsm/L; urine Na < 20 mEq/L; increased urine osmolality; increased BUN and creatinine
    - ▪ Management: correct underlying pathology and consult with MD concerning isotonic fluid replacement. If serum Na <125 mEq/L, discuss hospitalization with MD.
- • Hyponatremia with euvolemia can be related to various pathologies.
  - • SIADH
    - ▪ Characterized by serum Na < 135 mEq/L; urine osmolality > 100 mOsm/L; urine Na > 20 mEq/L; normal BUN (< 10); uric acid < 4 mg/dL; normal thyroid, renal, adrenal, and hepatic function
    - ▪ Management: correct underlying pathology and institute fluid restriction. If serum Na < 125 mEq/L, consult with MD regarding need for hospitalization.
    - ▪ Increased dietary sodium and ADH inhibitors such as Demeclocycline (300 to 600 mg PO BID) or lithium have also been used in the treatment of SIADH. Consultation with the primary care physician is recommended before instituting therapies as Demeclocycline is associated with renal toxicity and lithium can precipitate thyroid dysfunction or psychogenic polydipsia.
  - • Management of hyponatremia associated with reset thermostat consists of correcting the underlying disorder.
  - • If psychogenic polydipsia or beer potamia: fluid restriction and behavioral counseling are recommended.
- • Pseudohyponatremia
  - • Pseudohyponatremia associated with hyperglycemia is managed by correcting the hyperglycemia.
  - • Pseudohyponatremia associated with hyperlipidemia or hyperproteinemia does not require specific intervention, but is treated with correction of the hyperproteinemia or hyperlipidemia.
  - • Hyponatremia associated with genitourinary irrigants require cessation of the offending irrigant.

Consultation/Hospitalization

- Physician consultation is recommended for serum sodium levels < 125 mEq/L, to discuss treatment options, and determine whether or not hospitalization is necessary. Consultation is also indicated for patients who do not respond to treatment.
- Hospitalization is indicated for patients with acute SIADH and serum sodium less than 115 mEq/L as IV hypertonic saline (3% NaCl) may be indicated. Hypertonic saline should be administered slowly to prevent central pontine myelinosis and brain damage.

Complications

- Quality of life issues related to fluid/dietary restrictions
- Seizures
- Coma
- Death

Education for Nursing Home/Rehabilitation Staff

- Explain etiology of hyponatremia and potential neurologic consequences.
- Discuss importance of weight measurements, fluid and dietary restrictions, and careful measurement of I&O.
- The side effects of medications should be discussed.
- The importance of frequent, good oral hygiene for patients on fluid restrictions should be discussed.
- The possibility of lowered serum sodium occurring in patients on genitourinary (GU) irrigation should be explained.

Patient/Family Education

- It is important that patients and families understand the nature of the disorder as well as treatments, particularly if fluid restriction is recommended.
- The side effects of any medications used in the treatment of hyponatremia should also be discussed.

HYPOKALEMIA

ICD-9: 276.8

Hypokalemia may be acute or chronic. It is most commonly related to diuretic therapy. Other more common causes of hypokalemia include decreased dietary intake, alcoholism, hypomagnesemia, endocrine disorders, and GI losses related

Adapted from Buttaro, T.M., et al. (Eds.). (2003). Hypokalemia and hyperkalemia. In *Primary care: A collaborative practice* (2nd ed). St. Louis, Mosby.

BOX 10-1	Causes of Hypokalemia

Alcoholism
11-β-hydroxysteroid dehydrogenase deficiency
Bartter's syndrome
Catecholamine excess
Congenital adrenal hyperplasia
Excess licorice ingestion
Familial periodic hypokalemic paralysis
Gitelman syndrome
Hyperaldosteronism (primary and secondary)
Hypertension: malignant, renovascular, or glucocorticoid induced
Hypomagnesemia
Leukemia
Liddle syndrome
Medications: antibiotics, β-adrenergic agents, insulin, and non–potassium-sparing diuretics
Osmotic diuresis
Renin-secreting tumor
Thyrotoxic hypokalemic paralysis
Trauma
Type I and type II renal tubular acidosis

---

to vomiting and diarrhea. Less common causes of hypokalemia should be considered if the more common causes are excluded (Box 10-1). Though serum potassium values may vary from one laboratory to another, mild hypokalemia is usually defined as 3.5 to 4 mEq/L, moderate hypokalemia as 3 to 3.5 mEq/L, and severe hypokalemia less than 3 mEq/L.

History and Physical Examination

Patients are often asymptomatic even with low-serum potassium levels. Frequently, however, patients will complain of fatigue or lower extremity weakness. A careful history including medication use (especially diuretics or laxatives), vomiting, diarrhea, co-morbid disease (diabetes or hypertension), or altered urinary output is important to ascertain.

Vital signs, including orthostatic changes, aid in determining volume status.

As low potassium levels can affect muscle strength, the neuromuscular system should be examined to determine the presence of any muscle weakness or respiratory distress related to the lowered potassium. It is also important to determine if the patient is hypertensive, normotensive, or has orthostatic changes.

Diagnostics

Diagnostic evaluation is individualized and based on the patient history, physical findings, and the differential diagnosis.

Laboratory Evaluation
- Serum electrolytes
- Serum glucose
- BUN and creatinine
- Serum magnesium: magnesium deficiency is associated with hypokalemia
- Serum bicarbonate*
- Plasma osmolality*
- Urinary potassium—random*
- Urine osmolality*
- 24-hour urine collection for potassium*
- Early-morning urinary pH*
- Plasma renin activity*: evaluate after hypokalemia is corrected.
- Plasma aldosterone*: evaluate after hypokalemia is corrected (spironolactone may cause elevated aldosterone level).

Other Diagnostics
- Electrocardiogram (ECG) to determine presence of ventricular arrhythmias, S-T segment depression, flattened or inverted T wave, and prominent U wave that may be present in hypokalemia but are not diagnostic for hypokalemia

Differential Diagnosis

Most often, hypokalemia is related to a medication. Alcoholism, vomiting, or excess licorice ingestion are other causes fairly easily recognized. If none of these seems to be associated with the hypokalemia, other causes need to be investigated. The differential is somewhat simplified by classifying the hypokalemia as follows:

- Hypokalemia associated with hypertension and increased renal potassium excretion (> 20 mEq/L)
  - Consider primary hyperaldosteronism if plasma aldosterone is elevated and plasma renin activity (PRA) is depressed
  - Consider secondary hyperaldosteronism if both PRA and plasma aldosterone are elevated
  - Liddle syndrome is suggested if both PRA and plasma aldosterone are depressed.

---

*If indicated.

- Hypokalemia associated with normal blood pressure and increased renal potassium excretion
  - If serum bicarbonate is decreased, consider diabetes ketoacidosis, metabolic acidosis, or renal tubular acidosis (RTA). Type 1 renal tubular acidosis should be considered if the hypokalemia is associated with hyperchloremic metabolic acidosis (morning urinary pH > 6 is a reliable indicator of type 1 RTA).
  - If serum bicarbonate is increased, consider Bartter's syndrome, a rare disorder associated with high PRA and plasma aldosterone.
  - If serum bicarbonate is normal, consider hypomagnesemia (common in alcoholic, chemotherapy, or malnourished patients).
- Hypokalemia associated with normal or decreased renal potassium excretion (< 20 mEq/L) is associated with GI losses (vomiting, diarrhea, villous adenoma), treatment with non–potassium-sparing diuretics, or laxative therapy.

Treatment Plan

Management includes establishing the etiology of the hypokalemia, treating the underlying cause, and correcting the hypokalemia. The potassium should be replaced to a serum potassium of 4 mEq/L, the goal of therapy. Oral replacement with a potassium chloride preparation is preferred. For patients with normal renal function, each 10 mEq of oral potassium chloride (KCl) will increase the sodium potassium approximately 01. mmol. Maintenance replacement therapy is usually 20 to 40 mEq PO once or twice daily, though some patients may require as much as 40 mEq PO four times a day. For patients with renal failure, potassium should be replaced cautiously. All patients receiving potassium replacement therapy must have serum potassium carefully monitored and the dose adjusted accordingly to avoid hyperkalemia. For patients with renal failure, a potassium-sparing duretic may be considered.

It is also possible to replace potassium IV if the patient is cannot take oral supplements. IV potassium concentration should not exceed 40 mEq/L and should not be infused faster than 10 mEq per hour. Cardiac monitoring and frequent assessment of the serum potassium are necessary (every 3 to 6 hours). Many facilities are unable to provide the required monitoring, thus requiring hospitalization.

Consultation/Hospitalization

- **Consultation with the physician is recommended for serum potassium levels < 3 mEq/L, when the cause of the hypokalemia is obscure, and if the patient also has renal failure (patients with renal failure require careful replacement to avoid causing hyperkalemia) or hypokalemia associated with diabetic ketoacidosis or nonketotic ketoacidosis.**
- Consultation with an endocrinologist is appropriate for patients with hyperaldosteronism or if the diagnosis remains unclear.

- Surgical consult is necessary for patients with an aldosterone-secreting tumor.
- Hospitalization is necessary for patients with severe signs of hypokalemia (e.g., progressive muscle weakness, flaccid paralysis, hypoventilation). Hospitalization should also be considered for patients requiring IV potassium replacement.

Complications

- Ileus, muscle weakness or paralysis, hypertension, and even stroke have been associated with hypokalemia.
- Other complications of hypokalemia include arrhythmias, conduction defects, sudden cardiac death, and renal injury.

Education for Nursing Home/Rehabilitation Staff

- Explain to the nursing staff the importance of promptly reporting abnormal electrolyte levels.
- The nursing staff should understand that giving oral potassium with food and fluids helps prevent esophageal and gastric irritation. Patient should be sitting up when taking oral potassium.
- Nurses need to understand that IV potassium infusions should not exceed 10 mEq/hour.
- Explain to nurses that overuse of laxatives is associated with below normal serum potassium levels.

Patient/Family Education

- The nature of the disorder should be explained to the patient and family.
- Patients should understand that oral potassium should be swallowed while sitting up with food and with adequate fluids.
- The need for frequent monitoring of serum potassium levels should be explained.

HYPERKALEMIA

ICD-9: 276.7

Hyperkalemia is defined as a serum potassium > 5 mEq/L and may be either acute or chronic. Most often, hyperkalemia is related to renal failure, but can also be related to volume depletion, hypoaldosteronism, medications (NSAIDs, ACE inhibitors, potassium-sparing diuretics, trimethoprim-sulfamethoxazole, heparin, cyclosporine), dietary indiscretion, salt substitutes containing potassium chloride, Addison's disease, infection, or trauma. Traumatic venipuncture or leukemia associated with leukocytosis may also cause pseudohyperkalemia.

History/Physical Examination

Irritability, weakness, and neuromuscular symptoms such as paresthesias or fasciculations are possible. Peripheral paralysis may occur, but the increased serum potassium primarily affects the cardiac conduction system. Patient history, including all medications (over-the-counter, as well as prescribed), dietary changes, and past medical history should be elicited. Vital signs, volume status, and skin changes should be determined, and the neuromuscular system assessed.

Diagnostics

Laboratory Evaluation
- Serum glucose, electrolytes, BUN, and creatinine: to assess volume and renal status.
- 24-hour urine for creatinine clearance*: if history of chronic renal failure but normal serum potassium
- Plasma aldosterone, plasma cortisol, and plasma renin activity*: to differentiate hypoaldosteronism and adrenal insufficiency
- Cosyntropin stimulation test*: if Addison's disease is suspected

Other Diagnostics
- ECG*: First-degree atrioventricular (AV) block may be present in early hyperkalemia; globally elevated T waves also are indicative of hyperkalemia. If the serum potassium exceeds 6 mEq/L the T waves become tall, peaked, and ST segments are not visible. If serum potassium exceeds 6.5 mEq/L, P waves flatten and widen. Serum potassium levels > 7.5 mEq/L can result in cardiac arrest or ventricular fibrillation.

Differential Diagnosis

Most often, elevated serum potassium levels are related to medications or renal failure. Occasionally, the hyperkalemia is falsely elevated. Other causes of hyperkalemia include the following:
- Pseudohyperkalemia
  - Severe leukocytosis
  - Traumatic venipuncture
  - Unspun serum specimen
- True hyperkalemia
  - Adrenal insufficiency (Addison's disease)
  - Burns
  - Congenital adrenal enzyme deficiency
  - Crush injuries

---

*If indicated.

- Familial hyperkalemic periodic paralysis
- Gordon's syndrome
- Hypoaldosteronism
- Insulin deficiency/uncontrolled diabetes mellitus
- Medications
    - ACE inhibitors
    - Bactrim
    - β-blockers
    - Cyclosporine
    - Digitalis overdose
    - Heparin
    - Pentamidine
    - Potassium sparing diuretics
    - Potassium supplements
    - NSAIDs
    - Succinylcholine
- Metabolic acidosis
- Renal failure
- Rhabdomyolysis
- Severe infections
- Sickle-cell anemia
- Systemic lupus erythematosus
- Hyperkalemic type 1 renal tubular acidosis
- Type IV renal tubular acidosis
- Tumor lysis syndrome
- Ureterojejunostomy

Treatment Plan

The elevated potassium level should be verified expediently (which may require hospitalization) and the underlying cause considered. In cases of mild hyperkalemia, the patient does not usually require hospitalization.

Acute Hyperkalemia

- Hospitalization for cardiac monitoring and IV administration of calcium (10 mL of a 10% calcium chloride solution over 2 to 3 minutes) is indicated if the serum potassium exceeds 7 mEq/L and widening of the QRS is evident. IV calcium does not correct the hyperkalemia, but temporarily counters the effects of the elevated potassium. If the patient is not hyperglycemic, IV administration of 50 g of 50% glucose and 10 units of regular insulin can then be utilized to shift extracellular potassium into the cell. An IV glucose solution should also be administered to prevent hypoglycemia.
- If the potassium is less than 7 mEq/L, the patient is able to take oral medications, and there are no life-threatening symptoms, sodium polystyrene sulfonate (Kayexalate), 15 g PO, is appropriate. Sodium polystyrene sulfonate

may also be used rectally but should not be used in patients who have recently had abdominal surgery.
- Sodium bicarbonate is used cautiously for hospitalized patients with hyperkalemia and metabolic acidosis.
- Therapy with a loop or thiazide (or both) diuretic is an appropriate therapy for patients with adequate renal function.
- Hemodialysis in extreme cases
- Closely monitor potassium level.

Chronic Hyperkalemia
- Low-potassium diet
- Kayexalate therapy: as indicated by serum potassium levels
- Diuretic therapy: if renal function is adequate
- For hyperkalemia related to Addison's disease, replacement hydrocortisone is indicated.
- For hyperkalemia related to hypoaldosteronism, treatment with fludrocortisone (Florinef), a mineralocorticoid, may be beneficial.

Consultation/Hospitalization

Hyperkalemia is often related to a medication, volume depletion, or uncontrolled hyperglycemia. For patients with renal failure or suspected hypoaldosteronism, or if the etiology is unclear, MD consultation is recommended.
- **Hospitalization is indicated for patients with life-threatening hyperkalemia.**
- Physician consultation is recommended for serum potassium levels > 6 mEq/L.

Complications

- Arrhythmias
- Cardiac conduction defects
- Peripheral paralysis
- Death

Education for Nursing Home/Rehabilitation Staff

- The signs and symptoms of hyperkalemia and the importance of reporting these findings should be discussed with the nursing staff.
- Nurses should understand the importance of recognizing abnormal lab values and reporting the values immediately.

Patient/Family Education

The nature of the disorder, treatment plan, dietary measures, and expected outcome should be explained to both the patient and family.

HYPOCALCEMIA

ICD-9: 275.41

A serum calcium < 8.5 mg/dL may be transient or chronic. Transient causes include burns, sepsis, frequent blood transfusions with citrated blood, acute pancreatitis, and medications such as anticonvulsants (impede calcium and Vitamin D absorption and metabolism), protamine, heparin, or glucagons. Chronic causes of hypocalcemia are more frequently seen in long-term care facilities and include hypoalbuminemia, chronic renal failure, hypoparathyroidism, pseudohypoparathyroidism, liver disease, malabsorption syndromes, vitamin D deficiency, decreased magnesium levels, and loop diuretics.

History

Patients can be asymptomatic, even with significant hypocalcemia. However, fatigue, irritability, restlessness, as well as numbness and tingling around the nose, earlobes, lips, and extremities are the complaints most commonly associated with hypocalcemia. Other symptoms include clumsiness, musculoskeletal and GI cramping, depression, psychosis, memory loss, muscle spasms, carpopedal spasm, seizures, and laryngospasm. Past medical history and a review of current medications aids in determining the underlying precipitant.

Physical Examination

A complete physical examination including vital signs is indicated, although often there are no significant findings. Positive findings may include any of the following:

- Mental status changes including lethargy, depression, mood changes, memory impairment, hallucinations, psychosis
- Skin: dry, scaly in chronic hypocalcemia with coarse, dry hair, patchy alopecia, and brittle nails
- Eyes: cataracts, papilledema; slit-lamp evaluation may reveal subscapular cataracts
- Pharynx: laryngospasm
- Cardiovascular: hypotension, bradyarrhythmias
- Pulmonary: bronchospasm
- Neuromuscular: movement disorders, muscle spasms
  - Facial muscle spasm indicated by positive Chvostek sign (tapping in front of ear elicits spasm of eyelid, nose, and lip)
  - Tetany: continuous tonic spasm of muscle manifested by positive Trousseau's sign (occlusion of brachial artery for 3 minutes with blood pressure cuff causes carpal spasm—thumb adducts, fingers contract)
  - Hyperreflexia of deep tendon reflexes

Diagnostics

Laboratory Evaluation

- Serum calcium
    - If initial serum calcium is low, serum calcium should be repeated and correlated with serum albumin
        - Corrected calcium (mg/dL) = measured Ca (mg/dL) – albumin (g/dL) + 4
        - If corrected serum calcium is still below normal, obtain ionized calcium
- Further diagnostics are dependent on patient presentation and history and are obtained to determine the underlying cause of the hypocalcemia.
    - Serum electrolytes, BUN, creatinine, phosphorus, and magnesium: renal disease, hypomagnesemia, and hyperphosphatemia are associated with hypocalcemia
    - Hypoparathyroidism and pseudohypoparathyroidism are suggested by elevated phosphorus and decreased calcium levels if renal failure or crush injury is not present. Vitamin D deficiency is suggested by hypocalcemia associated with hypophosphatemia.
    - Serum pH*: acidosis decreases amount of calcium bound to albumin, increasing amount of ionized calcium available; alkalosis increases the amount of calcium bound to albumin decreasing amount of available ionized calcium
    - Amylase*: if pancreatitis is suspected
    - Parathyroid hormone (PTH)*: to distinguish hypoparathyroidism
    - Vitamin D metabolites: 25(OH)D and 1,25(OH)$_2$D*: to detect vitamin D deficiencies

Other Diagnostics

- ECG*: increased QT interval and ST segment, block, ventricular arrhythmias
- Radiographs*: if malignancy is suspected
- Bone scan*: if malignancy is suspected

Differential Diagnosis

- Alcoholism
- Burns
- Frequent blood transfusions with citrated blood
- Hyperphosphatemia
- Hypomagnesemia

*If indicated.

- Liver disease
- Malabsorption syndromes
- Malignancy
- Malnutrition
- Medications: antiseizure medications (cause vitamin D deficiency), some chemotherapeutics, foscarnet, and loop diuretics
- Pancreatitis
- PTH deficiency
  - Idiopathic
  - Hypoparathyroidism
  - Pseudohypoparathyroidism
  - Radiation exposure
  - Surgery
- Renal disease
- Rhabdomyolysis
- Sepsis
- Tomorlysis syndrome
- Vitamin D deficiency

Treatment Plan/Consultation/Hospitalization

Consultation with the primary care physician or endocrinologist is indicated for symptomatic hypocalcemia or corrected calcium < 8.5 mg/dL. Acute, symptomatic hypocalcemia requires hospitalization for IV calcium therapy and cardiac monitoring.

Chronic Hypocalcemia

- Low serum calcium associated with low serum albumin often will not require calcium replacement.
- Hypocalcemia associated with hyperphosphatemia: if acute hyperphosphatemia, hospitalization is indicated; if chronic hyperphosphatemia, decrease dietary phosphorus and discuss phosphate-binding antacid therapy with physician.
- Hypocalcemia associated with hypomagnesemia: replete magnesium and correct underlying cause of hypomagnesemia
- Hypocalcemia associated with chronic renal failure: consult with physician regarding management of renal failure, prevention of hyperphosphatemia with a phosphate binder such as calcium carbonate, and 0.25 to 1 mcg calcitriol (1,25 dihydroxyvitamin D) daily. Patients require close monitoring.
- Hypocalcemia associated with vitamin D deficiency: consult with physician regarding daily calcium replacement and vitamin D supplementation
- Hypocalcemia associated with anticonvulsant therapy requires daily calcium supplementation. Discuss vitamin D supplementation with the

physician. Also discuss possible changes related to anticonvulsant therapy with the physician or neurologist.

- Hypocalcemia associated with malabsorption, hypoparathyroidism, or pseudohypoparathyroidism requires physician consultation.
- If hypocalcemia is related to diuretic therapy, calcium supplementation is indicated.

Complications

- Laryngospasm
- Airway obstruction
- Seizures
- Tetany
- Cardiac arrhythmias
- Coma
- Death

Education for Nursing Home/Rehabilitation Staff

- Nurses should be able to recognize the symptoms associated with hypocalcemia and recognize the importance of discussing these symptoms with the healthcare provider.
- Explain to nursing staff the importance of promptly notifying the healthcare provider of any laboratory abnormalities.
- Discuss with nursing the importance of vitamin and calcium supplementation.

Patient/Family Education

- The disorder, diagnostics, and therapy should be discussed with both patients and families.
- The need to continuously take vitamins and calcium supplementation should be carefully explained to patients and families.

HYPERCALCEMIA

ICD-9: 275.42

A serum calcium level > 10.5 mg/dL is associated with hypercalcemia. This disorder is the most common metabolic emergency in cancer patients, but elevated serum calcium also occurs in familial hypocalciuric hypercalcemia, hyperparathyroidism, vitamin D toxicity, aluminum toxicity, renal tubular defects, and milk-alkali syndrome. Thiazides, lithium, and vitamin A intoxication are also associated with hypercalcemia.

History

A significant alteration in mental status is the most serious symptom associated with hypercalcemia. However, as with most electrolyte disorders, patients may have vague symptoms or even be asymptomatic. Often an abrupt increase in serum calcium may cause symptoms, whereas a more chronic increase will not. Fatigue, lethargy, depression, memory loss, confusion, inattentiveness, polyuria, polydipsia, nocturia, and GI symptoms such as weight loss, anorexia, nausea, vomiting, abdominal pain, bone pain, or constipation are other possible presenting complaints. A family history of hyperparathyroidism or personal history of head or neck radiation, peptic ulcer disease, or pancreatitis may be significant. A dietary and medication review may suggest milk-alkali syndrome, which is related to increased calcium intake.

Physical Examination

Unfortunately, the physical examination may also be unremarkable. Dehydration is possible, and, therefore, weight and vital signs (including postural signs) are indicated. The central nervous system is most likely affected by the elevated serum calcium, resulting in sensorium changes, weakness, tremor, ataxia, hyporeflexia, and stupor. The cardiovascular system may also be affected, causing cardiac irregularities.

Diagnostics

Laboratory Evaluation
- Serum calcium
  - If serum calcium is elevated > 10.5 mg/dL, it is necessary to repeat the test, then correlate the serum calcium level with the serum albumin: corrected calcium (mg/dL) = measured calcium (mg/dL) − albumin (g/dL) + 4.
- If the serum calcium is still elevated, further laboratory testing is based on history and clinical presentation. Slightly elevated levels may reflect hyperparathyroidism, whereas critically elevated serum calcium suggests malignancy.
  - Serum electrolytes, serum phosphorus, serum magnesium, and amylase
    - Low phosphorus suggests hyperparathyroidism or humoral hypercalcemia of malignancy; normal or elevated phosphorus levels suggest milk-alkali syndrome, vitamin D intoxication, thyrotoxicosis, granulomatous disease, metastatic bone cancer, or even immobilization
    - Elevated serum chloride: suggests hyperparathyroidism if serum bicarbonate is decreased
    - Decreased serum chloride: suggests milk-alkali syndrome if associated with metabolic alkalosis

■ Elevated amylase: associated with pancreatitis
- BUN and creatinine
- Alkaline phosphatase*: increased in malignancy, Paget's disease, and liver disease
- Serum protein electrophoresis*: to exclude multiple myeloma
- Intact PTH*: if elevated, indicates primary hyperparathyroidism; will also be elevated if patient is on lithium
- Vitamin D metabolites*: elevated vitamin D levels will cause hypercalcemia
- Urinary calcium*: elevated in hyperparathyroidism (may be high normal) or hypercalcemia of malignancy; decreased if related to thiazides, milk-alkali syndrome, or familial hypocalciuric hypercalcemia

Other Diagnostics
- ECG*: bradycardia, shortened QT interval, T wave inversion, or ventricular arrhythmias
- Chest radiograph*: to assess for malignancy and sarcoidosis
- Bone scan*: to evaluate for bony metastases and Paget's disease

Differential Diagnosis

The three most common causes of elevated serum calcium are primary hyperparathyroidism, malignancy, and milk-alkali syndrome. Usually, the history suggests the etiology of the hypercalcemia. Other causes to consider include:
- Addison's disease
- Drug toxicity (e.g., lithium, theophylline)
- Exogenous calcium intake (e.g., Tums, calcium supplement)
- Familial hypocalciuric hypercalcemia
- Granulomatous disease
- Primary and secondary hyperparathyroidism
- Pheochromocytoma
- Prolonged immobilization
- Malignancy
- Milk-alkali syndrome
- Paget's disease
- Renal failure
- Rhabdomyolysis
- Sarcoidosis or other chronic granulomatosis disease
- Thiazide diuretics
- Thyrotoxicosis
- Total parenteral nutrition (TPN)
- Vitamin A or D hypervitaminosis

*If indicated.

Treatment Plan

- Treatment is aimed at restoring the serum calcium levels to normal as well as treating the underlying pathology.
- Emergent therapy requires IV N/S (0.9%) to restore hydration and increase calcium excretion. Concurrent furosemide was frequently given in the past, but is now only recommended if the IV fluid induces fluid overload.
- Medications should be reviewed and offending medicines discontinued after consultation with the physician.
- Dietary calcium should also be limited to 1 g/day, but dietary sodium increased (if tolerated by the patient) and fluid intake encouraged to at least 2 L/day.
- Eliminate exogenous calcium.
- Consider oral phosphate therapy, 1 to 3 g PO daily, with monitoring to prevent phosphate levels above 4 mg/dL.
- Hyperparathyroidism-induced hypercalcemia is treated with biphosphonates, phosphates, loop diuretics, and, when indicated, surgery.
- Malignancy-induced hypercalcemia is treated with antineoplastic therapy and pamidronate, etidronate, or zoledronic acid, all biphosphonates that inhibit osteoclastic activity. Currently, zoledronate, 4 mg IV over 15 minutes, is recommended, although careful monitoring for renal failure is necessary. Oral risedronate is currently under investigation for use in hypercalcemia, and the biphosphonates are in some circumstances being given to cancer patients to prevent hypercalcemia. Calcitonin may also be used in combination with the biphosphonates for malignancy-induced hypercalcemia, although there is a significant risk for tachyphylaxis.
- Renal failure may require hemodialysis.
- Sarcoidosis and granulomatous disease are treated with a low-calcium diet and steroid therapy.

Consultation/Hospitalization

- **Physician consultation is indicated for serum calcium levels > 10.5 mg/dL (or ionized calcium > 5 mEq/L) and to discuss appropriate diagnostic testing and medical management.**
- Consultation with an oncologist is recommended for malignancy-induced hypercalcemia.
- An endocrinology consult is indicated for patients with hyperparathyroidism or thyrotoxicosis.
- Nephrology consultation is indicated for hypercalcemia related to renal failure.
- Hospitalization is indicated for severe hypercalcemia (> 12 mg/dL) requiring aggressive IV N/S hydration.

Complications

When appropriately treated, hypercalcemia is reversible, although in patients with advanced malignancy, patients and families may not desire aggressive treatment. Complications include ataxia, mental status changes, weakness, pathologic fractures, obstipation, ileus, cardiac arrest, renal failure, and death. Complications are also associated with some recommended therapies, and, therefore, careful monitoring is necessary.

Education for Nursing Home/Rehabilitation Staff

- Nurses should be able to recognize the symptoms associated with hypercalcemia and recognize the importance of discussing these symptoms with the healthcare provider.
- Explain to nursing staff the importance of promptly notifying the healthcare provider of any laboratory abnormalities.
- Explain to nursing staff that excessive antacid therapy (e.g., Tums) may cause hypercalcemia.

Patient/Family Education

- It is important to explain to both patients and families that symptoms associated with hypercalcemia often can be reversed with appropriate therapy. However, hypercalcemia associated with malignancy is an ominous sign.
- The suspected cause of the hypercalcemia as well as expected diagnostics and therapy should also be explained.

Bibliography

Adeleye, O., et al. (2002). Hypernatremia in the elderly. *Journal of the National Medical Association, 94*(8), 701-705.

Agus, Z.S., et al. (2004). Treatment of hypercalcemia. *www.uptodate.com*. Accessed January 3, 2004.

Agus, Z.S. (2004). Causes and treatment of hyperphosphatemia. *www.uptodate.com*. Accessed January 3, 2004.

Agus, Z.S. (2004). Treatment of hypocalcemia. *www.uptodate.com*. Accessed January 3, 2004.

Agus, Z.S., et al. (2004). Treatment of hypercalcemia. *www.uptodate.com*. Accessed January 3, 2004.

Fabian, T.J., et al. (2004). Paroxetine-induced hyponatremia in older adults: A 12 week prospective study. *Archives of Internal Medicine, 164*(3), 327-332.

Fried, L.F., & Palevsky, P.M. (1997). Hyponatremia and hypernatremia. *Medical Clinics of North America, 81*(3), 585-609.

Green, D.M., et al. (2002). Serum potassium levels and dietary potassium as risk factors for stroke. *Neurology, 59*(3), 314-320.

Gross, P. (2001). Treatment of severe hyponatremia. *Kidney International, 60*, 2417.

Kang, S.K., et al. (2002). Pathogenesis and treatment of hypernatremia. *Nephron*, 92(suppl 1), 14-17.

Kruse, J.A., & Carlson, R.W. (1990). Rapid correction of hypokalemia using concentrated intravenous potassium chloride infusion. *Archives of Internal Medicine, 150*(3), 613-617.

Major, P., et al. (2001). Zolendroic acid is superior to pamidronate in treatment of hypercalcemia of malignancy: A pooled analysis of two randomized, controlled clinical trials. *Journal of Clinical Oncology, 19*(2), 558-567.

Mandal, A.K. (1997). Hematuria and hypokalemia. *Medical Clinics of North America, 81*(3), 641-652.

Narins, R.G., & Krisha, G.G. (1998). Disorders of water balance. In Stein, J.H, et al. (Eds.), *Internal Medicine*, (5th ed.). St. Louis: Mosby.

Rose, B.D. (2003). Treatment of hyperkalemia. *www.uptodate.com*. Accessed December 31, 2003.

Rose, B.D. (2003). Treatment of hypokalemia. *www.uptodate.com*. Accessed December 28, 2003.

Rosner, M.H. (2004). Severe hyponatremia associated with the combined use of thiazide diuretics and selective serotonin reuptake inhibitors. *American Journal of Medical Science, 327*(2), 109-111.

HYPERMAGNESEMIA

ICD-9: 275.2

Magnesium stimulates most carbohydrate enzyme reactions and is needed for protein synthesis, neuromuscular function, and cell membrane transfer of sodium and potassium. Normal magnesium levels range from 1.8 to 3 mg/dL, and increased levels are uncommon. However, elevations do occur and are associated with parenteral magnesium infusions (particularly in patients with renal failure), end-stage renal disease, rhabdomyolysis, adrenal insufficiency, primary hyperparathyroidism, hypercatabolic states, theophylline toxicity, lithium ingestion, milk-alkali syndrome, and increased oral intake of magnesium compounds such as antacids or cathartics.

History

Determining the past medical history, history of the current illness, and a review of all medications (prescribed and over-the-counter) is essential. Vitamins, antacids, and cathartics often contain magnesium and will cause hypermagnesemia if renal function is compromised. Most patients are asymptomatic, although nausea, vomiting, and muscle weakness are possible complaints. Other presenting symptoms include headache and sedation.

Physical Examination

Elevated serum magnesium levels affect physical findings. Confusion, lethargy, flushing, diaphoresis, and weak or absent tendon reflexes are not uncommon with moderately elevated serum magnesium levels. At higher levels, hypotension, arrhythmias, bradycardia, muscle paralysis, decreased levels of consciousness, complete heart block, and respiratory arrest are possible.

Diagnostics

Laboratory Evaluation
- Serum magnesium
- Serum electrolytes, BUN, and creatinine: assess for renal failure or concurrent hyperkalemia or hypercalcemia
- Serum creatine phosphokinase (CPK): if suspected rhabdomyolysis or tumor lysis syndrome
- Urine myoglobin: if suspected rhabdomyolysis or tumor lysis syndrome
- TSH: to exclude hypothyroidism

Other Diagnostics
- ECG: increased PT interval, prolonged QRS and Q-T interval, T-wave elevation, or heart block

Differential Diagnosis

- Acute and chronic renal failure
- Milk-alkali syndrome
- Excessive IV magnesium or oral magnesium-containing compounds
- Rhabdomyolysis: causes increased release of intracellular magnesium
- Tumor lysis syondrome: causes increased release of intracellular magnesium
- Hypothyroidism: uncommon cause of increased serum magnesium
- Hypoparathyroidism
- Lithium intoxication
- Skeletal muscle neoplasm
- Adrenal insufficiency: may cause secondary hypermagnesemia
- Severe diabetic ketoacidosis

Treatment Plan

The underlying cause must be determined and corrected. IV 0.9% N/S and IV furosemide are used emergently to increase magnesium excretion. IV calcium gluconate may also be necessary in acute hypermagnesemia. Patients with renal failure may require peritoneal or hemodialysis.

Consultation/Hospitalization

Hospitalization and/or physician consultation is indicated for patients with serum magnesium levels higher than normal and/or for symptoms suggesting neuromuscular toxicity.

Complications

Neuromuscular toxicity: muscle paralysis, coma, respiratory/cardiac arrest

Education for Nursing Home/Rehabilitation Staff

- Discuss with nursing staff the importance of avoiding magnesium containing antacids and laxatives in patients with renal insufficiency.
- Explain to nurses the importance of providing a safe environment for patients with hypermagnesemia and accompanying muscle weakness.

Patient/Family Education

- Discuss with families and patient the cause of the disorder and expected treatment.
- Explain the importance of avoiding antacids containing magnesium.

Bibliography

Agus, Z.S. (2004). Causes and treatment of hypermagnesemia. *www.uptodate.com*. Accessed February 1, 2004.

HYPOMAGNESEMIA

ICD-9: 275.3

Normal serum magnesium levels range from 1.8 to 3 mg/dL. Lowered magnesium levels may be related to malnutrition, alcoholism, decreased intake, GI disorders, chronic diarrhea, endocrine disorders, intestinal bypass surgery or other major surgery, increased renal excretion, or medications (e.g., diuretics, aminoglycoside antibiotics, cisplatin, amphotericin B). There is often a coexisting hypokalemia or hypocalcemia. Low magnesium levels do not always correlate with physical signs or symptoms so it is important to maintain a high degree of suspicion for patients at risk for this disorder.

History

Symptoms associated with hypomagnesemia may be vague. Confusion or mental status changes are possible. Other symptoms include anorexia, nausea, vomiting, diarrhea, vertigo, lethargy, weakness, increased heart rate, muscle cramps, paresthesias, and neuromuscular changes. A careful symptom analysis and a review of the past medical history and current medications are indicated. Most often, a lowered serum magnesium level is associated with medication or GI or renal losses.

Physical Examination

Hypomagnesemia may affect the cardiovascular system as well as the neuromuscular system. Magnesium is regulated by the intestine and kidneys; therefore, weight and vital signs should be obtained. Physical findings may include the following:

- Weight loss
- Eyes: nystagmus
- Cardiovascular: elevated blood pressure, tachycardia, irregular heartbeat
- Neuromuscular: agitation, confusion, depression, hallucinations, ataxia, clonus, slow or involuntary movements, tremors, tetany, increased reflexes, seizures, positive Chvostek sign, positive Trousseau sign, or positive Babinski

Diagnostics

Laboratory Evaluation

- Serum magnesium: levels not necessarily reflective of intracellular magnesium stores, but below normal serum levels are significant
- Serum glucose and serum electrolytes: hypokalemia often related to hypomagnesemia
- Serum calcium: hypocalcemia associated with hypomagnesemia

Other Diagnostics

- ECG: nonspecific T wave changes, tachycardia, premature atrial contractions, premature ventricular contractions, prolonged QT interval, or ventricular fibrillation

Differential Diagnosis

- Medications: diuretics, digoxin, aminoglycoside antibiotics, cisplatin, cyclosporine, amphotericin B, or excessive calcium intake
- Decreased food intake associated with alcoholism or malnutrition
- Conditions associated with impaired magnesium absorption: GI disorders (bowel resection, gastric bypass surgery, chronic diarrhea, GI fistulas, chronic bowel disorders)
- Conditions associated with excessive fluid loss: diabetic ketoacidosis, diuretic therapy, major surgery, primary hyperparathyroidism, primary aldosteronism

Treatment Plan

Treatment consists of correcting the underlying cause of the disorder. If the cause is related to a medication, changing the medication should be considered. However, this may not always be practical. The serum magnesium must also be repleted: orally, intramuscularly, or IV. Hospitalization is usually recommended for IV replacement as continuous monitoring for decreased respirations, diaphoresis, flaccidity, and other signs of hypermagnesemia is essential. Slo-Mag

64 mg PO two to four times daily may be administered to patients with asymptomatic hypomagnesemia. Monitor magnesium levels and correct as necessary. (Some patients will require higher doses of magnesium daily.)

Consultation/Hospitalization

- **Physician consultation is indicated for serum magnesium levels < 0.5 mg/dL.**
- Hospitalization is indicated for patients with severe hypomagnesemia, neuromuscular symptoms, or cardiac arrhythmias.

Complications

- Digoxin toxicity is associated with low serum magnesium.
- Respiratory failure can occur with IV administration of magnesium.

Education for Nursing Home/Rehabilitation Staff

- Discuss with nurses the importance of reporting mental status changes, clonus, paresthesias, new tremors, involuntary writhing or twisting movements, tetany, or seizures.
- Discuss with nurses the importance of promptly reporting abnormal laboratory values.
- Explain to nurses the importance of continuously monitoring patients receiving IV magnesium and stopping the infusion immediately if untoward signs occur.

Patient/Family Education

- Explain to patients and families the importance of reporting new symptoms promptly.
- Discuss the cause of the lowered magnesium level and explain necessary treatments to patients and families.

Bibliography

Agus, Z.S. (2004). Diagnosis and treatment of hypomagnesemia. *www.uptodate.com*. Accessed February 12, 2004.

FLUID DISORDERS AND INTRAVENOUS THERAPY

ICD-9: 276.5 (DEHYDRATION)

Hypervolemia and the hypovolemic fluid disorders occur frequently in nursing home and rehabilitation settings. The origin of these fluid disturbances is multifactorial, but the resulting imbalance in both fluid and electrolytes is particularly harmful, especially for elderly patients.

HYPOVOLEMIA

Hypovolemia is commonly associated with bleeding from an injury or trauma. However, hypovolemia may result from any condition that causes a reduction in the amount of extracellular fluid: poor fluid intake, diaphoresis, vomiting, diarrhea, polyuria, excessive diuretic or laxative use, burns, bleeding, draining wounds, or third spacing from ascites, pancreatitis, or peritonitis. There are three types of hypovolemia associated with an extracellular fluid deficit: hypertonic hypovolemia, isotonic hypovolemia, and hypotonic hypovolemia. The consequence of these disorders is a decrease in tissue perfusion and its effect on the brain and other vital organs.

Dehydration, a hypertonic fluid deficit, is the most common fluid and electrolyte disorder in elders. Characterized by a serum sodium > 145 mEq/L and a serum osmolality > 295 mOsm/L, dehydration is associated with water loss and commonly occurs with fever and diaphoresis. Isotonic volume deficit or isotonic hypovolemia is most often related to vomiting and diarrhea and is distinguished by a normal serum sodium and normal serum osmolality. Hypotonic hypovolemia, the hypotonic fluid deficit, occurs in patients with renal fluid losses, is often caused by overzealous use of diuretic medications, and is differentiated by a lowered serum sodium (< 135 mEq/L) and lowered serum osmolality (< 275 mOsm/L).

Risk Factors

- Physiologic changes in elderly patients
  - Decreased amount of total body water
  - Reduced renal sodium conservation
  - Diminished ability to excrete water
  - Increased antidiuretic hormone
  - Increased atrial natriuretic factor
  - Impaired thirst perception
  - Decreased lean body mass
  - Decreased glomerular filtration rate (GFR)
- Increased vulnerability
  - Increased age (particularly in patients > 85 years)
  - Female gender
  - Immobility
  - Dietary restrictions
  - Chronic and acute illness
  - Medications: diuretics, laxatives
  - Dysphagia: poor oral intake

- Issues in rehabilitation and long-term care settings
  - Limited amount of fluid consumed in 24 hours
  - Poor oral intake between meals
  - Lack of social supports
  - Inattention to cultural and individual patient preferences for fluids and foods
  - Knowledge deficit of nursing assistants and staff who may not understand the importance of adequate hydration
  - Inadequate staffing ratios

History

The most common presenting symptom in elderly patients is a change in mental status or a decrease in activities of daily living (ADLs). Significant history necessary to elicit includes the source of fluid loss (vomiting, diarrhea, polyuria, fever), thirst, dizziness, syncope, fatigue, constipation, oliguria, or other symptoms, current medications, and past medical history.

Physical Examination

The patient's history and a thorough physical examination assist in diagnosis and management. Marked physical weakness and confusion/delirium can be associated with fluid deficits.

- If possible, the weight should be obtained, as an acute weight loss > 3 lb (or 3% to 5% of body weight) over 3 days is a significant sign of fluid deficit.
- Vital signs including temperature, postural blood pressure, and heart rate should be obtained.
  - Elderly patients can normally have orthostatic hypotension and thus postural changes may not be a reliable indication of fluid status.
  - Some elderly and immunocompromised patients will not have temperature elevation, despite infection.
- Skin: poor skin turgor can be an unreliable sign of hypovolemia in older patients, but dry skin, especially in the axilla, may be indicative of hypovolemia. In elderly patients, the more reliable areas to check skin turgor include the forehead and sternal area.
- Pharynx: lips and tongue are often dry, cracked, or furrowed.
- Cardiac: tachycardia may be present. Jugular vein pressure (JVP) is decreased.
- Pulmonary: respiratory rate may be increased.
- Abdomen: pain on exam may indicate ischemia from hypoperfusion or ascites.
- Rectal: test for occult blood.
- Extremities: cold, clammy, cyanotic extremities are a sign of hypoperfusion.

- Urine output may be < 30 mL/hour, or if polyuria (> 3L/24 hours) is present may be > than expected.

Diagnostics

Serum osmolality should be calculated (2[Na] + glucose/18 + BUN/2.8) to determine if patient has hypertonic, isotonic, or hypotonic fluid deficit. Suggested diagnostics include:
- Serum glucose
- Serum electrolytes
  - Serum Na is elevated in dehydration, normal in isotonic hypovolemia, and below normal in hypotonic hypovolemia.
  - Serum potassium is elevated in renal failure, adrenal insufficiency, and certain metabolic states; but lowered with increased renal or GI losses.
- BUN and creatinine: increased BUN: creatinine ratio (> 20:1) is suggestive of volume deficit.
- CBC/diff (hemoconcentration may cause elevated hematocrit)
- Urine for sodium, specific gravity, osmolality, urinalysis
- Arterial blood gases (ABGs)*: hypokalemia can cause metabolic acidosis

Differential Diagnosis

The differential diagnosis includes assessment of the serum osmolality and total water loss as well as establishing the etiology of the water deficit.
- Assessment of total body water loss is determined by calculating the fluid deficit (Box 10-2)
- The serum sodium and calculated serum osmolality facilitates differentiation of the water deficit as hypertonic, isotonic, or hypotonic (Box 10-3).

Treatment Plan

Treatment is based on assessment of total body water loss (see Box 10-2), serum electrolytes, and serum osmolality (2[Na] + glucose/18 + BUN/2.8), as well as the precipitating cause.

BOX 10-2	Calculated Fluid Deficit for Elders

For men: 0.5 × [current weight in kg] × [serum Na/140 − 1]
For women: 0.45 × [current weight in kg] × [serum Na/140 − 1]).

---

*If indicated.

BOX 10-3   Differential Diagnosis Fluid Deficits

Hypertonic hypovolemia
  Dehydration
Isotonic hypovolemia
  Renal losses
  Extrarenal losses
  Vomiting/diarrhea
Hypotonic hypovolemia
  Renal fluid losses
    Diuretics

- Mild dehydration is associated with a 1- to 2-L fluid loss. If the patient is able to take oral fluids and does not have a GI disorder:
  - Provide an extra 1000 to 1500 mL/day in addition to the recommended daily oral intake
  - Hold diuretics and laxatives
  - Monitor I&O, daily weight, and daily Chem 7 until patient is stable, laboratory values are normal, and patient is adequately hydrated for 48 hours.
  - Consider hypodermoclysis (Box 10-4): 500 mL to 1500 mL 0.9% N/S (0.45% N/S may also be used) subcutaneous fluid replacement may be given twice in 24 hours
    - Maximum amount of fluid infused in one site should not exceed 1500 mL/24 hours, but 3000 mL can be infused daily in two different sites.
    - Preferred rate of infusion is 1 mL/minute. (Hypodermoclysis is not appropriate for patients who are significantly dehydrated or hypotensive.)
    - For patients with associated hypokalemia, may add 20 to 40 mEq KCl per 1 L IV fluid.
    - Hyaluronidase, 15 units per 100 mL N/S (150 U/L), increases the subcutaneous absorption of the subcutaneous fluid.
- Significant fluid loss
  - Isotonic IV fluid (0.9% N/S) if patient is hypotensive, mildly hyponatremic, or normonatremic.
    - Hypotensive patients with obvious hemodynamic compromise (supine hypotension, tachycardia with weak pulse) should receive rapid infusion of IV 0.9% N/S until blood pressure is stabilized at baseline, tachycardia is resolved (< 100/minute), and urine output is approaching 30 mL/hour. Further fluid replacement should follow the guidelines that follow.
  - Hypotonic IV fluid (0.45% N/S or D_5W) if patient is hypernatremic.

BOX 10-4   Hypodermoclysis

- Supplies
  - Povidone-iodine solution
  - Sterile gloves
  - Occlusive dressing
  - 21- or 23-gauge butterfly needle
  - Intravenous (IV) fluid/IV tubing connected and primed with appropriate IV fluid
  - IV pump
- Procedure
  - Using aseptic technique, prepare an area with adequate subcutaneous tissue (abdomen, outer thigh, upper outer arm, or scapula area). Area should be carefully cleaned, then swabbed in a circular motion from center of site for at least 1 minute with povidone-iodine solution (if patient not allergic). A 21- to 23-gauge butterfly needle is then inserted at a 45- to 60-degree angle into the subcutaneous tissue (blood should not be present in needle; if blood is present, needle should be withdrawn and procedure restarted with new butterfly needle), connected to the intravenous solution and IV pump to run at maximum 1 mL/minute.
- Cover site with occlusive dressing, label with date and time, and check patient hourly for edema, erythema, or leakage at insertion site as well as for signs of fluid overload.
  - An area of edema at insertion site can be gently massaged to facilitate absorption, if necessary.
- IV tubing should be changed per institution policy (usually every 3 days)

Data from Sasson, M., & Shvartzman, P. (2001). Hypodermoclysis: An alternate infusion technique. *American Family Physician, 64,* 1575–1578.

- ■ 0.45% N/S is preferable for patients with diarrhea or other fluid deficits associated with both salt and water loss; D_5W can be used for patients with diabetes insipidus and other disorders associated with pure water loss, but hyperglycemia must be avoided with D_5W.
- ■ Maximum serum Na should be decreased is 0.5 mEq/L/hour.
- Replace maintenance fluids, plus $1/2$ deficit over the first 24 hours; the remainder of the deficit can be replaced over the next 48 to 72 hours. If patient has a history of CHF or is a frail elder, it may be prudent to replace 25% to 30% of deficit per day.
- Hold diuretics and laxatives
- Regular assessment of blood pressure, heart rate, and respiratory rate
- Accurate I&O and daily weight
- Daily serum glucose, electrolytes, BUN, and creatinine while on IV therapy to monitor electrolytes and serum osmolality.

- Replace potassium appropriately, but it is important to remember that the addition of potassium to IV fluid can change the osmolality of the IV fluid.

Consultation/Hospitalization

- Consultation with the physician is recommended if IV fluid resuscitation is necessary or if hypodermoclysis is a consideration.
- Hospitalization should be considered for patients with significant volume loss.

Complications

- Cerebral edema, manifested by acute confusion or other change in mental status, may occur if the serum osmolality is corrected too quickly.
- CHF may result from zealous IV fluid resuscitation.
- Hyponatremia and other electrolyte imbalances may occur with IV fluid resuscitation.

Education for Nursing Home/Rehabilitation Staff

- Discuss with nurses the importance of regularly monitoring patients receiving IV fluid for signs and symptoms of fluid overload (shortness of breath, dyspnea, cough, increased respiratory rate, hypoxia, cyanosis) and signs of infection at IV or hypodermoclysis insertion site.
- Explain to nurses that elderly patients often need assistance to drink fluids and that the minimum oral intake for most patients who are not ill is 1200 to 1500 mL/day. Patients who are ill require increased fluid intake.
- Discuss with nursing staff importance of accurate I&O, weights, and vital signs to monitor patient progress.

Patient/Family Education

It is important to explain the cause and treatment of the fluid deficit with the patient and family. Patient/family wishes for hospitalization should also be discussed.

HYPERVOLEMIA

Any disorder that causes fluid retention can result in fluid overload. Fluid volume overload may be related to several causes: increased sodium ingestion and retention, decreased cardiac output, hepatic or renal insufficiency, or hypothyroidism.

History

Medical history may be pertinent and should be elicited along with medication and allergy history. Patients may be asymptomatic or complain of increased fatigue, anorexia, paroxysmal nocturnal dyspnea (PND), shortness of breath, dyspnea on exertion, orthopnea, edema, or weight gain.

Physical Examination

Physical signs may be elusive as patients often have unrecognized hypervolemia, particularly in chronic heart failure. Thus, even subtle patient changes require a careful physical examination. *Possible* physical findings include:
- Change in mental status: inattentiveness or aphasia
- Weight gain
  - Mild fluid volume excess = 2% weight gain
  - Moderate fluid volume excess = 5% weight gain
  - Severe fluid volume excess = 8% weight gain
- Vital signs: hypertension, tachycardia, tachypnea, and hypoxia possible
- Decreased urinary output
- Skin: warm/moist/flushed, anasarca, jaundice (if liver failure), or spider angiomas
- Hair: coarse, thin hair or alopecia suggests hypothyroidism
- Eyes: periorbital edema/ptosis suggests hypothyroidism/myxedema
- Cardiac: tachycardia, S_3,S_4 gallop, or distended neck veins
- Pulmonary: wheezes or rales
- Abdominal: ascites or hepatomegaly
- Extremities: note peripheral pulses; unilateral edema suggests deep vein thrombophislebitis, lymphedema, filariasis, or lymphangitis; bilateral extremity edema more prevalent in cardiac failure, nephrotic syndrome, hypoalbuminemia, or cirrhosis.
- Neurologic: diminished mental status may indicate associated hyponatremia or hypothyroidism.

Diagnostics

Diagnostics are dependent on clinical presentation. A serum sodium < 135 mEq/L (rarely, hypervalemia is associated with an elevated level [> 145 mEq/L]) and serum osmolality < 275 mOsm/L suggest hypervolemia, as does a urine osmolality < the serum osmolality.

Laboratory Evaluation
- CBC/diff
- Serum glucose, serum electrolytes, and BUN and creatinine
- Calculation of serum osmolality: 2(Na) + Glucose/18 + BUN/2.8

- LFTs, including serum albumin and total protein
- TSH: to determine if hypothyroidism is present
- T$_4$*
- Urine for analysis and osmolality

Other Diagnostics
- Chest radiograph*
- ABGs*
- ECG*
- Ultrasound*

Differential Diagnosis

There are several causes of hypervolemia (Box 10-5). However, generalized edema suggests a cardiac, renal, hepatic, or nutritional etiology. Pretibial and/or periorbital edema may imply myxedema, although periorbital or facial edema can also reflect a nutritional abnormality, allergic reaction, or trichinosis. Facial edema accompanied by upper extremity edema may be a sign of superior vena cava obstruction. Localized edema suggests lymphedema, deep vein thrombosis, or obstruction. Hypernatremic hypervolemia is usually related to IV saline infusion, but it may be an effect of medication (e.g., ticarcillin).

BOX 10-5   Differential Diagnosis Hypervolemia

Cirrhosis
Congestive heart failure
Deep vein thrombosis (unilateral extremity edema)
Excessive salt intake
Hypoalbuminemia
Hypothyroidism (myxedemia coma)
Idiopathic
Intravenous therapy
Nephrotic syndrome
Obstruction of lymphatic or venous drainage
Parenteral nutrition
Renal failure
Renal insufficiency
Syndrome of inappropriate ADH

---

*If indicated.

Treatment Plan

Management is dependent on etiology and includes determination of serum sodium and serum osmolality. However, fluid and salt restriction are beneficial if the fluid overload is related to cardiac failure, cirrhosis, or nephrotic syndrome.

- Patients with CHF should be treated with diuretics and other medications as needed (see Chapter 5).
- Diuretic therapy may also be indicated in patients with cirrhosis or nephrotic syndrome, but this should be discussed with the physician.
- Patients with elevated TSH and suspected myxedema (hypothyroidism) require thyroid replacement therapy.
- Compression stockings may be used for comfort if the patient has adequate peripheral pulses.
- Fluid in the lower extremities may be reduced by having the patient lie in the supine position for 1 hour in the morning and 1 hour in the afternoon.
- Intake and output should be monitored.
- The cause of a lowered serum albumin should be determined. Procel, 1 scoop PO each day, ProMod 3 scoops PO each day, or another supplement may be helpful.
- For patients with hypervolemia associated with hypernatremia, correct the underlying cause. Discuss use of a loop diuretic to promote excretion of sodium and water with the physician.

Consultation/Hospitalization

- Hospitalization is indicated for patients with acute pulmonary edema, edema that suggests superior vena cava obstruction, and acute renal failure.
- Physician consultation is recommended if diuretic therapy is considered for treatment of nephrotic syndrome or cirrhosis.
- Hospitalization and therapy with IV levothyroxine are indicated for patients with myxedema coma.

Complications

- CHF/pulmonary edema/hypoxia
- Hydrothorax
- Neurologic changes
- Seizures
- Hypertension
- Skin breakdown from fluid retention

Education for Nursing Home/Rehabilitation Staff

- Explain to nursing staff importance of daily weights, salt and fluid restriction, and documentation of intake and output.

- Discuss with nursing staff importance of notifying healthcare provider if patient has a change in mental status.

Patient/Family Education

- Explain to patient and family the cause of the increased fluid volume and need for fluid and salt restriction.
- Discuss with patient and family treatment options and their associated risks and benefits.

Bibliography

Androne, A.S., et al (2004). Relationship of unrecognized hypervolemia in chronic heart failure to clinical status, hemodynamics, and patient outcomes. *American Journal of Cardiology, 93*(10), 1254-1259.

Kayser-Jones, J., et al. (1999). Factors contributing to dehydration in nursing homes: Inadequate staffing and lack of professional supervision. *Journal of American Geriatric Society, 47*(10), 1269-1270.

Post, T.W., & Rose, B.D. (2004). Clinical manifestations and diagnosis of volume depletion. *www.uptodate.com*. Accessed January 14, 2004.

Rose, B.D. (2004). Fluid replacement in volume depletion. *www.uptodate.com*. Accessed January 14, 2004.

Sasson, M., & Shvartzman, P. (2001). Hypodermoclysis: An alternative infusion technique, *American Family Physician, 64*, 1575-1578.

Singer, G.G., Brenner, B.M. (1998). Fluid and electrolyte disturbances. In Fauci, A.S., et al. (Eds.), *Harrison's principles of internal medicine* (14th ed). McGraw Hill.

CHAPTER 11

Hematologic Disorders

ANEMIA

ICD-9: 285.9

Anemia is fairly prevalent in nursing homes and rehabilitation settings, and is considered to be an indication of an underlying disorder. Patients may be symptomatic, but many times the lowered hemoglobin and hematocrit are found inadvertently. Patients are often asymptomatic until hemaglobin and hematocrit are very low. Once anemia is identified, it is vital to evaluate the cause, which, in some cases, may be multifactorial.

History

Prescribed herbals and over-the-counter (OTC) medications, as well as medical, employment, and family history should be reviewed, as the anemia may be long-standing or associated with work history, a medication, or ethnicity. Presentation may be acute and associated with bleeding or infection, or patients may be completely asymptomatic, particularly if the onset of the anemia is gradual. A sore mouth, fatigue, headache, tinnitus, angina, shortness of breath, dyspnea on exertion, constipation, diarrhea, and increased vulnerability to infections are common signs and symptoms.

Physical Examination

The physical examination may be unremarkable, but it is important to do a complete examination, because specific changes may aid in diagnosis. Weight and vital signs, including temperature and postural signs are essential. Possible findings (depending on etiology of anemia) may include:
- Weight loss or fever
- Skin: pale, jaundice, or petechiae

- Head, eyes, ears, nose, and throat (HEENT)
  - Eyes: pale conjunctiva or scleral icterus
  - Mouth: cheilosis, glossitis, or pale mucous membranes
  - Tongue: smooth and red in vitamin B_{12} deficiency; angular stomatitis or atrophy in iron deficiency anemia
  - Neck: masses or lymph nodes (enlarged, tender, or immobile)
- Cardiac: tachycardic even at rest; midsystolic or holosystolic flow murmur
- Lungs: tachypnea, rales (if congestive heart failure (CHF) is present)
- Abdomen: hepatomegaly; tender, enlarged spleen
- Rectal: positive occult blood or melena
- Extremities: spoon-shaped or brittle nails; palmar creases
- Musculoskeletal: bone pain or tenderness
- Neurologic: listlessness, irritability, inability to concentrate, confusion, decreased vibratory sense, poor finger coordination, hyperactive or hypoactive reflexes, positive Romberg's sign, and ataxia

Diagnostics

An anemia work-up should be expeditious and efficient. The complete blood count with differential (CBC/diff) is the most important test initially to evaluate the hemoglobin, hematocrit, white blood cell count, platelets, and mean corpuscular volume (MCV). Examination of the MCV differentiates the anemia as microcytic, normocytic, or macrocytic, although many anemias can be classified into more than one of these categories.

The peripheral smear and reticulocyte count also help differentiate anemias and should be part of the initial evaluation. An elevated reticulocyte count usually suggests acute blood loss or hemolysis unless the patient has an infection or problem that affects red blood cell production. A lowered reticulocyte count is consistent with hypoproliferative anemia (associated with bone marrow injury, iron deficiency, or diminished erythropoietin production) or a maturation disorder (microcytic or macrocytic anemia). Other tests that may be indicated include the following:

Laboratory Evaluation
- CBC/diff
  - Hemoglobin, hematocrit, red blood cell (RBC) count, RBC indices, white blood cell count with differential, and platelet count
- Peripheral smear
- Erythrocyte sedimentation rate (ESR)
- Reticulocyte count: to evaluate red blood cell production by bone marrow
  - Lowered in megaloblastic anemias
- Ferritin, serum iron, transferrin, and TIBC*: to evaluate iron stores

*If indicated.

- Ferritin: normal or increased in anemia of chronic disease; low in iron deficiency anemia; elevated in hemachromatosis, alcoholism, inflammatory disorders, and sometimes in anemia of chronic disease
- TIBC: increased in iron deficiency anemia; normal or decreased in anemia of chronic disease
- Serum iron: decreased in iron deficiency anemia and anemia of chronic disease
- Transferrin: may be acutely elevated in iron deficiency anemia; decreased with malignancy or infection
- Folate and B_{12}: deficient in macrocytic anemias
  - Methylmalonate and homocysteine levels*
    - May aid in diagnosis with borderline folate and B_{12} deficiency
    - Methylmalonate: elevated in B_{12} deficiency; normal in folate deficiency
    - Homocysteine: elevated in both folate and B_{12} deficiency
- Anti-intrinsic factor antibodies*: to identify pernicious anemia
- Thyroid-stimulating hormone (TSH)*: hypothyroidism is associated with pernicious anemia and diminished erythropoiesis
- Liver function tests (LFTs)*: increased aspartate transaminase and lactate dehydrogenase (LDH) in hypothyroidism (LDH increased in sickle cell disease)
- Coomb's (direct and indirect)*: hemolytic anemia
- Serum haptoglobin*: to detect hemolysis of red blood cells
- Creatinine*: chronic renal failure is associated with anemia of chronic disease myeloma
- Hemoglobin electrophoresis*: to identify hemoglobinopathies or thalassemias
- G6PD*: deficiency associated with hemolytic anemia
- Erythropoietin level*: decreased levels in anemia associated with renal disease
- Urinalysis*

Other Diagnostics
- Chest radiograph*
- Bone marrow aspiration*

Differential Diagnosis

As anemia is often multifactorial, it is essential to consider occult bleeding, hemolysis, iron insufficiency, and bone marrow suppression as potential causes. A careful history, physical examination, and laboratory review aid in determining the cause.

---

*If indicated.

Anemias are classified according to red blood cell morphology.
- Microcytic anemias (MCV < 80 fl)
  - Iron deficiency anemia
  - Thalassemia
  - Anemia of chronic disease (usually normocytic)
  - Myelodysplasia
  - Sideroblastic anemia
  - Hemoglobin E disease
- Macrocytic (megaloblastic) anemias (MCV > 100 fl)
  - Aplastic anemia
  - Alcohol abuse
  - Hypothyroidism
  - Myelodysplasia
  - Multiple myeloma
  - Acute myeloid leukemia
  - Vitamin B_{12} deficiency
  - Folate deficiency
  - Hemolytic anemia
  - Chronic liver disease
  - Medication induced (e.g., 6-mercaptopurine, hydroxyurea, methotrexate, AZT, some chemotherapeutic medications)
- Normocytic anemias (MCV 80 to 100 fl)
  - Acute blood loss
  - Anemia of chronic disease
    - Chronic renal disease or chronic infection; breast or lung cancer; Hodgkin's disease; rheumatoid arthritis and certain other noninfectious inflammatory disorders
  - Aplastic anemia
  - Iron deficiency anemia (typically microcytic)
  - Sickle cell disease
  - Hemolytic anemia
  - Endocrine disorders
    - Hypothyroidism
    - Adrenal insufficiency
    - Pituitary insufficiency
  - Myelodysplasia
  - Multiple myeloma
  - Myeloid metaplasia
  - Leukemia
  - Chronic liver disease (may also be macrocytic)

Anemia related to bleeding or hemorrhage
- Iatrogenic: repeated venesection
- Obvious
  - Hematemesis
  - Melena
  - Trauma

- Occult
  - Abdominal/retroperitoneal
  - Carcinoma
  - Polyp

Treatment Plan

Treatment of stable anemia is aimed at correcting the underlying condition. Severe anemia or anemia related to acute blood loss requires transfusion of erythrocytes and other supportive therapies to maintain blood pressure and tissue perfusion. Further treatment and recommendations are as follows.

Iron Deficiency Anemia

- Once the bleeding source in iron deficiency anemia is identified and corrected, supplemental iron should be given; the patient can begin taking ferrous sulfate 300 mg PO 30 minutes to 1 hour before eating. (Iron supplements are often given with vitamin C to enhance absorption.) Initially, the ferrous sulfate should be taken once a day, but can be increased by 2-week intervals to three times a day. Iron stores are usually replenished in about 6 months, although some patients may require lifelong treatment. Monthly evaluation of the hemoglobin, hematocrit, and ferritin is indicated. In patients with GI intolerance, ferrous gluconate or polysaccharide-iron complex (N.ferex) may be a better treatment. Patients who do not respond to treatment may require parenteral iron therapy. However, IV iron therapy requires careful continuous monitoring because side effects include anaphylaxis.

Normocytic Anemias

- Anemia of chronic disease
  - Anemia may be transient if related to an infection, but chronic renal insufficiency, chronic liver disease, and endocrine disorders are also associated with anemia of chronic disease.
  - Reticulocyte count low; iron and total iron-binding capacity (TIBC) are usually normal, but can be decreased; ferritin is normal or slightly elevated.
  - Treatment should be aimed at correcting the underlying disorder; otherwise, treatment is supportive and usually consists of erythro-poietin and periodic transfusions if indicated.
- Aplastic anemia, leukemia, myelodysplasia, or other suspected malignancies are associated with white blood cell and platelet abnormalities in addition to the anemia. If newly suspected, these disorders require immediate consultation with the physician or hematologist and may necessitate hospitalization.
- Hemolytic anemia occurs with many illnesses and may be autoimmune, idiopathic, or related to a medication.
  - Abnormally shaped red blood cells in association with a sudden decrease in hemoglobin, decreased serum haptoglobin, and increased LDH and indirect bilirubin strongly suggests hemolysis.

- If drug-induced, the offending drug must be avoided; other hemolytic anemias require evaluation by a hematologist.
- Folic acid is recommended for all patients with chronic hemolytic anemia.

Macrocytic Anemias

- B_{12} deficiency is associated with pernicious anemia, hydrochloric acid deficiency, gastrectomy, and autoimmune disorders. Treatment consists of 1000 mcg cyanocobalamin intramuscularly (IM) weekly for 2 months (8 weeks), followed by monthly injections. Oral cobalamin 1000 to 2000 mcg daily may be appropriate in some cases, but not in the presence of pernicious anemia. Sublingual and nasal forms of cobalamin are also available.
  - Serum potassium and phosphorus must be monitored and replenished during early stages of treatment.
- Folate deficiency may be related to hemolytic anemia, medication, nutritional status, or malabsorption and is treated with folic acid 1 mg PO daily. However, B_{12} deficiency must be excluded before treatment commences.
  - Folic acid 1 mg PO daily is indicated for patients with a history of partial/total gastrectomy.

Consultation/Hospitalization

- **Physician/hematology consultation and hospitalization are indicated for patients with active bleeding or anemia associated with postural vital sign changes.**
- Physician consultation is recommended for patients with coronary artery disease and hematocrit < 30%.
- Physician consultation is recommended for patients with suspected aplastic anemia, myelodysplasia, suspected malignancy, hemolytic anemia, or sickle cell crisis, or for patients who do not respond to treatment.
- Consultation with a hematologist is indicated for patients requiring parenteral iron therapy.
- Consult with physician and hospital to arrange transfusion with packed red blood cells when indicated. In elderly patients and patients with known heart disease, the goal hematocrit is > 26.

Complications

- Angina
- Arrhythmias
- CHF
- Falls
- Hypotension
- Myocardial infarction
- Pain: if sickle cell disorder

- Permanent neurologic injury can result from untreated or poorly treated B_{12} deficiency.
- Hypokalemia and hypophosphatemia may occur with treatment of B_{12} deficiency.
- Death

Education for Nursing Home/Rehabilitation Staff

- Discuss with nurses the importance of giving vitamin supplements as directed (e.g., before meals).
- Explain to nurses the importance of reporting signs and symptoms that might be associated with increased anemia.
- Explain the importance of monitoring stools for occult blood, as well as urine for hematuria.

Patient/Family Education

- Discuss with patients and families the nature of the anemia, expected diagnostics, and treatments.
- Patients need to understand the importance of reporting symptoms associated with anemia.
- Patients need to understand that treatment with oral cobalamin requires absolute adherence to the prescribed regimen.

Bibliography

Kuzminski, A.M., et al. (1998). Effective treatment of cobalamin deficiency with oral cobalamin. *Blood*, 92, 1191.

Mandell, E. (2003). Anemia. In Buttaro, T.M., et al. (2003). *Primary care: A collaborative practice* (2nd ed.). St. Louis: Mosby.

Schrier, S.L. (2004). Approach to the patient with anemia. *www.uptodate.com*. Accessed January 29, 2004.

Schrier, S.L. (2004). Diagnosis and treatment of vitamin B_{12} and folic acid deficiency. *www.uptodate.com*. Accessed January 31, 2004.

Smith, D. (2000). Anemia in the elderly. *American Family Physician*, 62(7), 1565-1572.

CHAPTER 12

Multisystem Disorders

FEVER

Fever may be related to infection, inflammation, or neoplasm. A temperature of 99.9° F or more is a common symptom of disease and is associated with many conditions. Very often, the cause of the fever is not immediately apparent. A fever higher than 101° F persisting beyond 3 weeks without a diagnosis despite intensive investigation is considered a fever of unknown origin (FUO).

In healthy people, temperatures are lowest around 6 AM and highest between 4 PM and 6 PM. Rectal temperatures, considered the most accurate, are approximately 1° higher than an oral temperature. However, many facilities no longer permit rectal temperatures and oral, axillary, or tympanic membrane temperatures are used. These temperatures are 1° to 2° lower than a rectal temperature.

Immunocompromised and elderly patients may not have elevated temperatures, despite severe infections. Although the most common infections in long-term care facilities are those of the respiratory or urinary tract, skin, or gastrointestinal (GI) systems, healthcare providers need to be aware of emerging and reemerging infections, such as food borne illnesses, human immunodeficiency virus (HIV), tuberculosis (TB), and drug-resistant microbes. The elderly and immunocompromised persons are particularly susceptible. Care should be taken to prevent the spread of infections, as well as manage patients with fever and prevent complications.

Risk Factors

- Age: elderly have impaired sweating mechanism and diminished ability to generate a temperature in response to illness
- Catheters: intravenous lines, indwelling catheters are a source of infection
- Flu season

- Ethnic origin: Mediterranean fever in Turkish, Arabic, Armenian, Sephardic Jews; recurring fevers in sickle-cell anemia in Africans, African Americans, Hispanics, and others whose ancestors originally lived in sub-Saharan Africa.
- Chemotherapy: compromised immune system
- Prosthetic devices, artificial joints, and artificial valves: increase risk for infection
- Poor dentition: mouth can be a major source of infection
- Impaired swallowing: increased risk for aspiration
- Feeding tubes: increased risk for aspiration
- HIV, cancer, and tumors: activity may cause increased temperature
- Intravenous (IV) drug use
- Malnutrition: adequate reserves to fight infection are depleted
- ETOH users: often malnourished
- Anemia: myelodysplasias can progress to an acute leukemia with fever
- Spinal cord injury or compromised mobility: increased risk for pneumonia, urinary tract infections (UTIs), pressure sores
- Other: peers/residents/family members/staff with contagious illness

History

Fevers are most often related to an infection, which, in some instances, may be dormant for many years. Malignancy and collagen-vascular disease are other common causes of fever. The history should include features of the fever as well as a review of allergies, medications (which can cause or relieve fevers), medical history, and possible recent or remote exposures. Pertinent aspects to consider include:

Onset
Onset may be related to a meal, injury, surgery, exposure, anesthesia, procedure, dental work, or catheter change. Recent antibiotic use may result in *Clostridium difficile* colitis, fungus, or drug reaction.

Characteristics/Course
- Intermittent temperature: returns to normal at least once a day
- Sustained daily temperature: common in viral or bacterial illness, non-infectious conditions, and chronic illness (e.g., TB, malignancy)
- Frequent temperature spikes: can be related to use of antipyretic or to abscesses
- Single temperature spike: can be related to blood transfusion or manipulation during a procedure
- Relapsing temperature comes and goes over several days or month-long cycles (common in lymphomas)

Accompanying Symptoms
- Night sweats: associated with TB
- Productive cough with yellow or green sputum: suggests respiratory infection

- Functional decline and mental status changes: common in the elderly
- Chills: common in bacterial infection
- Lymphadenopathy, myalgias, arthralgias, hemoptysis, headache, and masses: nonspecific symptoms associated with neoplasms, viruses, rheumatoid arthritis, and polymyalgia rheumatica
- Dysuria, hematuria, worsening incontinence, and frequency: may be present in UTI or renal cell carcinoma; increasing nocturia may suggest prostatitis
- Diarrhea or frequent, foul-smelling stool: common in C. *difficile* colitis
- Rash: may be present with herpes zoster, subacute bacterial endocarditis, or drug fever
- Nausea and vomiting: common in food-related infections, gastrointestinal infections, drug reactions, cholecystitis, pancreatitis
- Hyperglycemia: may be the only sign of underlying infectious process

Medical History

- Diabetes: are prone to UTIs; patients with diabetes are predisposed to trauma secondary to neuropathy; skin infections, otitis externa, and malignant otitis externa (an aggressive infection caused by *Pseudomonas*); and have associated vascular disease that may prevent adequate tissue repair
- COPD: at risk for exacerbation
- Dementia or cerebrovascular accident (CVA) with poor swallowing: dysphagia increases aspiration risk; immobility increases risk of pressure ulcers
- Prosthetic device: risk for infection
- Valvular disease: at risk for endocarditis
- Immunocompromised patients (HIV infection, chemotherapy, organ transplants, status post splenectomy) have increased infection risk
- Transfusion: reactions
- Prostate disease: at risk for obstruction with infection
- Chronic leukemia: may be associated with high fever
- Cancer: tumor activity generates fever
- Decubitus ulcer or open wound: at risk for infection
- Immunization status: question when last flu/pneumovax vaccine was given
- Malaria: recurring fevers
- Dental caries or recent dental work
- Recent surgery
- Medications: antipyretics mask temperature; drug fever may be related to diuretics, stool softeners, sleeping meds, antiarrhythmics, antibiotics, thyroid medications, and phenytoin; prednisone increases white blood cell count (WBC) and may cause low-grade temperature

Physical Examination

The physical examination must be systematic and thorough to determine the source of the fever as well as the patient's response to the fever. Important facets of the examination that may suggest a source of the fever include:

- Constitutional: mental status changes, shivering/rigors, diaphoresis

- Weight: weight loss may suggest dehydration, malignancy
- Vital signs
  - Degree of fever
  - Tachycardia: heart rate increases approximately four beats for every degree of temperature elevation
  - Tachypnea: frequent in pneumonia
  - Blood pressure: hypotension in dehydration and sepsis
- Head, eyes, ears, nose, and throat (HEENT) evaluation
  - Facial asymmetry present in cellulitis, dental infection, malignant otitis externa, and enlarged parotid
  - Eyes: scleral icterus associated with pancreatitis, hepatitis, cholycystitis, and obstruction in bile duct; conjunctival injection in presence of petechiae may signify drug reaction or conjunctivitis
  - Ears: otitis externa, otitis media, and mastoid tenderness
  - Nose: erythema, edema, and sinus tenderness
  - Mouth: dental abscesses, gingivitis, *Candida*, pharyngitis, parotid abscess
  - Neck: thyroid tender with sore throat, dysphagia, and thyroiditis; decreased range of motion (ROM) with encephalitis and meningitis; generalized lymphadenopathy with infections; isolated lymphadenopathy with malignancy
- Cardiac: regurgitant, new murmur in subacute bacterial endocarditis (SBE); pericardial friction rub; signs of high-output heart failure common with febrile illness
- Lungs: cough, decreased oxygen saturation, and decreased breath sounds; consolidation in pneumonia
- Abdomen
  - Increased bowel sounds with gastroenteritis
  - Decreased bowel sounds with obstruction or ileus
  - Hepatosplenomegaly with tenderness in hepatitis, splenomegaly with malignancy; mass in malignancy
  - Tenderness in right upper quadrant (RUQ) with cholecystitis or pancreatitis (common in elderly)
  - Tenderness with abscess, appendicitis, or diverticulitis
  - Abdominal rigidity with bowel, abscess, or appendix rupture
  - Costovertebral angle (CVA) tenderness with pyelonephritis
  - Ascites may be source of fever
  - Gentle rectal examination to exclude abscess or prostatitis
- Genitourinary (GU): suprapubic tenderness, hematuria, or cloudy urine
  - Indwelling Foley catheters increase risk for UTI and prostatitis
- Extremities
  - Check IV sites for erythema, edema, and lymphangitis
  - Unilateral edema and tenderness, suggesting deep vein thrombosis (DVT)

- Musculoskeletal
  - Joint effusions with erythema, tenderness, and/or edema in gout or septic joint
  - Spinal tenderness: possible tumor or abscess
- Neurologic: mental status changes or nuchal rigidity
- Skin: assess for cellulitis, folliculitis, rash, bullous lesions, splinter hemorrhages, petechiae, and herpetic lesions

Differential Diagnosis

- Infection: viral versus bacterial
  - Upper respiratory infection, sinusitis, pneumonia, UTI, skin infection, herpes zoster, cellulitis, flu, TB, wound infections (recent surgery or open area), prosthetic device such as knee or hip replacement, vascular graft, indwelling portal catheter, diarrhea (after antibiotic use with *C. difficile*), diarrhea (food poisoning, gastroenteritis), endocarditis, post-IV drug use (hepatitis, sepsis), diverticulitis (may be bloody stool), yeast infection, or parotitis
- Noninfectious: inflammation, thyroid toxicosis, systemic lupus erythematosus (SLE), rheumatoid arthritis (RA), polymyalgia rheumatica (PMR), giant cell arteritis (GCA), familial Mediterranean fever (people of Turkish, Arabic, Armenian, or Sephardic Jewish origin), inflammatory bowel, gout/ pseudogout, sarcoid, DVT, or anemia (sickle cell)
- Drug-related: diuretics, stool softeners, sleep medications, antiarrhythmic medications, antibiotics, thyroid medications, phenytoin (Dilantin), steroids, or immunosuppressants
- Neoplasm: leukemia, lymphomas, myelodysplasia, renal cell carcinoma, liver metastases, central nervous system metastases with disturbance in temperature-regulating mechanisms, or tumors
- Other
  - Environmental: recent hot drink or cigarette
  - Factitious: attention-seeking behaviors
  - Pulmonary embolus
  - Transfusion reaction
  - Status post head injury
  - Pheochromocytoma
  - Recent general anesthesia

Diagnostics

Depending on the patient's choice for care and the diagnostic availability (results may be difficult to obtain expeditiously) in the facility, the patient may need evaluation in the acute care facility.

If obtainable, immediate results from the following diagnostics can aid in diagnosis.

- Complete blood count (CBC) with differential: leukocytosis (WBC > 14,000) and left shift (bands > 6%) indicate bacterial infection; blasts may signify acute leukemia; neutropenia with associated fever suggests possible bacterial or fungal infection
- Serum glucose, electrolytes, blood urea nitrogen (BUN), and creatinine: determine renal status, dehydration; blood sugar may be elevated in infection; sodium increased in dehydration
- Urinalysis: dipstick if available; urine culture if positive leukocyte esterase and >10,000 WBCs; if patient ill and UTI is suspected, start antibiotic for 3 days while awaiting culture and sensitivities
- Blood cultures (aerobic and anaerobic) if rigors: usually two to three sets drawn at different times from different sites; antibiotic therapy may be indicated after blood cultures are drawn while awaiting results
- Joint aspiration culture and sensitivity*
- Chest radiograph: rule out pneumonia (if patient dehydrated, pneumonia may not be visualized), atelectasis, TB, sarcoidosis, tumors, and heart failure
- Computed tomography (CT) scan*: for abdominal tenderness
- Magnetic resonance imaging (MRI): if suspected cranial infection
- Nasal swab: for flu

If patient is not acute and diagnosis is unclear, consider:

- LFTs, amylase, and lipase*: to exclude cholecystitis, pancreatitis
- Erythrocyte sedimentation rate (ESR): although nonspecific, may suggest PMR or RA in presence of muscle/joint pain
- HIV antibody assay and HIV viral load*: for patients at risk for HIV infection (must have patient consent)
- Antinuclear antibody (ANA): if connective tissue disease is suspected
- Rheumatoid factor: if RA is suspected
- Uric acid: if gout is suspected
- Sputum culture*
- Stool *C. difficile* toxin × 3: if diarrhea is related to history of antibiotic therapy
- Stool culture: if no history of antibiotic use and severe, persistent diarrhea
- PPD: to exclude TB
- Lumbar puncture: if meningitis is suspected
- Kidney, ureter, and bladder (KUB) x-ray; abdominal, pelvic, or renal ultrasound; or abdominal CT: to determine presence of abdominal abscess, hepatobiliary disease, and kidney or abdominal tumors
- Doppler ultrasound: if DVT is suspected
- Biopsy
  - Temporal artery: if GCA is suspected
  - Liver biopsy: if sarcoid is suspected

*If indicated.

- Lymph node biopsy: if lymphoma or malignancy is suspected
- Bone marrow biopsy

Treatment Plan

An elderly patient with an acute temperature greater than 103° F should be sent to an acute care facility. For patients who can be cared for in the facility or refuse acute care hospitalization, it is important to determine an underlying, treatable cause of the fever while keeping the patient comfortable.

- Decrease temperature.
    - Tylenol 650 mg PO or PR every 4 hours PRN (use with caution if following fever trend)
    - Cool environment with fans and/or air conditioning
- Judicious use of antibiotics
    - If suspected UTI and patient able to drink and take oral medications: see Chapter 7
        - Ciprofloxacin 250 to 500 mg PO BID × 7 days (dosage dependent on creatinine clearance) *or*
        - Bactrim DS 1 PO BID × 7 days (monitor fluid status and BUN and creatinine)
    - If suspected *C. difficile* colitis: see Chapter 6
    - If suspected pneumonia: see Chapter 4
    - If suspected flu: see Chapter 4
- If suspected drug-related fever: stop potential causative medications for 72 hours and monitor temperature
- If suspected PMR: see Chapter 12
- If suspected gout: consider nonsteroidal antiinflammatory drugs (NSAIDs), colchicine (caution with renal function) or steroids
- Hydration: may need IV fluid (see Chapter 10)
- Nutrition: as patient can tolerate
- Monitor temperatures until patient has been afebrile 48 to 72 hours.
- Isolation per institution protocol

Consultation/Hospitalization

- If fever does not respond to treatment, consult with MD and consider hospitalization if patient/family agree.
- If diagnosis indicates abdominal process requiring surgery, consult with surgeon and hospitalize.
- Hospitalization is indicated for sepsis/shock, especially if patient exhibits lethargy or mental status changes and if patient/family agree.
- Consult with physician to determine if hospitalization is indicated for infection with resistant organisms.
- Hospitalization is indicated for infective endocarditis, necrotizing fasciitis, bacterial meningitis, acute viral encephalitis, and acute leukemia because rapid deterioration may occur.

- Consider GU evaluation for a male patient with a UTI.
- Consultation with a rheumatologist is recommended if joint aspiration is indicated.
- If diagnosis is obscure and patient is not acting ill, consult physician for referral and further workup. Diagnostics that should be included are:
  - Transesophageal ECHO: if endocarditis is suspected
  - Bone marrow biopsy: if abnormality in CBC
  - Liver biopsy: if indicated
  - Temporal artery biopsy: if GCA is suspected
  - Bone scan or biopsy: if osteomyelitis is suspected
  - Positron emission tomography (PET) scan: if indicated
  - MRI/CT: if a tumor is suspected
- If available, consider consult with infectious disease specialist for questions regarding antibiotic therapy.

Complications

- Sepsis
- Dehydration
- Delirium
- Seizures
- Falls
- Shock
- SBE can occur if initial infection is not treated promptly and effectively in susceptible patients.
- Heart failure: infection stresses a weak cardiovascular system
- Decrease in function secondary to fatigue
- Death

Education for Nursing Home/Rehabilitation Staff

- Explain importance of monitoring patient for functional decline (e.g., not eating, constipation), mental status changes, diarrhea, and/or restlessness and notifying healthcare provider.
- Discuss the rationale for removing oxygen before taking PO temperatures.
- Review the importance of universal precautions and good handwashing.
- Discuss importance of proper equipment and Foley catheter care, with particular emphasis on cleanliness.
- Review vital signs and implications of elevated temperature, tachycardia, tachypnea, lowered or elevated blood pressure, lowered oxygen saturation. Reiterate the importance of notifying the healthcare provider with changes.
  - Check temperature daily if patient is on chemotherapy, immuno-suppressed, or taking chemotherapeutic drug. Report temperature rise immediately. Discuss with nurses the fact that elders' baseline temperature may be lower than normal; thus, a 2° increase in temperature (even if temperature is now only 99°) may be significant.

- Emphasize the importance of activity, good hygiene, and adequate hydration to prevent infections.
- Initiate an infection control program with the nursing staff to isolate infected persons and materials.
  - Attempt to keep contagious persons away from patients during flu season.
  - Try to keep people with coughs out of dining room and social areas.
- Review decubiti care and prevention with staff.
- Explain the value of good mouth care.
- Update flu and Pneumovax immunizations, as well as PPD testing.

Patient/Family Education

Discuss with patients and families the importance of:
- Good dental care
- Hydration to prevent UTI and to treat infections
- Good hygiene to prevent UTI
- Exercise and sleep to enhance immune system

Educate patients and families about:
- Antibiotic use and their associated side effects
- The risk of resistant organisms
- Deferring patient visits if there is a risk of illness
- The importance of handwashing
- Antibiotic prophylaxis if risk of SBE

Bibliography

American Geriatrics Society. (2001). Practice guideline for evaluation of fever and infection in long-term care facilities. *http://www.americangeriatrics.org*. Retrieved April 14, 2004.

Freshman, M. (2003). Fever. In Buttaro, T.M., et al. (2003). *Primary care: A collaborative practice* (pp. 1156-1159). St. Louis: Mosby.

Glaser, V. (2000). Emerging infections. New pathogens and changing resistance patterns. *Patient Care for the Nurse Practitioner, 34*(7), 24-40.

Morrison, R.E., Lewis, J.B. (2004). Fever: Sorting out the potentially dangerous causes. *Consultant, 44*(2), 245-255.

POLYMYALGIA RHEUMATICA

ICD-9: 725

PMR is an inflammatory synovitis seen most often in persons older than age 50. This disorder is more common in white females in northern Europe and northern United States and may last several weeks or several years. Inflammation occurs in proximal joints and periarticular structures. The recurrent and chronic disorder is characterized by the following: pain and stiffness in the neck, shoulders, and hips; constitutional symptoms in a third of cases; an elevated ESR; and a speedy, dramatic response to corticosteroids. About 15% to 20% of patients with PMR have giant cell arteritis (GCA) or temporal arteritis, a medical emergency related to the risk of vision loss. Providers must be alert to assess for GCA, considered to be a similar inflammatory process that affects the arteries.

Risk Factors

- GCA: 40% to 50% of patients with GCA have symptoms of PMR
- Age: 90% of patients with PMR are older than 60 years of age.
- Gender: affects up to twice as many women as men
- Race: more common in white women
- Multiple environmental and genetic factors influence susceptibility and severity
- Family history

History

The symptom analysis is crucial. The onset of PMR can be abrupt or prolonged. The disorder is characterized by early morning stiffness (lasting 1 to 3 hours) and stiffness after rest. There is symmetric pain and stiffness in the neck (50% to 70% of cases), shoulders (70% to 90% of cases), and hips (50% to 70% of cases), as well as gelling (slow initiation of mobility after a period of rest).

Accompanying symptoms include:

- Fever, malaise, weight loss, anorexia, fatigue, muscle pain, and headache
- Headache, jaw claudication, and visual changes (may indicate temporal arteritis [GCA])
- Limited mobility and limited activity, difficulty rising from a chair, difficulty dressing, and difficulty turning in bed

Physical Examination

Positive physical findings are variable. Important features to determine include:

- Constitutional: fatigued look
- Vital signs: low-grade temperature
- Eyes: disc pallor; cotton wool spots; retinal hemorrhages possible with GCA
- Musculoskeletal
  - Observe for edema in wrists, hands, feet, and ankles, not accompanied by erythema; gelling or stiffness when arising from chair.
  - Palpation: muscle tenderness is nonspecific and nondiagnostic; synovitis present in up to a third of patients, usually in wrists or knees
  - ROM: carpal tunnel syndrome is common; frozen shoulder is common; decreased ROM in neck, shoulders and hips, usually symmetric, with pain; pain prevents patient from holding arms in horizontal position
- Peripheral vascular: temporal arteries may be tender with diminished or absent pulses in GCA; carotid bruits may be present with GCA.

- Neurologic: no change in muscle strength; no muscle atrophy
- Functional changes

Differential Diagnosis

- RA: difficult to differentiate when rheumatoid factor is negative. Patients with symmetric synovitis of proximal interphalangeal (PIP), metacarpal (MCP), and metatarsal (MTP) joints are not likely to have PMR. Radiograph may show joint erosion strengthening the diagnosis of RA.
- Polymyositis: muscle weakness, muscle atrophy, and abnormal muscle enzymes
- Multiple myeloma: abnormal serum protein electrophoresis
- Hypothyroid: abnormal thyroid function test (TFT) with fatigue, lethargy, and often weight gain
- Fibromyalgia: more common in younger persons; presence of irritable bowel syndrome (IBS); trigger point pain; normal ESR
- Degenerative joint disease (DJD): usually morning stiffness that does not last longer than 30 minutes
- Parkinson's disease: patient has tremors and cogwheel rigidity; normal ESR
- SLE: often accompanied by pleuritis, pericarditis, leukopenia, thrombocytopenia, and a positive ANA
- Paraneoplastic syndrome
- Infective endocarditis: suggested by continued fever and new onset heart murmur
- Bursitis
- Tendonitis
- Amyloidosis
- Synovitis: joint fluid shows infection
- Spondyloarthropathy: differentiated on radiograph
- Lyme disease

Diagnostics

Laboratory Evaluation

- CBC/diff: mild to moderate normocytic, normochromic anemia
- ESR: 7% to 20% of cases have ESR elevation (often > 100 mm/hr), but PMR may be present even with ESR < 40; when > 40, patient usually has more systemic symptoms
- RF and ANA: absent
- LFT: mild elevation of alkaline phosphatase in 33% of patients
- C-reactive protein: considered a sensitive indicator of active disease; when elevated, is a marker of inflammation
- Thyroid-stimulating hormone (TSH): to rule out hypothyroidism
- Serum levels interleukin-6: persistently increased even when symptoms improve
- Creatine phosphokinase (CPK): if indicated to exclude myopathy

- Serum electrophoresis: if no response to steroids to exclude multiple myeloma, systemic amyloidosis

Other Diagnostics

- X-ray of joints: to rule out erosion as in RA and nerve impingement
- Ultrasound of shoulders: shows proximal synovitis and subacromial/subdeltoid bursitis, which is the most frequent lesion in PMR
- Temporal artery biopsy: if GCA is suspected
- Other: if no response to prednisone, consider occult infection workup, occult malignancy workup, synovial fluid analysis, muscle biopsy, or nerve conduction studies

Treatment Plan

There is no specific diagnostic test for PMR. Diagnosis is based on patient's age (age > 50), ESR (elevation > 40 mm/hr) or elevated CRP, and the presence of symmetric aching/stiffness for at least 30 days in two or three of the following body areas: the neck/torso, shoulders/proximal arms, and/or hips/ proximal thighs. Symptoms that abate quickly with corticosteroid therapy also suggest PMR.

Nonpharmacologic Therapy

- Daily weight-bearing exercise
- Rest
- Adequate nutrition and hydration
- Possible water aerobics in warm water
- Emotional support until diagnosis is made and symptoms improve

Pharmacologic Therapy

- Tylenol 650 mg PO every 6 hours PRN for pain *or*
- Enteric-coated Naprosyn 500 mg PO BID (use cautiously in elders; monitor for GI bleed and lower extremity edema with sodium retention)
- Steroids: most patients started on prednisone 10 to 20 mg PO daily, usually for 2 to 4 weeks or until symptoms disappear (usually in 2 to 3 days) or ESR decreases; for most patients, symptoms are dramatically reduced within 24 to 48 hours, although some patients may continue to have bedtime stiffness that can be controlled with BID dosing or an increase in the daily dose.
  - After the pain and stiffness have been controlled for a month (and the ESR is within an acceptable range), the prednisone should be slowly tapered by 10% of the daily dose every 2 weeks or once a month. The patient should monitor symptoms closely, and the ESR must also be monitored (goal ESR is to remain within normal limits during the taper). Once the prednisone daily dose is 10 mg, the dose should only be decreased 1 mg/month. The final taper may be better tolerated with BID prednisone dosing. The ESR and patient's function should still be monitored monthly as relapse can occur, requiring increased steroid therapy. Maintenance therapy of 5 to 10 mg PO daily may be required

for several years. Because steroid therapy may be associated with GI bleeding, a proton pump or H_2 blocker is usually indicated.

- Managing steroid side effects
  - Baseline bone mineral density (BMD)
  - Osteoporosis prevention: total daily calcium intake (food and supplementation) should not exceed 1500 mg; vitamin D 400 to 800 IU daily (may need to monitor patient for hypercalcemia); consider raloxifene (Evista) 60 mg PO daily or alendronate (Fosamax) 70 mg PO weekly or risedronate (Actonel) 35 mg PO weekly (used cautiously with gastroesophageal reflux disease [GERD]). Proton pump inhibitor, H_2 blocker, or antacids may be necessary.
  - Monitor serum potassium
  - Monitor serum glucose (and, if indicated, HbA1C). Initiate therapy for steroid induced diabetes, if indicated

Consultation/Hospitalization

- Consult physician in all suspected cases of PMR.
- Any patient with suspected GCA should be seen emergently by an ophthalmologist.
- Consult with surgeon for expeditious temporal artery biopsy if temporal arteritis is suspected.
- If no immediate response to steroids, refer to rheumatology.
- Refer to physical and/or occupational therapy for exercise program.

Complications

- Patients with PMR may develop GCA, a medical emergency with risk of sudden and irreversible blindness.
- Side effects of corticosteroids include osteoporosis, infection, cataracts, slowly healing wounds, hypertension, hypokalemia, glucose intolerance, GI bleed, insomnia, and euphoria.
- Spontaneous exacerbation occurs in 30% to 50% of patients, usually in the first 2 years and independent of corticosteroid regimen.

Education for Nursing Home/Rehabilitation Staff

- Explain side effects of steroids and the importance of monitoring stools for occult blood.
- Discuss the importance of monitoring weight and blood sugars.
- Explain the importance of monitoring the patient for signs of infection, and regularly assessing for skin breakdown.
- Discuss the benefit of increased activity and the need to encourage activity.
- Explain the importance of good hygiene and good mouth care (to lessen risk for *Candida*).

- Describe the need to monitor patients for complaints of headaches, visual changes, and/or difficulty chewing (jaw claudication) and notifying health-care provider immediately if these symptoms occur.

Patient/Family Education

- Explain the risk for GCA so that patients/family understand the importance of reporting a new headache, change in vision, scalp tenderness, and difficulty chewing.
- Explain the risks/benefits of steroid therapy as well as side effects of steroids.
- Explain the importance of wearing a medical alert bracelet.
- Discuss the symptoms and signs of diabetes mellitus and hyperglycemia and the need to notify the healthcare provider.
- Explain why steroids should be taken with food and why gastric upset should be reported to the healthcare provider.
- Educate patient about watching for dark stools or blood in the stool.
- Explain the bone changes that occur with steroid therapy and the importance of continuing biphosphonate, calcium, and exercise regimen.
- Explain why steroid therapy should not be stopped abruptly.

Bibliography

Brown, J.B., et al. (1999). *Gerontological protocols for nurse practitioners*. Philadelphia: Lipppincott Williams & Wilkins.

Hoch, S. (2003). In Buttaro, T.M., et al. (2003). *Primary care: A collaborative practice* (pp. 1125-1129). St. Louis: Mosby.

Narvaez, J., et al. (2001). Musculoskeletal manifestations in polymyalgia rheumatica and temporal arteritis. *Annals of the Rheumatic Diseases*, 60(11), 1060-1063.

Salvarani, C, et al. (2002). Polymyalgia rheumatica and giant cell arteritis. *New England Journal of Medicine*, 347(4), 261-271.

Weyand, C., & Gorozny, J. (2003). Giant-cell arteritis and polymyalgia rheumatica. *Annals of Internal Medicine*, 139(6), 505-515.

CHAPTER 13

Mental Health Disorders

ANXIETY

ICD-9: 300.02 (GENERALIZED ANXIETY DISORDER);
300.0 (ANXIETY STATE UNSPECIFIED)

Anxiety may be related to the physical, emotional, and financial concerns that accompany illness or may be associated with depression. In older persons, anxiety may be a harbinger of cognitive decline. The symptoms of generalized anxiety disorder may be difficult to distinguish from physical illnesses. The *Diagnostic and Statistical Manual of Mental Disorders—Fourth Edition* (DSM-IV) describes criteria for generalized anxiety disorder as "excessive anxiety and worry" present daily for at least 6 months and associated with three or more of the following symptoms: restlessness, difficulty with concentration, irritability, muscle tension, sleep disturbance, and decreased energy. The symptoms must be associated with distress or functional impairment, but should not be related to another psychiatric disorder, substance abuse, or medical condition. Other anxiety disorders—panic, phobias, obsessive-compulsive disorder (OCD), and post-traumatic stress disorder (PTSD) (a concern in older combat veterans and Holocaust survivors)—can emerge in these facilities but are less prevalent.

Risk Factors

- History of alcohol or substance abuse, depression, or anxiety
- Chronic illness
- Recent loss: change in lifestyle; decline in function
- Stimulant medications, caffeine, or anticholinergics

263

History

Eliciting the history may be challenging, as patients may have difficulty discussing symptoms, history, or current concerns. The nursing staff and patient's family may be helpful in determining the onset of symptoms and the medical and psychiatric history. Fatigue, insomnia, forgetfulness, and physical complaints (e.g., dyspnea, palpitations, gastrointestinal symptoms, sleep problems, or nervousness) are important considerations requiring investigation to differentiate a medical disorder. In elders, an abrupt onset of these symptoms may suggest a physical problem.

Physical Examination

The patient should be observed for cognitive dysfunction, agitation, trembling, or restlessness and postural vital signs must be obtained. Next, a thorough physical examination is necessary to determine if there is an under-lying physical problem associated with the symptoms.

Diagnostics

Laboratory and other diagnostic tests are dependent on presentation and physical findings. Diagnostic tests are performed to exclude a medical cause for the patient's symptoms. Anxiety assessment scales (e.g., Beck Anxiety Inventory, Hamilton Anxiety Rating Scale) may be helpful in some patients, but they are not necessarily diagnostic.

Laboratory Evaluation
- Complete blood count with differential (CBC/diff): determine presence of anemia or infection.
- Serum glucose, serum electrolytes, blood urea nitrogen (BUN), and creatinine: to exclude hypoglycemia, hyperglycemia, electrolyte disorders, and dehydration
- Thyroid-stimulating hormone (TSH) and T_4: to exclude hyperthyroidism and hypothyroidism

Other Diagnostics
- Electrocardiogram (ECG): if chest pain or palpitations

Differential Diagnosis

The signs and symptoms of anxiety are similar to those of some medical conditions. Caffeine use, cardiac arrhythmias, chest pain, hyperthyroidism, anemia, hypoglycemia, medication effects, pulmonary emboli, asthma, chronic obstructive pulmonary disease (COPD), pheochromocytoma, and even partial seizures cause similar clinical presentations and should be considered in the differential diagnosis. Psychiatric disorders to be considered in the differential diagnosis include:

- Depressive disorders
- Generalized anxiety disorder
- Adjustment disorder
- Somatization disorder
- PTSD
- Acute stress disorder
- Panic disorder
- Phobic disorder
- Bipolar disorder
- Alcohol/substance abuse

Treatment Plan

Anxiety is a treatable condition. Treatment must be individualized for each patient. Organic causes for the symptoms should be addressed and, if possible, treated. Benzodiazepines are not usually recommended for older adults and may even contribute to cognitive decline when used for an extended time. However, there may be some circumstances in which the cautious short-term use of short-acting benzodiazepines is indicated for patient comfort. Patients with acute anxiety may benefit initially from a combination of a short-acting benzo-diazepine, such as a low dose of lorazepam (Ativan), with a selective serotonin reuptake inhibitor (SSRI). The SSRI should be gradually increased to the maximum effective dose, then the benzodiazepine slowly tapered. In these situations, the patient should be monitored closely for untoward symptoms.

SSRIs are indicated for patients experiencing generalized anxiety, panic attacks, OCD, and PTSD. SSRIs and venlafaxine (Effexor XR), a serotonin and noroepinephrine reuptake inhibitor, are the most common pharmacologic agents recommended for patients with anxiety disorders associated with depression (see later in this chapter). Tricyclic antidepressants have anticholinergic properties and may be cardiotoxic, and, therefore, are not appropriate for older adults, although they may be appropriate for younger patients who fail SSRIs. Other antidepressants that are indicated for anxiety and may be appropriate for patients who do not respond to the SSRIs include mirtazapine (Remeron) or buspirone (Buspar).

Exercise, relaxation techniques, and nonpharmacologic therapies (i.e., counseling, cognitive therapy) are reasonable in receptive patients who are cognitively intact. Although there is conflicting evidence suggesting the benefit of these therapies, most studies advocate combined treatment.

Consultation/Hospitalization

- **Immediate psychiatric consultation is indicated for patients with suicidal or homicidal ideation.**

- Psychiatric consultation is recommended for patients with complicated presentations or suspected psychosis, and for patients who are not responding to therapies.
- Psychiatric consultation is recommended for patients with a long history of benzodiazepine therapy if benzodiazepine taper is indicated.
- Consultation with a psychologist and/or social worker may be helpful for counseling patients.
- Referral to a social worker is indicated for patients with financial concerns.

Complications

- Untreated or undiagnosed anxiety may impact quality of life.
- Benzodiazepine dependence may occur with long-term use.
- Elderly patients are susceptible to medication side effects and are at greater risk for falls, impaired judgment, and cognitive changes related to medications.

Education for Nursing Home/Rehabilitation Staff

- Educate the nursing staff about the signs and symptoms of anxiety.
- Discuss with the nursing staff the benefit of listening to patients talk. Discussing concerns is often helpful for patients.
- Explain to the nursing staff the benefits of exercise and relaxation techniques (music, breathing exercises) for patients experiencing anxiety.
- Encourage the patient to participate in activities.

Patient/Family Education

- Patients and families should be educated about anxiety and the benefit of adequate sleep, a nutritious diet, exercise, and pharmacologic treatment.
- Educational materials about the benefits of relaxation and other non-pharmacologic therapies should be provided to patients and families.
- Patients and families should be educated about the potential for drug-drug interactions and hepatotoxicity with herbal supplements (i.e., Kava).
- Patients and families should understand that abrupt cessation of antidepressants or anxiolytics can result in return of symptoms or other untoward effects.

Bibliography

American Psychiatric Association. (1994). *Diagnostic and Statistical Manual of Mental Disorders—Fourth Edition*. Washington, DC: American Psychiatric Association.

Ciechanowski, P., & Katon, W. (2004). Overview of generalized anxiety disorder. *www.uptodate.com*. Accessed April 24, 2004.

Framptom, K.K. (2004).The state of geriatric mental health services in LTC. *Caring for the Ages*, 5(4), 47-50.

Kogan, N.J., et al. (2000). Assessment of anxiety in older adults: Current status. *Journal of Anxiety Disorders, 14*(2), 109-132.

Paterniti, S., et al. (2002). Long-term benzodiazepine use and cognitive decline in the elderly: The epidemiology of vascular aging study. *Journal of Clinical Psychopharmacology, 22*(3), 285-293.

Sinoff, G., Werner, P. (2003). Anxiety disorder and accompanying subjective memory loss in the elderly as a predictor of future cognitive decline. *International Journal of Geriatric Psychiatry, 18*(10), 951-959.

DEPRESSION

ICD-9: 296.2 (MAJOR DEPRESSION)

Everyone periodically experiences depression to some extent. Many patients with depression have a coexisting anxiety disorder. Illness, disability, pain, economic stresses, and aging increase the likelihood of depressive symptoms and may exacerbate anxiety. Symptoms may be obscure and, in institutionalized, ill, or elderly patients, attributed to other factors. As a result, depression and anxiety may be overlooked in these populations. In rehabilitation and long-term care facilities, patients should be screened for depression upon admission and again if there is a change that suggests possible depression. Studies have shown that most patients with depression are undertreated.

Although some patients may admit to a depressed mood, it actually may be the nursing or rehabilitation staff who first suspects that the lethargy or irritability a patient is experiencing represents depression rather than an underlying illness. Unfortunately, undiagnosed and untreated depression is associated with increased mortality, impacts rehabilitation, increases the risk for malnutrition, complicates medical management, and may be associated with suicide.

Risk Factors

- Age > 65 years
- Female gender
- Previous personal or family history of depression
- Chronic pain
- Medical illness
- Anemia, vitamin deficiencies, or malnutrition
- Endocrine disorders: Addison's disease, Cushing's disease, diabetes, hyperparathyroidism, hyperthyroidism, and hypothyroidism
- Stress
- Metabolic disorders
- Disability
- Recent loss or bereavement
- Previous personal or family history of psychiatric illness

- Alcohol or drug abuse
- Medications (prescribed and over-the-counter): Beta-blockers, steroids, and antihypertensives are commonly associated with depression, but depression many be associated with other medications too.
- Lack of social supports

History

The patient may not recognize the symptoms of depression, believing that the symptoms, often vague or atypical, are associated with illness or related to aging. Nurses or family members may relate anhedonia, poor appetite, cognitive changes, inability to concentrate or make decisions, weight loss or gain, malaise or restlessness, irritability or anxiousness, lethargy or sleep disturbances, constipation, fearfulness, hallucinations, suicidal ideation, and/or diminished functional capacity. Symptoms that may be associated with depression must be present for at least 2 weeks, cause distress or dysfunction, and not be related to a medication or medical disorder. A review of the DSM-IV and consultation with the psychiatric specialist are helpful to determine the type of depression (Box 13-1) and to guide treatment.

When possible, further history should be elicited from the patient and include a determination of psychotic thoughts and persistent thoughts of death or suicide. It is also necessary to determine a history of alcohol or drug abuse, history of depression or bipolar disease, recent bereavement, allergies, and medications, as well as a history of neurologic disorder (e.g., Parkinson's disease) or other comorbid disease.

Physical Examination

Most often, the diagnosis of depression is made clinically and based on the patient's history and clinical presentation. Although a physiologic cause for the

---

BOX 13-1   Types of Depression

Major depressive disorder
Minor depression
Dysthymic disorder
Mixed anxiety depression
Substance-induced depressive disorder
Psychotic depression
Bipolar depression
Atypical depression
Seasonal affective disorder
Postpartum depression

symptoms must be sought, it is important to remember that depression and medical illness frequently coexist. The physical examination is essential in evaluating the patient for signs of dementia, anxiety, confusion, lethargy, psychomotor agitation, hallucinations/psychosis, or organic signs of illness. Weight, vital signs, and a complete neurologic examination (including a mental status examination) are necessary.

Diagnostics

When indicated, diagnostics are helpful in screening for endocrine and metabolic abnormalities as well as for malignancy or other disease states. A CBC, TSH, and electrolytes are obtained to exclude anemia, electrolyte abnormalities, and hypothyroidism. Further testing is dependent on history and physical findings.

Differential Diagnosis

- Neurologic disorders: multiple sclerosis, Parkinson's disease, epilepsy, encephalitis, Alzheimer's disease, normal pressure hydrocephalus, or cerebral vascular accident
- Nutritional deficiencies
- Anemias
- Cancer: brain tumor, pancreatic tumor, or other cancers
- Carcinoid
- Cardiovascular disease: angina, myocardial infarction (MI), or cardiomyopathy
- COPD
- Electrolyte abnormalities: hypernatremia and hyponatremia, hyperkalemia and hypokalemia, and hypercalcemia
- Endocrine disorders: Cushing's disease, diabetes, hyperthyroidism and hypothyroidism, hyperparathyroidism and hypoparathyroidsm, and Addison's disease
- Infectious diseases: acquired immunodeficiency syndrome (AIDS) and viral infections
- Medication related
- Multisystem disorders: rheumatoid arthritis and temporal arteritis

Treatment Plan

Cognitive therapy combined with nonpharmacologic and pharmacologic therapy may be helpful. The choice of medication to treat depression must be individualized. Current medications and potential drug interactions must be considered. In older patients, the pharmacokinetics and pharmacodynamics of the medication must also be carefully gauged. General guidelines are as follows:

- Encourage daily excercise (5 to 30 minutes) to promote well-being.

- Facilitate socialization with other patients and staff who have similar interests.
- The recommendation for an antidepressant should be discussed with the patient and/or family, and specific symptoms (e.g., insomnia, hypersomnolence, loss of appetite) targeted.
- If the patient had a good response (and tolerable side effects) to an antidepressant in the past, it is reasonable to restart that antidepressant.
- Monoamine oxidase inhibitors (MAOIs) are not usually prescribed, as there are significant interactions with many medications and foods.
- Tricyclic antidepressants and SSRIs are equally effective. Tricyclic antidepressants are not indicated in patients with coronary artery disease and are associated with anticholinergic and orthostatic side effects that are not well tolerated in elderly patients.
  - Amitriptyline (Elavil): start at 10 mg PO at bedtime.
  - Desipramine (Norpramin): start at 10 to 25 mg PO daily; maximum dose is 150 mg daily.
  - Nortriptyline (Pamelor). Start at 10 mg PO at bedtime and increase if necessary by 10 mg weekly to a maximum dose of 75 mg daily.
- In general, the SSRIs, which are indicated for anxiety as well as depression, are better tolerated and, for most patients, are the initial drug of choice. There is no evidence that one SSRI is superior to another, although individual patients may respond better to one drug than another. The medication should be started at the lowest dose for 1 week, then slowly increased to relieve symptoms. Usually, SSRIs should be given in the AM, as insomnia has been associated with dosing later in the day. SSRIs include:
  - Paroxetine (Paxil): indicated for depression, anxiety, panic disorder, and OCD. Start at 5 mg PO daily and increase by 5 to 10 mg weekly to optimal dose; maximum daily dose is 40 mg in elderly patients.
  - Fluoxetine (Prozac): Start at 5 mg PO daily and increase by 5 to 10 mg weekly. Use cautiously in elders because longer half-life is a concern for older patients. This medication is contraindicated if there is a history of seizures, mania, or hepatic or renal disease.
  - Sertraline (Zoloft): indicated for depression. Start at 25 mg PO daily and possibly increase by 25 mg increments every 3 to 7 days.
  - Citalopram (Celexa): may have fewer drug-drug interactions as a weaker inhibitor of the CYP450 enzyme system than other SSRIs; start at 10 mg PO daily and increase by 10 mg weekly to a maximum dose of 40 mg PO daily.
  - Escitalopram (Lexapro): start at 5 to 10 mg PO daily and possibly increase to a maximum of 20 mg PO daily.
- Other medications for depression include the following:
  - Bupropion (Wellbutrin) inhibits dopamine, serotonin, and norepinephrine reuptake and is contraindicated in patients with a history of anorexia, bulimia, or seizures. Start at 50 mg PO daily. Medication may be increased every 3 to 5 days to a total of 300 mg daily.

- Venlafaxine (Effexor) strongly inhibits serotonin and norepinephrine while weakly inhibiting dopamine and is indicated for generalized anxiety disorder or major depression. The extended release form should be started at 37.5 mg PO daily and increased weekly to a maximum dose of 225 mg daily. Venlafaxine is associated with increased blood pressure and seizures.
- Mirtazapine (Remeron), a $5HT_2$ and HT_3 antagonist, is especially helpful for depression associated with insomnia or weight loss as it is sedating and increases appetite. Start 7.5 mg PO at bedtime and increase every 2 weeks, if necessary, to a maximum dose of 45 mg daily. This medication is associated with orthostatic hypotension and agranulocytosis. Regular monitoring of CBC is recommended.
- Methylphenidate (Ritalin) is sometimes used for depression in elderly patients and is often beneficial for patients with diminished appetite. The starting dose is 2.5 mg PO before breakfast. The dose can be increased weekly by 2.5 mg, and total daily dose is 20 mg in divided doses. Consultation with a psychopharmacologist is recommended.
- The medication should be changed if the patient has not responded in 6 to 8 weeks.
- Antidepressants should not be stopped abruptly. To avoid the anxiety, dizziness, and other symptoms associated with "discontinuation syndrome," SSRIs should be gradually tapered by 25% per week. If symptoms suggesting increased anxiety or depression occur during the taper, the taper should not be continued and the physician or psychopharmacologist consulted.
- Elders and patients with a past history of major depression will probably require life long maintenance therapy while for others pharmacologic therapy may not be necessary after 9 to 12 months.
- Benzodiazepines are generally not recommended for elderly patients or for patients with a medical history of substance abuse, and they may be addictive/habit forming.
- Electroconvulsive treatment (ECT) may be considered for patients with resistant depression.

Consultation/Hospitalization

- **Immediate psychiatric evaluation is indicated for patients with suicidal or homicidal ideation.**
- Hospitalization may be indicated for suicidal or psychotic patients.
- Consultation with a psychopharmacologist is indicated for suicidal and/or psychotic patients, for patients with a substance abuse disorder, and for patients with a suspected bipolar disorder.
- Psychiatric consultation is indicated if diagnosis is unclear and for patients with continued depression despite maximum therapy.
- Consultation with a psychopharmacologist is indicated for patients requiring augmentation therapy (the use of one or more antidepressant).

- Consultation with the social worker is recommended for patients with financial, medical insurance, or housing concerns.
- Arrange physical and occupational therapy consult to promote independence.
- Arrange consult with an appropriate religious leader, if indicated, for spiritual guidance.
- Consultation with the Activities Director is recommended to encourage socialization.

Complications

- Drug-drug interactions are possible with any antidepressant.
- SSRIs have been associated with tremors, hyponatremia, increased falls, serotonin syndrome, weight gain, and weight loss in a small percentage of patients.
- Increased risk for dementia: associated with untreated depression
- Impaired cognitive, physical, and social function
- Suicide

Education for Nursing Home/Rehabilitation Staff

- Discuss with the nursing home staff the importance of monitoring depressed patients for suicidal ideation.
- Discuss nursing interventions for depression.
  - Provide a safe environment.
  - Encourage regular meals, elimination, exercise, and sleep patterns.
  - Provide pain management and promote patient comfort.
  - Encourage socialization, relaxation, recreational, and reminiscence programs.
  - Encourage family/friends visits, home visits.
  - Provide emotional support for patients and families.
  - Utilize guided imagery.
- Explain the side effects of treatment and the need to provide precautions to prevent falls.
- Discuss the importance of monitoring and recording the patient's response to interventions.

Patient/Family Education

- Explain to patients and families that the symptoms of depression may include physical symptoms or may be quite vague. It is also necessary to explain that depression is an actual illness commonly associated with aging and illness, and that some research suggests that depression may be related to neurotransmitter changes in the brain.

- Inform patients that treatment for depression is beneficial, but that medications may take 14 to 21 days before the patient notices a difference.
- Discuss the risk/benefits of pharmacologic treatment, potential side effects, and the importance of not discontinuing antidepressant medications abruptly.
- Encourage patients to consider counseling.
- Encourage patients and families to report medication side effects.
- Explain to patients and families that there can be acute interactions with prescribed, herbal, and/or over-the-counter medications.

Bibliography

Butler, R., et al. (2003). Depressive disorders. *www.clinicalevidence.com*. Retrieved March 31, 2004.

Cole, M., & Dendukuri, N. (2003). Risk factors for depression among elderly community subjects: A systematic review and meta-analysis. *The American Journal of Psychiatry*, *160*(6), 1147-1156.

Greenless, B.A., & Heister, T. (2004). The effects of antidepressants on cognition in the elderly. *Long-Term Care Interface*, *5*(3), 56-60.

Hirsch, M., Birnbaum, R.J. (2004). Pharmacology and use of antidepressants. *www.uptodate.com*. Accessed March 31, 2004.

Kalpan, B., & Levenson, S. (2002). Managing depression in long-term care. *Caring for the Ages*, *3*(6), 24-29.

Paulsen, R.H., et al. (2004). Treatment of depression. *www.uptodate.com*. Accessed March 31, 2004.

The Postoperative Patient

POSTOPERATIVE CARE

The length of stay for patients hospitalized for acute medical and surgical problems continues to decrease. As a result, postoperative patients are transferred to rehabilitation and skilled nursing settings before returning to the community. These patients may need specialized wound care, continued intravenous (IV) therapies, pain control, and ongoing evaluation and treatment of comorbid conditions.

Discharge Information

Patients transferred from the hospital are required to come with a discharge summary and referral forms, including a Page One (medical director [MD] orders), a Page Two (nursing information), and a Page Three (used for physical therapy/occupation therapy/speech therapy [PT/OT/ST] or social work updates). It is not uncommon to find discrepancies between discharge summaries and Page One referral forms, as they may be written by different providers, often at different times during the patient's hospital stay. Medications may have been added, deleted, or changed; for example, IV antibiotics are changed to oral antibiotics on the day of discharge; cardiac medicines are often started or changed on the day of discharge; or pain regimens are altered. A careful review of the accompanying paperwork is critical to ensure a safe transition across settings. If necessary information is not available at the time of admission, it is important to contact referring physician or hospital unit.

Communication

It is important to have clear contact information for the attending surgeon or surgical team. All questions specific to the surgical condition should be directed to the surgical team. Surgical teams involved in patient care in the hospital may include other physicians, advanced practice nurses, or physician assistants. These healthcare providers are a valuable resource for consultation and advice regarding the expected trajectory of recovery, as well as approaches to common postoperative problems. Some hospitals also have designated clinics or programs that families, patients, and providers can access for postoperative information and advice.

In general, all patients have a scheduled postoperative appointment with the surgeon, usually within 1 to 4 weeks. If the visit occurs while the patient is still hospitalized on the subacute/rehabilitation unit, the healthcare provider can send a copy of a recent note as well as specific questions with the patient. The surgeon can answer in writing, by telephone, or by e-mail (if available).

Suspected wound infections should also be discussed with the surgeon before starting the patient on antibiotic therapy. Wound infections usually require evaluation by the surgeon, although, in some instances, a phone conversation with the surgeon will suffice.

Complications of Hospitalization

Older adults are at risk for the adverse consequences of hospitalization. These complications, which include nosocomial infections, falls, incontinence, surgical complications, adverse medication effects, nutritional and fluid imbalances, and altered mental status, affect functional status and quality of life. In addition, these complications present challenges for rehabilitation. It is important to determine the patient's pre-illness/surgical baseline and to systematically identify any new behavior or limitations. Disturbances in the sleep-wake cycle, as well as depression and anxiety, may also occur; all of these may interfere with the patient's recovery.

Special Considerations

Anticoagulation

Practice parameters for post-interventional or post-surgical anticoagulation can vary greatly and are dependent on the nature of the specific procedure, and the preference of the referring provider. It is important to establish at admission to the subacute/rehabilitation setting what the international normalized ratio (INR) goal is for the patient's specific condition. For example, anticoagulation for an orthopedic patient may be a daily aspirin, low–molecular-weight heparin, or Coumadin therapy for 4 to 6 weeks. Some orthopedic patients may be on fixed dose Coumadin and not require INR monitoring; for other patients, specific ranges for the INR may necessitate prothrombin time (PT)/INR monitoring. Postinterventional cardiology patients may be receiving combination therapies of platelet inhibitors and anticoagulants. It is also necessary to establish which provider will be managing the anticoagulation; some hospitals have anticoagulation clinics/programs that are specifically designed to oversee all aspects of anticoagulation, even during the subacute stay. See Chapter 16 for more information regarding Coumadin dosing and management.

Intravenous Therapy

Patients may be discharged from the acute care setting with a peripherally inserted central catheter (PICC) or midline for continued IV therapy. The facility's policy and procedure manual provides specific guidelines for PICC line flushes, frequency of dressing changes, and local care. However, the healthcare provider may be asked to discontinue a PICC line at the completion of therapy. Removal of a PICC line is determined by the duration and type of therapy, the presence of an infectious or inflammatory process, and improper positioning of the catheter. Principles of PICC line removal are as follows:

- Gather all necessary supplies, including gloves, sterile gauze, antiseptic solution, antimicrobial ointment, sterile occlusive dressing, and a tourniquet.
- Place the patient in the supine position.
- Wash hands and apply gloves.
- Carefully remove dressing and tape and discard appropriately.
- Clean the area with antiseptic solution, and let it dry.
- In one hand, hold sterile gauze to be placed over the insertion site when the catheter is removed; with the other hand, grasp the hub and main catheter. While the patient inhales, slowly pull the IV device toward you, keeping it flush with the skin. Use relaxation techniques (e.g., deep breaths) to calm patient.
- Stop pulling if resistance is felt. Resistance during removal could indicate a knot in the catheter, a clot, or spasm. Do not stretch or pull a PICC against resistance. Redress and apply heat along the vein for 15 to 20 minutes, and try again. If still unsuccessful, the patient may need to have the PICC line removed in interventional radiology.
- Upon PICC line removal, apply pressure, antiseptic ointment, sterile gauze, and a sterile occlusive dressing.
- Inspect the PICC and its tip and measure to be certain the entire catheter has been removed; check against documentation from the hospital made upon device insertion. If the length of the PICC is shorter than the length documented, and you suspect that the PICC has broken, immediately apply a tourniquet to the proximal end of the extremity (upper arm), occluding only venous flow, and arrange for the patient to be immediately transported to an acute care setting for further evaluation.
- Document the PICC line removal in the patient's record.

Sutures and Staples

Instructions for the date of suture or staple removal should be identified on the discharge summary or Page One. If the information is not clear, call the surgeon or surgical team for specific instructions regarding suture/staple removal, including which provider is to remove them. Some surgeons schedule patients for follow-up visits to inspect the wound and remove the staples or sutures. The length of time that sutures/staples are left in place can vary significantly based on the location on the body, amount of tension on the wound, and surgeon preference. In general, sutures on the face are in place for 4 to 5 days, sutures on other parts of the body are in place for 5 to 7 days, and sutures across a joint or sutures on the scalp may be left in place for 7 to 14 days. Guidelines for suture and staple removal follow.

Sutures

- Obtain supplies: suture removal kit, Steri-Strips, alcohol wipes, dry sterile dressing (DSD), and tape.
- Explain procedure to patient: the patient may feel a slight "tugging" or "pulling" as each suture is removed.
- Wash hands and apply clean gloves.
- Remove dressing, if any, and clean (soap and water, alcohol, or normal saline) and gently dry the incision.
- Grasp suture at the knot with forceps and lift suture away from skin.
- Place curved tip of suture removal scissors under the suture, and cut one side of the suture close to the skin. Do not cut both sides of the suture, as a portion of the suture will be left under the skin.
- With forceps, pull the suture out in one piece.
- Discard suture.
- Remove every other suture.
- If no dehiscence occurs, remove the remaining sutures.
- Apply Steri-strips if needed. Cover with clean dry gauze or Band-Aid for patient comfort.
- Document suture removal, number of sutures removed, and wound appearance in the patient's record.

Staples

- Obtain supplies: staple removal kit, Steri-Strips, alcohol wipes, DSD, and tape.
- Explain procedure to patient: the patient may feel a slight "tugging" or "pulling."
- Wash hands and apply clean gloves.
- Remove dressing, if any, and clean (soap and water, alcohol, or normal saline) and gently dry the incision.
- Place both curved tips of the staple remover under the first staple.
- Gently close the staple remover down on the staple. The staple should open. Lift staple out of skin.
- Discard staple, usually onto piece of gauze.

- Remove every other staple.
- If no dehiscence occurs, remove the remaining staples.
- Apply Steri-Strips if needed. Cover with clean, dry gauze or Band-Aid for patient comfort.
- Document staple removal, number of staples removed, and wound appearance in the patient's record.

Specific Surgeries/Procedures
Coronary artery bypass surgery
Coronary artery bypass surgery is a commonly performed surgery. Patients who have coexisting comorbidities or who have complicated postoperative courses and are in need of additional care may be discharged to the subacute setting from the hospital. Specific concerns in this population include:
- Infections of sternal or leg incisions
  - Discuss with surgeon/surgical team if there is a need for a change in wound-care protocols or a need for antibiotic thereapy (elderly, patients with diabetes, and malnourished patients are at greatest risk for infection).
- Sleep disturbance
  - Promote optimal sleep-wake cycle by minimizing interruptions during sleep, adequately controlling pain, and alleviating anxiety.
- Cognitive impairment (short-term memory loss)
- Poor appetite
- Depression
  - Identify patient's preoperative status.
  - Ensure adequate control of sleep-wake cycle, pain, and anxiety.
  - Refer to social work or psychiatry as needed.

Interventional procedures (angioplasty and/or stenting)
Percutaneous coronary revascularization procedures include atherectomy, balloon angioplasty, or stenting. Most patients undergoing these procedures are discharged home after brief hospital stays, but those who have major complications or comorbid conditions requiring additional evaluation and treatment may be discharged to the subacute setting. Post-procedure concerns include:
- Groin hematoma at the puncture site: may present with localized pain edema, or tenderness, lower-extremity edema, or lower-extremity neurologic symptoms. Patients need emergent ultrasonography or computer tomography (CT) scan of the area to confirm the diagnosis.
- Retroperitoneal hematoma: may present with significant flank, abdominal, or back pain, along with hypotension or unexplained drop in hematocrit; requires emergent evaluation.
- Groin pseudoaneurysm: may present with groin tenderness, pulsatile mass, or bruit; requires emergent evaluation.
- Anticoagulation: unless allergic to aspirin (ASA) all patients who have undergone angioplasty or stenting will be on oral ASA, with doses ranging from 81 to 325 mg daily indefinitely. In addition, patients who have

undergone stenting with bare-metal stents will also receive clopidogrel (Plavix) for 4 weeks to prevent stent thrombosis. For patients who have stenting done with drug-eluting stents, Plavix therapy is extended for 3 to 6 months. The ASA and Plavix regimen should not be interrupted for episodes of minor bleeding or elective invasive or surgical procedures during the first 4 weeks postprocedure.

- Chest pain: patients who complain of angina like chest pain/discomfort at rest in the days to weeks postprocedure need emergent transport to an acute care facility for evaluation of stent occlusion.

Education for Nursing Home/Rehabilitation Staff

- Review importance of assessing wound sites for erythema, warmth, edema, drainage, and pain, as well as notifying healthcare provider with findings suggestive of infection.
- Review deep vein thrombosis (DVT) prophylaxis measures, including early mobilization/ambulation, compression stockings, use of anticoagulation, and associated bleeding precautions.
- Discuss importance of good pulmonary regimen, including coughing and deep breathing exercises, use of incentive spirometry, and early mobilization.
- Review importance of scheduled vital signs, including monitoring and reporting temperatures above 100° F.
- Explain importance of monitoring and recording intake and output, weights, and pedal pulses.
- Review importance of a thorough pain assessment, including response to pain medication. The importance of reporting unusually increased complaints of pain should be emphasized.
- Explain importance of ensuring optimal sleep with modifications in the physical environment to minimize interruption and noise; offer sleep aids where appropriate.
- Review importance of adequate nutrition with supplementation or nutrition consult if needed.
- Review importance of ongoing discharge teaching with patient and family concerning medication, exercise, diet, and nutrition.

Patient/Family Education

- Encourage family participation in promoting the patient's self-care.
- Provide anticipatory guidance on usual trajectory of recovery.
- Provide ongoing preparation for discharge.

Bibliography

American College of Cardiology/American Heart Association (ACC/AHA). (2004). Guideline update for coronary artery bypass graft surgery. *Circulation*, *110*(14), e340-e437.

Intravenous Nurses Society. (2000). Infusion nursing standards of practice. *Journal of Intravenous Nursing*, S1-S85.

Levine, G., et al. (2003). Management of patients undergoing percutaneous coronary revascularization. *Annals of Internal Medicine*, 139(2), 123-136.

McCrone, S., et al. (2001). Anxiety and depression: Incidence and patterns in patients after coronary artery bypass surgery. *Applied Nursing Research*, 14(3), 155-164.

Moureau, N. (2002). How to remove a PICC with ease. *Nursing*, 2(5), 30.

Suture and staple removal. (2004). *www.spaceref.com/iss/medical/8641.suture.staple. removal.pdf*. Accessed June 10, 2004.

CHAPTER 15

Functional Concerns

FALLS

Falls are a significant cause of morbidity and mortality and can be related to aging, functional status, illness, or even a medication. For patients admitted to a nursing or rehabilitation facility, a previous history of falls (within the last month to year) is a concern. Some risks are identifiable and modifiable. The admission history and physical assessment should identify risk factors. A care plan can then be implemented to encourage mobilization and prevent injury.

Risk Factors

- Age > 65
- History of falls within the past year
- Environmental hazards: loose rugs, poor lighting, lack of safety equipment, slippery surfaces, poor foot coverings
- Sensory impairment: decreased vision, hearing, and peripheral and proprioceptive sensation
- Medications: antidepressants, antihistamines, antiarrhythmics, anxiolytics (particularly benzodiazepines), antihypertensives, antiseizure medications, digoxin, diuretics, hypoglycemics, hypnotics, laxatives, narcotics, neuroleptics, sedatives, psychotropics, muscle relaxants, vasodilators, or polypharmacy
- Cardiovascular disorder: aortic stenosis, arrhythmia, or syncope
- Fluid or electrolyte disorder
- Musculoskeletal disorder: amputation, arthritis, deconditioning, gait disorder, or pain
- Neurologic disorder: transient ischemic attack (TIA); cerebrovascular accident (CVA); Parkinson's, Shy-Drager, or other motor disease; peripheral neuropathy; seizure

- Incontinence or nocturia
- Acute illness
- Delirium or dementia with wandering

History

If possible, the cause of the fall must be discerned to determine if the fall was related to an environmental factor, or an underlying medical or psychological problem. History should include any symptoms noted before the fall, the time of the fall, loss of consciousness, injuries, and current symptoms. Activity and symptoms both before and after the fall should be elicited as the timing of meals, a position change, micturition, head turning, dizziness, lightheadedness, a sense of imbalance, or symptoms suggestive of an infection are significant. Unfortunately, often falls are not witnessed, and the patient may not recall the incident. The area where the fall occurred should be inspected to discover environmental factors that may have contributed to the fall. Medications must be reviewed.

Upon admission to the facility, a previous history of falls (particularly within the past month to year) must be elicited. A history of wandering, medications, or comorbid conditions associated with falls place the patient at increased risk for falls.

Physical Examination

The admission physical examination and yearly physical assessment should include an evaluation of the patient's ability to change from a sitting to standing position and gait/balance impairment (if appropriate); conditions associated with falls must also be assessed. Mental status assessment, orthostatic vital signs, visual acuity and the cardiovascular, musculoskeletal, and neurologic systems require particular emphasis. Feet should also be evaluated, assessing for neuropathy and podiatric abnormalities.

The "Get up and Go Test" (which determines a patient's ability to rise from a chair without using hands, walk 10 to 20 feet, turn 360 degrees, and return to the chair) is helpful in assessing the patient's gait, balance, use of assistive devices (if applicable), and ability to turn. Other tests of mobility include the Functional Reach Test and the Tinetti Balance and Gait Evaluation. The Functional Reach Test assesses the patient's ability to reach for something while maintaining balance, and the Tinetti Balance and Gait Evaluation actually measures the patient's balance and gait to determine fall risk.

If a patient does fall, a thorough physical examination may be necessary to determine injuries and the cause of the fall. The etiology of the fall may multifactorial, and patient injuries may occur to any part of the body. Essential factors to consider include:

- Vital signs, including oxygen saturation and blood sugar: assess for presence of fever, hypoglycemia, orthostatic blood pressure, or heart rate changes (postural vital signs should be assessed first with the patient lying down, then again 3 minutes after standing)

- Skin: presence of lacerations, abrasions, or contusions
- Head, eyes, ears, nose, and throat (HEENT): evaluate mental status; visual and auditory acuity; tongue for lacerations or edema; tracheal deviation (which indicates pneumothorax); carotid bruits and neck stability; and lacerations, bruising, and deformities.
- Cardiac: assess for arrhythmias, murmurs, rate abnormalities, and congestive heart failure (CHF)
- Lungs: determine presence of abnormal breath sounds suggestive of pneumonia or CHF
- Musculoskeletal: determine skeletal abnormalities, podiatric irregularities, muscle strength, gait/balance (if possible)
- Neurologic: assess mental status, cranial nerve function, Romberg with sternal push, proprioception, peripheral nerves, and cerebellar and extrapyramidal function.

Diagnostics

Diagnostics are dependent on presentation. For example, a head injury accompanied by loss of consciousness after a fall will require a computer tomography (CT) scan; musculoskeletal injury may require radiographs. Laboratory and radiographic assessment after a fall may be indicated if a urinary tract infection, pneumonia, or dehydration is considered as possible cause of the fall.

Differential Diagnosis

The differential diagnosis is based on clinical presentation, history, and risk factors. In addition to diagnosing the injuries that were incurred, the cause of the fall must be determined to prevent further falls and injuries.

Treatment Plan

Treatment after a fall consists of caring for the injury, preventing further falls, and determining the cause of the fall. Fall distance in institutionalized patients is usually less than 15 feet. Thus, the injury usually reflects the body area impacted by the fall. All falls have the potential to be quite serious. Airway, breathing, and circulation should always be assessed first. If the patient does not require basic life support, the patient can then be evaluated for injuries. Patients with suspected head or spinal injuries, neurologic deficits, facial injuries, headache, cervical or thoracic spinal pain or tenderness, nausea, dizziness, lightheadedness, loss of consciousness or change in sensory or motor function should not be moved or allowed to move. Stabilization of the cervical spine and immediate transfer to the emergency department are indicated. Other considerations include the following.

For patients without a head or neck injury, a thorough physical examination is indicated to determine injuries, treatment, and cause of fall. Obvious musculoskeletal injuries (e.g., fracture) require emergency room evaluation, but skin tears and small lacerations can usually be cared for in the facility. If the patient does not require emergency department evaluation, neurologic and vital signs should be assessed every 15 minutes, for 1 hour, then every 30 minutes for 1 hour, and then every hour for 2 hours. Any change in consciousness warrants an emergency department evaluation.

No single intervention has been proven to prevent falls, but the Centers for Medicare and Medicaid Services (CMS) recommend individual patient-risk assessment and fall management. Underlying medical conditions should be treated appropriately. Medications should be reviewed as sedatives, antihypertensives, and other medications may increase the risk for falls. If it is possible to decrease the dosage or eliminate unnecessary medications, this should be considered. However, patients with a long history of benzodiazepine use will require a slow, long taper. Other medications may require similar tapering. Other suggestions for fall and related injury prevention include:

- Physical/occupational evaluation and treatment for assistive ambulatory devices (canes, walkers [Zimmer frames]), adaptive devices, gait and balance training. Collaborative discussions with all caregivers may be particularly beneficial in identifying risk factors and implementing fall prevention strategies.
- Recommendation of proper footwear: walking shoes with low-resistance soles
- Exercise to strengthen muscles and help reduce the patient's fear of falling
  - Tai chi or other balance training may be helpful in some patients, but the benefit is still unclear
- Adaptation of environment to reduce falls
  - Call bells always within reach
  - Proper lighting
  - Reduce clutter
  - Beds locked and low
  - Stationary furniture
  - Wheelchairs should be correct height for patients (feet on floor if patient can use feet to propel)
  - Wheelchair anti-tippers
  - Signage and adequate lighting for bathrooms
  - Bedside commode, if indicated
  - Bed bumpers (i.e., rolled blanket or body pillow) rather than bedrails
  - Bed and chair alarms for at-risk patients
  - Bedside floor mattress
  - Appropriate transfer equipment for each patient (i.e., trapeze, slideboard)
- Vision examination to correct visual defects; auditory examination to improve hearing
- Treatment for hypotension; possible decrease in antihypertensives if systolic blood pressure is less than 120 mm Hg
- Treatment of cardiovascular disorders
- Nutritional supplements, such as fortified foods, protein snacks, if indicated, to help improve body strength

- Routine toileting
- Hip protectors are frequently recommended for patients at risk for falls, although the efficacy of this recommendation is uncertain.
- Encourage smoking cessation if applicable.
- Consider Anodyne therapy for patients with diabetic peripheral neuropathy (*www.anodynetherapy.com*).

Consultation/Hospitalization

- Physical therapy/occupational therapy for exercise, gait, and balance training; assistive devices and wheelchair or walker evaluation; and home safety evaluation may be indicated.
- Consultation with a cardiologist is recommended for falls related to cardiac abnormality.
- Consultation with a neurologist is indicated for falls related to neurologic defects.
- Visual impairment requires consultation with an ophthalmologist.
- Hearing deficit requires consultation with an audiologist.
- Consultation for esthetics and orthotics may be indicated.

Complications

- Abrasions
- Anxiety
- Concussion
- Contusions
- Decreased quality of life
- Fear of repeat falls
- Hemorrhage
- Impaired mobility
- Lacerations
- Loss of consciousness
- Loss of independence
- Musculoskeletal injury: dislocation, fracture, sprain
- Rhabdomyolysis
- Subdural hematoma

Education for Nursing Home/Rehabilitation Staff

- Educate nursing staff about importance of monitoring patients closely and reporting any change in mental status (which might indicate infection, dehydration, or other fall-related risk factors).
- Educate staff about management of patient with an acute fall.
- Discuss each patient's risk for falls with staff and modify care plan to reduce fall risk.
- Educate nursing staff on safe patient transfers, appropriate use of assistive

devices, proper clothing and footwear for patients, and relationship of falls to restraint use.
- Transfer to a room close to the nursing desk for patients at high risk for falls should be discussed with nursing staff.
- Explain the importance of daily exercise to improve endurance, balance, muscle strength, and flexibility in preventing falls.

Patient/Family Education

- Discuss concerns about the patient's fall risks and safety interventions with the patient and family.
- Explain medication changes.
- Discuss the importance of taking biphosphonates as directed to prevent esophageal irritation.
- Discuss the benefit of regular exercise (even in wheelchair-bound) to improve endurance, balance, muscle strength, and flexibility.

Bibliography

American Geriatrics Society. (2001). Guideline for the prevention of falls in older patients. *www.americangeriatrics.org/products/positionpapers/abstract.shtml*. Accessed April 28, 2004.

Duncan, P., et al. (1990). Functional reach: A new clinical measure of balance. *Journal of Gerontology, 45*(6), M192-197.

Ettinger, B., et al. (1999). Reduction of vertebral fracture risk in postmenopausal women with osteoporosis treated with raloxifene: Results from a 3-year randomized clinical trial. Multiple Outcomes of Raloxifene Evaluation (MORE) Investigators. *JAMA, 282*(7), 637-645.

Kiel, D.P. (2004). Overview of falls in the elderly. In *www.uptodate.com*. Accessed April 24, 2004.

Mathias, et al. (1986). Balance in elderly patients: The "Get Up and Go" test. *Archives of Physical Medicine and Rehabilitation, 67*(6), 387-389.

Skidmore-Roth, L. (2004). *Mosby's drug reference*. St. Louis, Mosby.

Tinetti, M. (2003). Clinical practice: Preventing falls in elderly persons. *New England Journal of Medicine, 348*(1), 42-49.

FEEDING ISSUES

ICD-9: 787.2 (DYSPHAGIA); 783.3 (FEEDING DIFFICULTY); 263.9 (MALNUTRITION); 783.21 (WEIGHT LOSS)

Feeding issues are a frequent source of concern in older patients, as well as in patients with specific illnesses. The causes are multifactorial and include aging changes, gustatory dysfunction, dental and gastrointestinal (GI) disorders, cultural differences, depression, dementia, disease, and medications. Unfortunately, the resulting anorexia, dysphagia, aspiration, malnutrition, and weight loss impact patient care and well being. Although some weight loss is expected with aging, anorexia and weight loss may indicate a new illness or feeding problem. Patients with weight loss require careful evaluation, as malnutrition is a significant, often overlooked problem in older patients, particularly in those who are hospitalized or residing in subacute or nursing home settings. Estimates of malnutrition range from 37% to 75% in institutionalized elders. The cause may be an acute or chronic illness, but in some instances is unidentified. Prompt treatment is essential to prevent the anemia, falls, pressure sores, and other sequelae associated with malnutrition.

Risk Factors

- Comorbid disease: cancer, CHF, collagen disease, chronic obstructive pulmonary disease (COPD), CVA, dysphagia, end-stage renal disease, HIV, neuromuscular disease (amyotrophic lateral sclerosis, myasthenia gravis, multiple sclerosis, muscular dystrophy, Parkinson's, polyneuropathies), rheumatoid arthritis, or tuberculosis (TB); many of these conditions actually induce cachexia
- Chronic drug use
- Dentition
- Dysphagia
- Endocrine disorders: adrenal insufficiency, diabetes mellitus, hypercalcemia, hypothyroidism, or hyperthyroidism
- GI disorders: atrophic gastritis, constipation, diarrhea, intestinal ischemia, nausea, reflux, or vomiting
- Immobility
- Infection
- Malabsorption syndromes: celiac disease or Whipple's disease
- Medications: digoxin, selective serotonin reuptake inhibitors [SSRIs], hydralazine, aspirin, antibiotics, or theophylline
- Movement disorders
- Pain
- Poverty
- Psychologic disorders: anxiety, delirium, depression, or psychosis
- Sensory deficits: hearing, sight, smell, or taste disorder
- Social/cultural isolation
- Vitamin deficiencies
- Xerostomia

History

The family or nursing staff may be the first to notice a change in a patient's weight or appetite, or the patient may complain of anorexia. Often, however, patients are unaware of a diminished appetite or weight loss. A thorough review of systems is necessary, but it is also important to determine actual weight loss, what the patient's previous highest and lowest weight has been, and if there has been a change in appetite. A medication review is necessary, as many medications affect taste, swallowing ability, and/or appetite. History also helps determine whether dysphagia is contributing to weight loss and helps classify the dysphagia as oropharyngeal dysphagia (trouble passing foods from mouth to esophagus often requiring multiple swallowing attempts or a sensation of food stuck in the throat), odynophagia (pain with swallowing), or esophageal dysphagia (difficulty passing food through the esophagus to the stomach).

Physical Examination

It is helpful to observe the patient eating and drinking, because the ability to feed oneself, the amount and types of foods of consumed, and chewing or swallowing problems can be easily observed. The observation may also reveal restlessness, agitated behavior, or movement disorder.

- Current height and weight and body mass index (ideal range is 23 to 25 kg/m^2; < 20 kg/m^2 is concerning)
- Vital signs, including postural blood pressure and pulse
- Skin: check for pallor, temporal muscle wasting, loss of subcutaneous fat, poor wound healing, decubiti, and edema.
- HEENT: assess for hair thinning or loss; facial asymmetry or weakness; lips for cheilosis; mouth for candida, lesions, glossitis, or dental condition; and neck for masses or lymphadenopathy.
- Cardiac: determine presence of CHF, which may affect appetite.
- Lungs: assess for adventitious sounds; determine presence of COPD, which may affect appetite.
- Abdominal: ascites, epigastric discomfort, tenderness, or hepatomegaly may affect appetite. Rectal examination is necessary to determine occult blood and masses.
- Neuromuscular: assess cognitive status, cranial nerves, muscular strength, rigidity, cogwheeling, and gait to determine presence of neuromuscular disease impacting eating or swallowing.

Diagnostics

Diagnostic testing may be helpful, but it is primarily the history, physical examination, and careful monitoring that identify the problem. Appropriate diagnostics should be ordered when indicated.

- Complete blood count with differential (CBC/diff)
- B$_{12}$ and folate
- Transferrin
- Serum glucose, electrolytes, BUN, and creatinine
- Serum calcium, magnesium, and phosphorus
- Lipid profile
    - Fasting cholesterol < 156 mg/dL suggests malnutrition.

- Liver function tests (LFTs)
- Serum protein, albumin, prealbumin
  - Albumin level < 3.2 mg/dL is concerning and in elderly patients may predict a poor prognosis.
- Thyroid profile
- Prothrombin time (PT) and partial thromboplastin time (PTT)
  - Elevated levels may reflect a liver disorder or malnutrition.
- Mini Nutritional Assessment
- Geriatric Depression Scale*
- Mini-Mental State Examination*
- Subjective Global Assessment*
- Speech/swallow evaluation*
- Barium swallow radiography*
- Videofluoroscopy*: if aspiration with swallowing is a concern
- Endoscopy*: if esophageal mass or stricture

Differential Diagnosis

Feeding problems, dysphagia, weight loss, or malnutrition may be related to numerous causes.

- Anxiety/restlessness
- Dementia
- Dysphagia
- Endocrine disorders: uncontrolled or undiagnosed diabetes, Cushing disease, or thyroid disorder
- Gastroesophageal reflux disease (GERD)
- Esophagitis
- Immobility or inability to feed oneself
- Chewing or swallowing difficulty
- Illness
- Malabsorption syndromes
- Malignancy
- Medications
- Neurologic disorders
- Neuromuscular disorder
- Structural disorder

Treatment Plan

When possible, the underlying cause should be identified and treatable issues addressed. If anorexia or weight loss is related to dysphagia, the etiology of the dysphagia must be sought and, if possible, corrected. Illness, as well as medications and some physical disorders, will also affect swallowing ability and their

*If indicated.

relationship to the problem should be considered and addressed. Discussion with the patient, family, and staff addresses each patient's food preferences as well as considered interventions (i.e., medications, dietary recommendations, feeding tubes). Careful documentation of the feeding problem, attempted remedies, and discussions with patients, families, and healthcare providers are essential.

All institutionalized patients can benefit from a vitamin and mineral supplement. Patients at risk for osteoporosis require both calcium and vitamin D supplements. Documented vitamin deficiencies such as thiamin, B_{12}, and folate deficiency require appropriate vitamin replacement. Fortified foods, supplemental feedings, and attention to personal and cultural preferences may also be beneficial. Other interventions include:

- Liberalize dietary restrictions.
- Consider fortified foods.
- Encourage personalized dining room experiences (e.g., some patients may prefer a quieter experience).
- Encourage a well-lit, unhurried dining experience.
- Encourage family and friends to visit and eat with patient.
- Encourage patient cooking activities with activities director.
- Enhance the dining experience (e.g., winter barbecue night, dining music on special occasions).
- 6 to 8 small meals per day may be better tolerated.
- Consider a restorative feeding program, frequent finger foods, and assistance with meals.
- Promote healthy snacks and bedtime snacks.
  - Coffee, teas, carbonated beverages, and spicy foods may cause indigestion.
- With dysphagia, swallowing ability is variable and dependent on many factors in debilitated patients or older adults. Although a swallowing evaluation may be helpful, a patient's ability to swallow improves or declines from day to day and dysphagia management has not proven beneficial in preventing pneumonia. Swallowing ability may have no relation to the patient's risk for aspiration. In addition, dietary modifications are often unpalatable for patients resulting in weight loss, dehydration, malnutrition, and diminished quality of life.
  - Use dietary modifications; soft or semi-soft foods may be easier for patients with dental problems and some types of dysphagia.
  - Educate to improve swallowing: that is, following solids with liquids, using a straw or special cup.
  - Maintain 1:1 staff to patient ratio during mealtime, if indicated.
  - Referral to speech therapist for therapy to learn swallow techniques for oropharyngeal dysphagia may be helpful for patients with neurogenic disorders.
- Liquid supplements between meals (but not closer than 1 hour before a meal) may be helpful in some, but not all, patients.
- Treat anxiety/depression.
  - Consider SSRI or Remeron (Mirtazapine), 7.5 mg PO at bedtime (may be slowly increased), *or*

- Ritalin (Methylphenidate HCl), 2.5 mg PO before breakfast (may be increased to before breakfast and lunch; dose may also be slowly increased)
- Consider appetite stimulant. The following medications have been useful for patients with cancer and AIDS patients, but no medication has yet been approved explicitly for geriatric anorexia.
  - Marinol (Dronabinol), 2.5 mg at bedtime has been used for cancer and AIDs patients successfully for weight gain and control of both nausea and vomiting. Additionally, reports suggest patient agitation may be decreased with dronabinol. Dosage can be gradually increased in divided doses, but monitor for delirium.
  - Megace (Medroxyprogesterone acetate), 40 mg PO before meals, can improve appetite and has produced weight gain in some, but not all studies (contraindicated if there is a history of thromboembolic events).
  - Periactin (Cyproheptadine), 2 to 4 mg PO QID may improve appetite, but has not improved weight gain in elders.
  - Other considerations include recombinant human growth hormone; oxandrolone, an oral anabolic steroid; or testosterone. However, studies are limited.
- Enteral feedings may be appropriate for a small number of patients. However, there is little evidence that enteral feedings improve quality of life or prolong life, particularly in elders.
  - Nasoenteric feeding tubes are appropriate for short-term use, although they are frequently removed inadvertently by patients.
  - A radiograph must be obtained after nasoenteric feeding tube placement (and replacement) to verify placement. Goal of placement is adjacent to or beyond ligament of Treitz. Feedings must not be started until proper tube placement is verified via x-ray. The numerical marking of the nasoenteric feeding tube at the nares should be documented. The nasoenteric tube must be secured appropriately to cheek or nose.
  - Placement of nasoenteric tubes must be frequently monitored and documented as tubes migrate; vomiting and diarrhea are signs of tube migration.
  - A jejunostomy or gastrostromy tube is necessary for a patient requiring long-term enteral feedings (> 1 month).
  - Pump-controlled feedings are indicated for jejunostomy and gastrostomy feedings. Gravity feedings may be used for nasogastric (NG) tube feedings, but continuous feedings seem to help prevent tube blockage.
  - A jejunostomy tube may be beneficial for patients with recurrent G-tube aspiration pneumonia.
  - Fast bolus feedings increase risk of aspiration, thus, continuous feedings are preferred over bolus feedings.
  - Tube feedings should be started slowly and patients monitored for inability to tolerate the feeding amount.
  - Monitor gastric aspirate if there is abdominal distention or vomiting.

- Irrigate enteral infusion tubes with 30 mL water every 4 hours and before and after medication. Do not use juices for irrigation fluid.
- A jejunostomy tube should be irrigated with 10 to 20 mL normal saline (0.9%) each shift. Irrigant should not be aspirated for jejunostomy tube.
- Aspiration precautions are indicated for all patients with feeding tubes. Head of bed should be raised 30 to 45 degrees during feeding and for at least 1 hour after feeding ends.
- Monitor fluid and electrolyte status regularly to determine fluid needs and appropriate tube feeding preparation. Some patients will require significant amounts of free water.
- Monitor tube site and tube for signs of deterioration and displacement.
- Consider parenteral feedings for patients in whom enteral feedings are not appropriate (e.g., those with ileus, bowel obstruction, GI hemorrhage, short bowel syndrome, peritonitis).

Consultation/Hospitalization

- Consult with dietitian about appropriate enteral feedings for each patient and for complications associated with feedings (e.g., diarrhea, hyponatremia, hypernatremia, hyperglycemia, increased BUN).
  - The selection of enteral feedings is based on each patient, although the formulas are similar. Usually, the nutritional requirements range between 1.2 to 1.5 gm/kg/24 hours. Some patients may not be able to tolerate the nitrogen balance (BUN and creatinine must be monitored routinely in patients on any tube feeding); others may require increased calories. Specific formulas are available for patients with diabetes, diarrhea, constipation, or lactose-intolerance.
- Consult with physician, gastroenterologist, and surgeon for gastrostomy or jejunostomy placement.
- Consult with physician regarding appropriate referral for parenteral nutrition.
- Daily physician consultation is necessary for patients receiving parenteral nutrition.
- Consult speech therapy for appropriate patients.

Complications

- Complications of poor nutritional intake
  - Anemia
  - Anergy
  - Aspiration
  - Cognitive changes
  - Decreased immunity
  - Dehydration
  - Edema

- Fatigue
- Hip fracture
- Impaired wound healing
- Infection
- Orthostatic hypotension
- Pressure ulcers
- Enteral feeding tube complications
  - Aspiration
    - Bolus feedings in particular increase chance of aspiration
  - Clogged tube (electric/battery pump feedings help prevent clogging)
  - Diarrhea
  - Erratic drug absorption: tube feedings must be turned off for a period of time with some medications (i.e., phenytoin)
  - Fluid and electrolyte abnormalities
  - GI irritation and bleeding
  - Hyperglycemia
  - Infection
    - Bacterial
    - Fungal
    - Tube feedings can also become contaminated, causing infection
  - Leakage of feedings or GI contents around stoma site: indicates improper tube placement requiring reinsertion.
  - Pressure necrosis at insertion site
  - Tube decay/corrosion (requiring replacement)
- Parenteral feeding complications
  - Fluid and electrolyte imbalance
  - Hyperglycemia
  - Infection

Education for Nursing Home/Rehabilitation Staff

- Discuss with nursing staff importance of respecting patient/family preferences.
- Encourage staff to have patient be able to feed self with finger foods or other easily handled foods.
- Explain to nursing staff the importance of recognizing and reporting changes in patient's eating habits.
- Stress the importance of maintaining aspiration precautions in susceptible patients. Feed patient with HOB elevated to 90 degrees, (Ideally, patients should be out of bed and sitting in a chair for all meals.)
- Educate nurses about enteral feedings and the care of enteral feeding tubes.
  - For feeding tube care, wash daily and as needed around site with gentle cleaner, pat dry, apply protective ointment (not petroleum based). Assess tube placement and be certain tube is well secured.
  - Change pump tubing daily.
  - Opened enteral feeding formulas should be discarded after 24 hours; dated and refrigerated after opening.

- Formula should be at room temperature at time of administration, but should not be opened/administered for longer than 8 hours at room temperature.
- Liquid medications are preferred over pills. Medications should not be added to feeding formulas.
- Check gastric aspirate per physician orders (usually before feedings or every 4 hours). Reinstill gastric aspirate. Usually feedings are held for an hour if aspirate is over 200 mL or patient has abdominal distention, nausea, or discomfort, but orders for each patient should be clearly understood.
- Discuss the nature of swallowing abnormalities with nursing staff, explaining that many patients will be able to eat safely.
- Educate nursing staff about the benefits of good mouth care.
- Discuss importance of notifying the healthcare provider if patient has nausea, vomiting, abdominal distention, constipation, or diarrhea.
- Educate the nursing staff about the importance of monitoring and recording patient weights each month. All patients should be weighed and height measured on admission to the facility. Thereafter, the patient should be weighed at the same time of day each month, preferably in the early morning before breakfast, and be dressed in the same clothing (pajamas and no slippers or shoes).
- Patients on tube feedings should initially be weighed every other day: weight gain of 2 lb or more in 2 days should be reported to the healthcare provider.
- Explain to nursing staff that patients on tube feedings, even if they are to take nothing by mouth (NPO), can rinse their mouths out with pleasant drinks (or even foods), then expectorate the substance, as this may improve quality of life (tasting foods/fluids).

Patient/Family Education

- Encourage patient socialization in activities associated with foods patient might be interested in eating.
- Discuss with families the progression and associated eating changes with aging, dementia, and so on.
- Explain the risks and benefits of thickened liquids and soft, pureed diets.
- Ongoing discussions with patients and families are recommended to explore preferences, risks/benefits, and issues concerning survival rates and quality of life if enteral feedings are a consideration.

Bibliography

Collier, S., & Duggan, C. (2004). Overview of parenteral and enteral nutrition. *www.uptodate.com*. Accessed March 15, 2004.

Henkel, G. (2004). Nutrition basics for LTC. *Caring for the Ages*, 5(1), 20-22.

Kirby, D.F., et al. (1995). American Gastroenterological Association technical review on tube feeding for enteral nutrition. *Gastroenterology, 108*(4), 1282-1301.

Levinson, S., & Crecelius, C. (2003). Common versus evidence-based practice: The facts about dysphagia and swallowing studies. *Caring for the Ages, 4*(2), 17-18.

MacKenzie, D., et al. (2004). Care of patients after esophagectomy. *Critical Care Nurse, 24*(1), 16, 18-31.

Morley, J., et al. (1998). Nutritional deficiencies in long-term care. Part I. *Annals of Long-Term Care, 6*(5), 183-191.

Morley, J., et al. (1998). Nutritional deficiencies in long-term care. Part II. *Annals of Long-Term Care, 6*(8), 250-258.

CHAPTER 16

Special Considerations

INSOMNIA

Insomnia is a symptom characterized by an inadequate quantity and quality of sleep that affects daytime functioning. One of every three adults complains about a sleep problem and nearly half of elderly persons report transient sleep difficulties. Changes in sleep quality occur in normal aging as rapid eye movements (REM) and deep restorative sleep diminish. Medications, as well as physical and psychological illnesses, may also affect sleep. Both insomnia and primary sleep disorders affect quality of life. It is important to thoroughly assess sleep patterns and make every effort to manage insomnia without medications. Drug use should always be short term and used with caution because of the risk for falls in the elderly.

Risk Factors

- Psychiatric illness
- Adjustment disorders
- Stress: divorce or death of a spouse, new environment, or illness
- Older age: elderly have increased frequency of apnea without the diagnosis of sleep apnea
- Female sex, especially postmenopausal
- History of insomnia
- Medical illness; endocrine disorders
- Medications
- Obesity: associated with sleep apnea
- Habits: caffeine, cigarettes, drugs, or alcohol

History

It is important to elicit a complete history in an attempt to diagnose and treat insomnia. Current medications and a description of the sleep problem are helpful in determining the cause of the insomnia. Issues to be explored include the following:

- Onset: sudden onset may be related to a change in sleep environment, stress, or acute illness versus long-term, chronic sleep disorder.
- Description of problem: difficulty with sleep initiation may indicate poor sleep hygiene, delayed phase sleep, or restless leg movement; sleep maintenance: may be related to drugs, alcohol, poor sleep hygiene, advanced sleep phase, psychiatric issues, primary sleep disorder, or depression with early morning awakening
- Aggravating factors: stressors such as death; environmental changes such as being moved from home, noise, heat, pain, or snoring
- Accompanying factors: fatigue, headache, appetite loss, weight gain, nocturia, frequency, dysuria, low energy, sadness during winter (suggests seasonal affective disorder [SAD]), or preoccupation with sleep
    - Nocturia, dysuria, or uninary frequency, may be related to congestive heart failure (CHF), urinary tract infection (UTI), or prostate disease.
- Alleviating factors: walking around eases discomfort associated with restless leg syndrome (RLS); sitting up relieves dyspnea)
- 2-Week sleep log: helps clarify the problem
    - Time getting into bed: in delayed sleep phase, a person falls asleep very late and awakens midday; in advanced sleep phase, person goes to sleep early and awakens very early
    - Habits at bedtime: food, drink, medications, activities, content and use of television
    - How long does it take to fall asleep; when do lights go off?
    - Number of awakenings during night? What causes awakening (e.g., nocturia, shortness of breath, choking, RLS)?
    - How long does patient stay in bed after awakening?
    - Time of arising
    - Daytime alertness: does patient take naps or doze off during the day?
    - Drug use: alcohol (fragmented sleep), over-the-counter (OTC) medications, diuretics, bronchodilators, seizure drugs, steroids, levodopa, thyroxine, central nervous system stimulants, tobacco, or caffeine are commonly associated with insomnia
- Medical conditions that affect sleep
    - Heart failure: nocturia, paroxysmal nocturnal dyspnea (PND), or diuretic use
    - Pulmonary disease: shortness of breath, or orthopnea
    - Pain: cancer, headaches, arthritis, fibromyalgia, peripheral vascular disease, or neuropathy
    - Gastroesophageal reflux disease (GERD)

- Obesity with sleep apnea
  - Pruritus
  - Diarrhea
- Psychiatric illness that affect sleep
  - Psychosis
  - Anxiety
  - Depression
  - Dementia
- Family history: RLS or circadian rhythm disorders, such as delayed sleep phase syndrome or advanced sleep phase syndrome
- Interview of bed partner or roommate regarding snoring and RLS

Physical Examination

Sleep disturbances may be related to medical as well as psychiatric illness. The following physical findings may suggest a physical cause for insomnia.
- Constitutional: sleepiness; pain affects sleep; obesity related to sleep apnea
- Vital signs: hypertension commonly related to sleep apnea
- Mouth: petechial hemorrhage of soft palate and enlarged tonsils present in sleep apnea
- Neck: thyroid enlargement (overactive or hyperthyroid affects sleep)
- Respiratory: asthma in sleep apnea; CHF
- Prostate examination: enlarged prostate causes frequent urination
- Neurologic: mental status, dementia workup, neuropathy, symptoms of depression, or anxiety

Differential Diagnosis

Less than 1 month:
- Acute transient insomnia: change in environment (particularly present on admission to rehab or long-term care unit), noise, temperature, stressors, acute illness, stimulants, medication, SAD, alcohol
Greater than 1 month:
- Chronic persistent
  - Primary sleep disorders
    - Sleep apnea
    - Periodic limb movement: involuntary upper and lower extremity movements interrupting sleep; may occur with RLS
    - RLS: intense sensation to move legs associated with leg discomfort; occurs with rest or inactivity, in early evening as well as during sleep; alleviated by movement
  - Medications associated with insomnia
    - Theophylline, amphetamines, selective serotonin reuptake inhibitors (SSRIs), sympathomimetics, psychotropics, hypnotics, caffeine, or other stimulants result in wakefulness.

- Anticholinergics, antihistamines, antihypertensives, and antidepressants can cause daytime somnolence.
- Anti-Parkinsonian drugs, β-blockers, quinidine, steroids, and tricyclics may cause nightmares.
- Diuretics interrupt sleep by causing nocturia.
- Benzodiazepines and alcohol may cause rebound insomnia.
- Doxepin and anticholinergics (Benadryl) may cause urinary retention.
- Benzodiazepines and narcotics may cause agitation in some patients.
- Blindness: misses cues associated with light
- Circadian rhythm disorders: goes to sleep late or early or awakens late or early
- Psychiatric illness: substance abuse, obsessive-compulsive disorder, stress, depression with early morning awakening, difficulty initiating sleep, anxiety with nightmares, panic attacks, posttraumatic stress syndrome (PTSS), schizophrenia with prolonged sleep onset latency, akathisia, withdrawal of alcohol or sedatives, or SAD
- Medical disorders associated with chronic, persistent insomnia
  - Cardiac: nocturnal angina or heart failure
  - Pulmonary: chronic obstructive pulmonary disease (COPD) or asthma
  - Gastrointestinal: gastroesophageal reflux
  - Genitourinary: benign prostatic hypertrophy or overactive bladder
  - Musculoskeletal: degenerative joint disease, rheumatologic disease, or fracture
  - Neurologic disease: dementia/delirium with day/night sleep reversal or neuropathy
  - Skin: pruritus from scabies, malignancy, renal or liver failure or skin rashes
  - Endocrine: hyperthyroidism or polyuria
  - Chronic pain
- Psychophysiologic: poor sleep hygiene, sleep state misperception (patient complains of poor sleep without objective evidence), or night fears

Diagnostics

Testing is often not indicated. However, specific clinical presentations may suggest a need for diagnostic evaluation.
- CBC with iron studies: renal failure, iron deficiency anemia, and low serum ferritin levels are a common cause of RLS
- Blood urea nitrogen (BUN), creatinine, and serum electrolytes: renal failure with pruritus associated with insomnia
- Urinalysis with urine culture: to exclude infection

- Thyroid-stimulating hormone (TSH): to exclude thyroid disease
- Sleep apnea study: if indicated

Treatment Plan

Nonpharmacologic
- Treat medical or psychiatric illness as appropriate
- Sleep hygiene
  - Regulate sleep schedule: keep consistent bedtime and wake time; do not stay in bed longer than you sleep; keep midday nap to less than 90 minutes *or* avoid daytime naps; use bedroom only for sleep; stay out of bedroom during the day; get out of bed after trying to fall asleep for 20 minutes and return when sleepy.
  - Improve sleep environment: quiet, with earplugs if necessary; white noise with air conditioner or fan; proper temperature (cool), humidifier; face clock so face cannot be seen (to decrease worry about time); dark room, nightlight below level of bed; elevate head of bed if necessary with two or more pillows if GERD, cardiovascular problems, COPD; use audiotapes.
  - Phototherapy: may need referral to reset sleep rhythm if exposure to light in the morning is not effective.
  - Attempt to expose patient to bright sunlight in midday or use phototherapy.
  - Improve bedtime behavior: warm bath 2 hours before bedtime, light bedtime snack with warm milk and low-carbohydrate, low-fat foods; eat on regular schedule; relax before bedtime; read; avoid intense mental activity, worrying or vigorous exercise within 2 hours of bedtime. No television when in bed; avoid caffeine, nicotine, alcohol, tea, chocolate, amphetamines, cocaine, corticosteroids, decongestants, bronchodilators at bedtime; decrease fluid intake in afternoon and evening; go to bed only when sleepy; no bed restraints.
- Review all medications and time of administration: e.g., Prozac should be given early in day; change time of diuretic; give medications with side effect of somnolence at bedtime (e.g., phenytoin [Dilantin], acetaminophen [Tylenol], β-blockers; may need to change antidepressant to a more sedating alternative); slowly taper benzodiazepines and barbiturates.
- Relaxation therapy: encourage massage, music therapy, warm milk, or warm sheets at bedtime.
- Encourage exercise in the early morning (not before bedtime).
- Reassure.
- For circadian rhythm disorders, move bedtime and arising time slowly; use bright lights in the morning.
- Sleep apnea: weight loss, keep patient from lying on back, nasal dilator, oxygen if saturation low, and CPAP if indicated

Pharmacologic
- Hypnotic drugs should only be used to complement nonpharmacologic therapy. Restrict sleep medications to less than 4 weeks or 1 to 2 nights per week. Use cautiously with renal, hepatic, or pulmonary disease.
- Restless leg syndrome
  - Ferrous sulfate, 325 mg PO with vitamin C 500 mg PO, is recommended TID if ferritin is < 18 mcg/L or iron saturation < 20%. Monitor labs and discontinue ferrous sulfate if iron saturation > 50%.
- Sleep medications: consider one of the following:
  - Trazodone 25 to 50 mg PO at bedtime; caution with men (can cause priapism) or with concurrent SSRI
  - Ambien, 5 mg PO every third night
  - Melatonin, 2 to 3 mg PO at bedtime, may correct circadian rhythm disorders, but it is not regulated and not well studied
  - Tylenol, 1000 mg PO at bedtime, often effective
- Manage pain
  - Tylenol, 1000 mg PO qhs for bone and joint pain
  - Neurontin, 300 to 800 mg PO qhs for stabbing, neuropathic pain
  - Nonsteroidal antiinflammatory drugs (NSAIDs) cautiously for arthritis pain
  - Consult with neurologist/primary care physician for pergolide or other dopaminergic agent, anticonvulsant (gabapentin [Neurontin], carbamazepine [Tegretol]), sedative-hypnotic agents, or tramadol (Ultram), 25 to 50 mg PO at bedtime.

Consultation/Hospitalization

- Combined use of cognitive and behavioral therapy and pharmacologic interventions better than either single intervention alone
- Psychiatrist, psychologist, or social worker for behavioral therapy and neuropsychologic tests; biofeedback if sleep hygiene changes ineffective after 3 weeks
- Phototherapy referral, if appropriate, for SAD
- Neurology consult for RLS
- Pulmonary consult for suspected sleep apnea or lung disease
- Sleep study when other interventions have been ineffective after 6 months and there is no apparent medical or psychiatric cause
- Oropharyngeal surgery for snoring/sleep apnea

Complications

- Sleep deprivation may affect immune response to illness.
- Sleep has major quality of life implications.

Education for Nursing Home/Rehabilitation Staff

- Explain to nurses how aging and disease can affect sleep patterns for patients.
- Discuss with nursing staff and aides the physical signs associated with insomnia: hypertension, irregular breathing, snoring, daytime somnolence, confusion in morning, observed periodic limb movements, or complaints about leg discomfort.
- Control patient environment with attention to interruption of sleep: privacy, talking, and other noise. Encourage nurses to minimize patient stimulation during the night or interruption of patient sleep.
- Discuss with nurses and staff the benefit of wearing soft-soled shoes to minimize noise during the night.
- Keep patient busy and entertained during day.
- Provide a relaxing environment for sleep (e.g., be certain patient is warm or cool enough).
- Discuss with staff risks of medication use for sleep.
- Discuss with staff the importance of scheduling medications appropriately (e.g., give diuretic in morning).
- Encourage facility to order *Getting your ZZZZs: How Sleep Affects Health and Aging* from *www.ilcusa.org/pub/books/htm*.

Patient/Family Education

Discuss with patient/family:

- Realistic expectations of sleep and potential untoward effects of sleeping medications
- Sleep hygiene
- Changes of aging related to sleep
- Benefits of continuous positive airway pressure (CPAP) in appropriate clinical situation

Bibliography

Brown, D. (1999). Managing sleep disorders. *Clinician Reviews, 9*(10), 51-71.

Cefalu, C. (2004). Evaluation and management of insomnia in institutionalized elderly. *Annals of Long-Term Care, 12*(6), 25-32.

Chokroverty, S. (2004). Evaluation and treatment of insomnia. *www.uptodate.com*. Retrieved April 10, 2004.

Cochran, H. (2003). Diagnose and treat primary insomnia. *Nurse Practitioner, 28*(9), 13-27.

Folks, D. (1999). Management of insomnia in long-term care. *Annals of Long-Term Care, 7*(1), 7-13.

Venugopal, M., & Susman, J. (2000). Insomnia in the elderly. *Consultant, 40*(6), 1234-1243.

PAIN

ICD-9: 780.9 (GENERALIZED PAIN)

Pain, which may be acute or chronic, is an unpleasant sensory and emotional experience associated with actual or potential tissue damage. Acute pain usually has an identifiable injury or disease. It is a symptom. Chronic pain is less well defined and may actually become the illness, although effective management of acute pain can reduce the risk of the pain becoming chronic. Chronic pain can be malignant or nonmalignant and is, by definition, intermittent or continuous and present for more than 3 months duration. Pain can also be affected by psychosocial issues.

The prevalence of painful conditions increases with age. This is reflected by the large number of patients in nursing homes suffering with pain. Nonpharmacologic measures and both nonopioid and opioid medications should be used to manage pain. Unfortunately, the elderly are predisposed to the side effects of drugs because of the physiologic changes of aging. Function, quality of life, and safety need to be considered when managing drug regimens.

Risk Factors

Acute Pain
- Postoperative pain
- Cancer
- Acute event: trauma, myocardial infarction, angina, or urinary tract infection

Chronic Pain
- Undertreated acute pain
- Depression, anxiety: complaints of pain may be a symptom
- Chronic illnesses leading to pain: diabetic neuropathy, postherpetic neuralgia, peripheral vascular disease (PVD), degenerative joint disease (DJD), or cancer
- Fall: may precipitate pain or be a side effect of pain medication
- Inadequate access to health care: neglected treatment of initial pain
- Genetic predisposition for abnormal processing of sensory input resulting in pain
- High pain intensity levels: important risk factor for developing chronic pain

History

The most accurate and reliable evidence of pain and its intensity is the patient's report. A thoughtful symptom analysis should elicit the location, quality, intensity, onset, frequency, and duration of the discomfort, as well as exacerbating and

relieving factors. Other helpful information to consider includes the following:
- Pain log
- Use of pain scale: at least once per shift and when pain medication is administered
- Medical history
  - Cancer recurrence or recent diagnosis
  - Recent surgery: acute pain postoperatively
  - Gout: painful joints
  - Depression: pain worse in AM; possible psychomotor agitation
  - Heart failure: may be precipitated by NSAIDs, which should be used cautiously
  - Vasculitis: accompanying myalgias or arthralgias
  - Osteoporosis
  - Falls
  - DJD
  - GI pathology: may inhibit absorption of oral medications; limits use of NSAIDs
  - Kidney or liver disease: require caution with morphine use (morphine metabolized by the liver and excreted by the kidney); NSAIDs affect kidney function
  - Herpes zoster: may result in postherpetic neuralgia
  - Cerebrovascular accident (CVA): limb pain may occur
  - Decreased libido, irritability, fatigue, and physical deconditioning from inactivity or isolation: may be related to pain
  - Coping techniques: assists in writing a plan of care
  - Surgeries: multiple surgeries at the same site can lead to nerve damage and scar tissue.
  - Medication use: OTC pain medications
- Functional health patterns: appetite, sleep, socialization, and mobility may be affected by pain.
- Behavioral changes: moaning, groaning, crying, or personality changes may indicate pain.
  - Interview family members and staff for baseline behavior.
  - If possible, elicit history of emotional or sexual abuse or a posttraumatic stress disorder (PTSD).

Physical Examination

Treatable causes of pain should be excluded before chronic pain is diagnosed. A complete physical examination as well as depression and mini-mental evaluation are helpful to assess the pain. Other necessary information should include:
- General appearance: facial expressions, verbalizations, splinting with position change, gait disorder, diaphoresis, or other nonverbal signs suggesting pain

- Vital signs
  - Increased temperature may indicate infection, vasculitis, polymyalgia rheumatica (PMR), or other inflammatory disorder.
  - Tachycardia, tachypnea, and hypertension are associated with pain, but hypotension and bradycardia may also be present with severe pain.
- Pain scale: large print for elderly, bright paper for visually impaired, and pictures for those with dementia
  - Quantifying pain is challenging in a patient with cognitive deficits.

Differential Diagnosis

Pain can be acute (associated with an identifiable injury or disease) or chronic. It is helpful to both classify and differentiate the type of pain to guide treatment. Usually, pain is classified with an analog scale on a scale of 1 to 10: 0 to 3, mild pain; 4 to 6, moderate pain; 7 to 10, severe pain. Types of pain include:

- Nociceptive: damage to soft or bony tissue; inflammatory disorders; treated more easily than neuropathic pain
- Somatic: aching, throbbing, stabbing pressure from skin or bone (e.g., rheumatoid arthritis, osteoarthritis, gout, fibromyalgia, ischemia)
- Visceral: gnawing, crampy, aching, sharp discomfort from internal organ involvement
- Neuropathic pain: damage or pressure on nerves or neural tissue causing continuous burning or paroxysmal stabbing, knifelike pain; related to postherpetic neuralgia, diabetic neuropathy, post-stroke pain, phantom limb, or radiculopathies
- Mixed: unknown mechanisms, as in chronic headache
- Psychologically based: uncommon in elders; associated with somatization disorders and hysteria; morphine usually ineffective
- Incident pain: related only to activity; may need increased medication 30 to 60 minutes before activity

Diagnostics

Diagnostic testing is helpful in monitoring physiologic response to pain medication as well as determining the most appropriate medication.

Laboratory Evaluation

- Complete blood count (CBC): to determine hematologic status if considering NSAID therapy
- Liver function test (LFT): baseline evaluation, because morphine is metabolized by the liver
- Renal function: assess renal function; morphine excreted by the kidneys
- Erythrocyte sedimentation rate (ESR)*: to rule out acute inflammatory disease

*If indicated.

- Uric acid: if gout is suspected
- Rheumatoid factor, antinuclear antibodies (ANA): if acute, inflamed joints
- Prothrombin time/international normalized ratio (PT/INR): if patient on warfarin, because acetaminophen (Tylenol) and other medications may increase INR
- Urinalysis and culture and sensitivity (C&S): if urinary tract infection (UTI) suspected

Other Diagnostics
- Radiographs*: to rule out fracture, intestinal obstruction, and so on
- Electrocardiogram (ECG)*: to rule out myocardial infarction (MI)
- Bone scan*: to detect infection, fracture, tumor, or bone disorder
- Electromyelogram (EMG)*: to assess neuromuscular function
- Magnetic resonance imaging (MRI): to diagnose disk herniation if patient shows neurologic deficits

Treatment Plan

Nonpharmacologic
- Assistive devices: cane, crutches, wheelchair, or walker
- Application of heat to increase blood flow or decrease stiffness (use cautiously), or application of cold to reduce inflammation, edema, and muscle spasm
    - Heat or cold pack must be used cautiously (i.e., wrapped and not applied to skin directly).
    - Apply heat or cold only 15 minutes every 30 to 60 minutes.
- Rest with elevation of extremity, if appropriate
- Activity: socialization diverts mind from pain
- Exercise: strengthens ability to perform and stimulates endorphins
- Weight reduction: if appropriate
- Water therapy: good for painful joints
- Massage: a back rub
- Consider referral for relaxation therapy, biofeedback, acupuncture, aroma therapy, massage, or PT/ OT.

Pharmacologic
Acute joint event: if appropriate, NSAID for 3 to 7 days; may be used in conjunction with acetaminophen (Tylenol). NSAIDs must be used cautiously, monitored carefully, and should not usually be used long-term because of GI, renal, and cardiovascular side effects (monitor for S&S gastric distress, weight gain, peripheral edema). May need to also give proton pump inhibitor to protect stomach.
- NSAIDs
    - Ibuprofen (Advil, Motrin) 200 to 400 mg PO every 6 to 8 hours with food for 3 to 7 days

*If indicated.

- Salsalate (Disalcid) 500 mg PO BID for 3 to 7 days
- Acetaminophen (Tylenol): maximum dose 4 g/day, but long term use should not exceed 3000 mg/d (maximum dose if on warfarin is 2500 mg PO daily). Doses should be scheduled rather than prn for maximum effect.
- Consider low-dose prednisone or colchicine for acute gout flare.
- If no effect, use immediate response opioids (see later).

Chronic Pain: Classify Pain as Mild, Moderate, or Severe (See Differential Diagnosis)

- Nonopioids:
  - Acetaminophen: maximum 1 g PO QID (not to exceed 4 g daily) for mild to moderate pain; if liver disease or on warfarin (Coumadin), lower dose is necessary; follow LFT every 6 months; potentiates effect of narcotics; can be given in suppository form if patient unable to tolerate oral route
  - NSAIDs: short-term use (see above)
  - Steroids for bone pain: consider oral prednisone 40 to 80 mg/daily; duration of therapy is unclear, but steroid therapy should be discontinued if patient does not respond within 1 week
  - Calcitonin for bone pain: effectiveness takes a few weeks; calcitonin-salmon nasal spray (Miacalcin) 200 international units daily: one nostril one day, other nostril next day; consult with physician regarding injectable Calcitonin
  - Pamidronate for bone pain: 90 mg intravenous (IV) over 2 to 3 hours monthly; follow calcium levels carefully

Neuropathic Pain

- Neurontin: start with 100 mg PO at bedtime; increase to 300 mg/day or higher; side effects include sedation, fatigue, and edema; reduce dose in renal failure
- Lidoderm patch: 5% for a 12-hour period; only to intact skin (monitor skin carefully)
- Capsaicin cream: 0.025% TID to QID to intact skin; use gloves when applying
- Nortriptyline: 25mg PO TID *or* 40 mg PO 2 hours before bedtime: affects neurotransmitters input to spinal cord; caution with cardiovascular disease; anticholinergic side effects
- Clonidine: 0.1 mg PO BID *or* transdermal patch up to 0.6 mg/daily; side effects are hypotension and bradycardia
- Tocainide: 400 mg PO every 8 hours; must be used cautiously because of cardiac effects; may need cardiology consult

Muscle Spasms

- Baclofen: 5 mg PO TID; monitor liver function carefully
- Opioids: Continue with nonopioids if no adverse reactions; may need to use alone when adverse reaction to nonopioids; avoid codeine, propoxyphene, and meperidine

Mild to Moderate Pain

- Tramadol (Ultram): 25 mg to 50 mg PO every 6 hours; not to exceed 400 mg PO/daily

Moderate Pain

- Immediate release oxycodone: 5 mg PO every 4 to 6 hours; increase dose as needed

Severe Pain

- Morphine: 5 to 15 mg PO every 4 to 6 hours; immediate release until sustained release (MS Contin 15 to 30 mg PO [do not crush or chew] every 12 hours) is effective *or*
- Oxycontin: 10 mg PO every 12 hours *or*
- Fentanyl patch, 25 mcg, change every 3 days; rotate sites as may cause skin reaction; not effective on patient with minimal subcutaneous (subQ) tissue; should not be used as initial narcotic on opiate naïve patients

Malignant Pain

- Start with immediate-release opioid. Schedule doses and assess response to pain. Once pain is managed, start sustained release opioid (see earlier) while continuing PRN immediate-release opioid
- Reassess pain every 24 hours until pain is well controlled.
- If more than four PRN doses used in 24-hour period, increase sustained-release medication by 25% for mild pain, 50% for moderate pain, and 100% for severe pain.
- May need morphine subQ, intramuscular (IM), or IV in the short term for acute exacerbation of pain until sustained-release dose increased and effective. If possible, instead of parenteral route, treat escalated pain with sublingual (SL) morphine IR (Roxanol) 20 mg/1 mL, 2 mg SL every 15 minutes until comfortable while increasing dose of sustained release.
- For end of life, use SL morphine IR or morphine suppositories.
- At end of life, escalating pain may be related to disease progression, tolerance to current opioid, and/or partial or total bowel obstruction. Consider antiemetics, scopolamine patch, and increase sublingual (or parenteral) IR morphine until comfortable *or* can change opioid, delivery route, or both.

Special Considerations for Pain Management

- Identify underlying process and type of pain.
- Balance symptom relief with drug side effects.
- Set realistic therapeutic goals with the patient and family.
- Improve function and enhance quality of life.
- Reduce morbidity and cost associated with untreated or inappropriately managed pain.
- Make every effort to use nonpharmacologic measures along with non-opioids and, if necessary, opioids.

- Route of administration should be oral or transdermal if possible. Use parenteral route only if absolutely necessary.
- Provide around-the-clock relief, on schedule, not as-needed.
- Use a stepwise drug approach.
- Start low, go slow.
- When using opioids, start with immediate release and assess if patient will benefit from sustained release.
- Use drugs from different groups in combination. Avoid single drug from two groups (like Percocet), which limits ability to increase dosing of one of the drug components.
- If one opioid is ineffective, may change to different opioid or add another drug.

Consultation/Hospitalization

- If appropriate, obtain orthopedic, rheumatology, or neurology consultation.
- Consultation is indicated for steroid injection into a joint.
- Consult physical therapy (PT) for exercise regimen, transcutaneous electrical nerve stimulation (TENS), or water therapy.
- Consult pain clinics if problems managing medication regimen or side effects are intolerable; patient may need nerve block or trigger-point injection. For end of life care, epidural or intrathecal access for pain management may be necessary.
- Hospitalization is unusual but must be considered if pain is unresponsive to interventions.
- Consult occupational therapy (OT) to improve independence.
- Consult psychology or psychiatry for cognitive, behavioral therapy, and biofeedback.
- Acupuncture can be affective for musculoskeletal conditions, cervical or lumbar spondylosis, postherpetic neuralgia, low back pain, and osteoarthritis.
- Consider aromatherapy, touch therapy, hypnosis, and yoga.
- Massage may enhance immune function.
- Chiropractor: caution in elderly
- Radiation therapy for intractable bone pain related to cancer
- Relaxation response can modify pain perception.

Complications

- Falls: if oversedated
- GI bleeding or CHF from NSAIDs: consider proton pump inhibitor for increased GI protection
- Urinary retention: review medications; straight catheterization for residual if urinary retention is suspected
- Constipation: give senna with each opioid dose or twice daily; Dulcolax PO

or PR; enema or prunes/prune juice to ensure bowel movements every 48 hours
- Nausea: order prn Compazine PO or PR
- Sedation and confusion: review medication regimen
- Abnormal INR with risk of bleeding if patient on warfarin
- Reflex sympathetic dystrophy: chronic pain syndrome associated with intense burning pain affecting skin, muscle, and bone; related to nerve injury

Education for Nursing Home/Rehabilitation Staff

Discuss with nursing staff:
- Medication side effects: constipation, risk of falls, signs and symptoms of heart failure, or renal failure
- Safety measures
- Nonpharmacologic pain management measures: ambulation, activity, backrubs, socialization, and positioning
- Importance of bowel regimen and monitoring bowels daily
- Necessity of recording breakthrough pain and notifying healthcare provider
- Benefits of medicating patient prior to activity, communicating with PT/OT
- Importance of assisting patient/family with transition to end of life care
- Nonverbal communication of pain or change in functional status
- Importance of addressing pain in documentation and care plan

Patient/Family Education

Explain to patient/family:
- Importance of exercise
- Support regarding pain medication use and tolerance
- Importance of quality of life rather than cure approach
- Importance of hydration, bowel regimen, activity
- Self monitoring of pain with use of pain scale
- Safety measures to prevent falls
- Necessity of assessing mood and function
- Importance of patient participation in pain management

Bibliography

American Geriatric Society Clinical Practice Guidelines. (1998). The management of chronic pain in older persons. *Journal of the American Geriatric Society*, 46(5), 635-651.

Battista, E.M. (2002). The assessment and management of chronic pain in the elderly, a guide to practice. *Advance for Nurse Practitioners*, November, 29-32.

Brown, J., et al. (1999). *Gerontological protocols for nurse practitioners*. Philadelphia: Lippincott, Williams and Wilkins.

Collett, B.J. (2002). The use of chronic opioid therapy for patients with nonmalignant pain. *Annals of Long-Term Care, 1011*, 53-58.

Freedman, G. (2002). Chronic pain: Clinical management of common causes of geriatric pain. *Geriatrics, 7*(5), 36–41.

Kumar, K., & Demeria, D. (2003). The role of opioids in the treatment of chronic nonmalignant pain in the elderly. *Annals of Long-Term Care, 11*(3), 34-40.

Miller, K.E., et al. (2003). Challenges in end of life pain management. *Annals of Long-Term Care, 11*(4), 26-32.

Wells-Federman, C.L. (2000). Care of the patient with chronic pain: Part II. *Clinical Excellence for Nurse Practitioners, 4*(1).

PALLIATIVE CARE

There is often little discussion concerning end of life care. Medicine has made such advanced strides that we forget that just as life has a beginning, there is an end. Frequently, it is an acute illness or injury that forces patients and families to think about the end of life. Sometimes, it is advanced age and a gradual decrease in the level of functioning that confronts us with this issue. Thus, some decisions at the end of life become reactive rather than proactive.

Over the years, much has been written about terminal cancer care and the benefits of hospice. Hospice provides comprehensive spiritual, psychological, social, and physical care by a team of skilled professionals: physicians, nurses, aides, volunteers, social workers, and pastoral workers. Medicare and many insurance plans will pay for hospice services at home or in the skilled nursing facility. Hospice agencies have criteria to accept patients for care. Usually, although not always, the patient has agreed to a "do not resuscitate" order. The benefit of hospice is the interdisciplinary care provided to families as well as patients, end of life comfort for terminally ill patients, and decreased expense of medications and equipment to the patient and family. Patients may choose to access their Medicare hospice benefit while in a long-term care facility; when they do, orders for care are still written by the healthcare provider in consultation with the hospice agency.

The palliative care movement, which started in Britain, has grown in response to consumers choosing to be included in decisions regarding end of life care. The World Health Organization (WHO) defines palliative care as "the active total care of the patient whose disease is not responsive to curative treatment." Palliative care addresses patient and family concerns regarding disease treatments and decisions while providing symptom control and psychological care. The focus is on comfort, advanced directives, planning psychosocial support, and quality of life. This requires intensive communication and understanding of the patient's and family's cultural, religious, and spiritual values as well as an understanding of the patient's and family's awareness of the disease progression. It is an essential component of providing care to frail individuals with chronic, debilitating illness as well as those with terminal disease.

Hospice care and palliative care are currently not the same. Palliative care can be provided without the patient accessing their hospice benefit and without being part of a hospice agency. Palliative care, which does not have the same Medicare reimbursement restrictions as hospice care, provides patients with symptom relief and psychologic care while permitting exploration of all treatment options. The patient's decisions about care are respected and followed. The concept of palliative care should be a fundamental component of the care provided to patients and families in both the subacute and long-term care environments. The admission process may identify some patients and families who would benefit from this philosophy of care. Patients with functional decline, failure to thrive, or terminal medical conditions during the continuum of care should be identified also. However, although healthcare providers may recognize the benefit of palliative care for a patient, it is important to allow families and patients to discuss their wishes and allow them to guide the transition to palliative care. Often, it is the immobility, fatigue, and functional changes combined with physical symptoms that precipitate the transition to palliative care. Each patient and each family has had different life experiences and begins the journey differently. A respectful, supportive approach enables the patient and family to maintain control and dignity while recognizing the need both patients and families have for support in participating in end of life care.

Nurse practitioners, clinical nurse specialists, and physician assistants in collaboration with primary care physicians, nurses, chaplains, and social workers have the unique opportunity to coordinate palliative care and address the complex issues related to caring for patients with both chronic and terminal illness. Addressing the patient's wishes for comfort, dignity, and medical treatments as well as respecting the decisions of the healthcare proxy are imperative. Continued assessment and healthcare provider presence are essential for the treatment of physical, psychologic, spiritual, and social issues at life's end.

History

The history should determine patient concerns and family or nursing observations about the patient. Additionally, it is important to determine the patient's medical history to learn if there are comorbid conditions that could contribute to pain or other symptoms. Assessing pain, nutritional intake, bowel function, and sleep, as well as cultural, psychologic, spiritual, and social issues are essential. The admission interview is an opportunity to discuss and document patient wishes for care if their health should fail further (e.g., advanced directives, feeding tube if unable to eat). Other considerations include, but are not limited to the following:

- Cognitive status
    - Is there evidence of cognitive dysfunction (delirium, dementia, or depression) or anxiety?
    - Is the patient able to participate in healthcare decisions? Has a healthcare proxy been designated?

- Weakness/fatigue/dizziness
- Food/fluid preferences
- Difficulty or painful swallowing; dry mouth
- Chest discomfort
- Palpitations
- Dyspnea
- Cough
- Nausea
- Vomiting
- Sadness/suicidal tendency

Physical Examination

The patient's wishes must be respected. Although a weight may be helpful in assessing weight loss or nutritional status, obtaining the weight may be uncomfortable for the patient. As a patient may not be able to adequately describe or even complain of pain or other concerns, a complete physical examination is usually indicated. Carefully monitoring of the patient during the physical examination is helpful in determining if the patient has discomfort or other distress. Aspects of the examination to consider include:

- Functional assessment
- Vital signs: assess for fever, hypertension/hypotension, tachycardia, tachypnea, and hypoxia
- Skin: monitor for edema and skin breakdown
- Oropharynx: evaluate for dry membranes, painful lesions, and infection
- Cardiac: assess for heart rate, rhythm, extra heart sounds, murmurs, and rubs
- Lungs: assess for respiratory distress, hypoxia, rales, wheezes, rhonchi, and rubs
- Abdomen: determine presence of distention, bowel sounds, and abdominal pain
- Rectal examination: assess for impaction
- Neuropsychiatric: evaluate cognitive status, attention, activity, and presence of tremors

Diagnostics/Differential Diagnosis

Appropriate diagnostic testing is based on the clinical presentation, physical findings, and differential diagnosis. Discussion with the patient and/or healthcare proxy about recommended radiographic or laboratory studies is essential as the patient's wishes are paramount.

Treatment Plan

Treatment addresses spiritual and social concerns and is intended to relieve any distressing symptoms. The underlying cause of any symptom should be identified, if possible, and treatment offered to alleviate patient suffering. The risks and benefits of treatments must be discussed with the patient and/or family. Common physical concerns and suggestions for management include the following:

- Altered skin integrity is a significant potential problem related to nutritional factors, immobility, circulatory disturbances, and declining health. All patients are at risk for developing pressure ulcers, but patients with terminal illnesses or declining health are even more susceptible. Prevention of pressure sores is paramount. Pressure relief; frequent, careful positioning; and fastidious skin care (especially in incontinent patients) are essential components of care (see Chapter 13).
- Anorexia may be related to the disease process, but it is also often related to a medication. Thus medications should be reviewed and, if possible, changed.
  - Small, frequent feedings with foods and liquids the patient prefers may be helpful, but anorexia may be the body's protective mechanism against nausea.
  - Diet should be liberalized.
  - Megestrol acetate, cryptoheptadine, alcohol, or other stimulants can be tried.
  - Socialization with family, friend, or staff member at mealtimes may be helpful.
- Anxiety (see Chapter 13)
  - Often, the most helpful treatment is listening and trying to address the patient's concerns.
  - For patients unable to describe symptoms, anxiety may be a sign of discomfort.
  - Attentiveness to physical and environmental comfort is essential. Music, repositioning, or a back rub may be helpful.
  - Pharmacologic interventions include:
    - Lorazepam 0.25 to 0.5 mg PO or SL every 4 to 6 hours if needed
    - If indicated, morphine 2 mg SL every 2 to 4 hours may be helpful, particularly if anxiety is related to pain; long-acting morphine (MS Contin) may be more appropriate in some patients.
- Bowel obstruction
  - Treatment is dependent on patient wishes. Hospitalization may be indicated, but often stopping oral fluids, initiating intravenous fluids and antiemetics are helpful for partial bowel obstructions. More severe obstructions require placement of nasogastric tube to alleviate the gastric distention and discomfort. IV metoclopramide may aid in peristalsis.
- Constipation
  - Bowel function should be continually assessed and an aggressive bowel protocol should be initiated to prevent constipation or bowel obstruction especially in patients receiving narcotics for pain. When possible, constipating medications should be changed.

- Patients receiving narcotics for pain need an aggressive bowel protocol to prevent constipation. "Smooth Moves Tea," a tea with senna, may be more palatable for some patients.
- A Dulcolax suppository, enema, or disimpaction may be necessary for some patients.
- Consider other causes of constipation, such as fluid, electrolyte or endocrine abnormalities or complications of malignancy (e.g., spinal cord compression, obstruction).
- Delirium: sudden, acute, vacillating confusional state
  - Consider fluid, electrolyte, or metabolic dysfunction; infection; hypoxia; and pain; and treat if appropriate.
  - Explain to nurses and family that delirium may be related to medications, infection, hypoxia, or dehydration or may be a form of restlessness that accompanies the transition from life to death.
- Depression
  - Encouraging the patient to talk with a social worker, chaplain, or psychologist allows the patient to talk about their life experiences. Encouraging reminiscing, reviewing old photographs, and family stories may be helpful for some patients and families.
  - If appropriate, an antidepressant medication may be helpful. The medication should be chosen based on the patient's history and accompanying symptoms (e.g., Remeron may be helpful for depressed, anxious patients and may aid sleep and appetite).
- Dysphagia
  - Some patients with dysphagia may have feeding tubes, but want to eat or drink. Discussion regarding risks/benefits and quality of life is necessary: for some patients, eating/drinking improves quality of life and the benefit outweighs the risk of aspiration.
- Dyspnea
  - Treat the underlying cause (e.g., pain, pneumonia, heart failure, pleural effusions, anemia, anxiety), although sometimes dyspnea is not related to a specific cause.
  - Give oxygen if indicated.
  - Opioids
    - Morphine elixir, 1 to 2 mg PO or SL every 4 to 6 hours if needed
  - Anxiolytics
    - Lorazepam, 0.25 to 2 mg PO or SL every 4 to 6 hours
  - Corticosteroids may be indicated for some patients with cancer, asthma, and COPD.
  - Nonpharmacologic interventions include providing a cool, but serene, peaceful environment, careful positioning (usually in a high Fowler's position), and personal support. They may also include fans, peaceful music, and guided imagery.
- Fatigue and weakness are common in chronic illnesses, particularly when the illness is end-stage. Causes are usually multifactorial. Medications should be reviewed and anemia, fluid, electrolyte or metabolic disturbances,

depression, and organ failure considered. Treatment is supportive and individualized, but for some patients methylphenidate or even steroid therapy may be indicated.

- Incontinence is not an uncommon problem in older patients. Urinary incontinence may be transient or chronic. Transient urinary incontinence may be related to infection, medications, or change in cognitive status. Chronic urinary incontinence is classified as functional, stress, urge or overflow incontinence and is often exacerbated by declining health. The type of incontinence should be identified and addressed.
- Nausea/vomiting
  - Review and eliminate offending medications.
  - Prevent constipation.
  - Minimize unpleasant odors.
  - Consider PRN or regularly scheduled antiemetic.
- Pain (see earlier in this chapter)
  - Determine if pain is acute (sudden onset) or chronic; if it is mild (0 to 3 rating), moderate (4 to 6), or severe (7 to 10); and if it is somatic, neuropathic, or visceral.
  - Assess for treatable cause of discomfort (e.g., constipation, infection).
  - Nonpharmacologic nursing interventions should be tried first, particularly if pain is chronic and mild to moderate in severity: sitting and being with patient, repositioning patient, back rubs, and modalities (e.g., cool/warm packs, topical capsaicin or muscle cream).
  - Consult with physical therapy for appropriate exercise, positioning, joint supports, or other appropriate interventions.
  - Pain management must be individualized and the patient should be asked frequently if more pain medication would be helpful and the patient's wishes respected.
    - Generally, NSAIDs should be used judiciously or avoided in elderly patients with a history of warfarin therapy, renal insufficiency, heart failure, or bleeding. If NSAIDs are prescribed, the lowest dose possible should be used and the duration of treatment should be limited. The patient must be carefully monitored for untoward effects.
  - Pain medication, when desired or necessary, should be scheduled with breakthrough pain medication available.
    - Nonopioid medications are indicated initially for mild or moderate pain.
    - Low dose opioids are necessary for severe pain or moderate pain that has not responded to other interventions.
      - Avoid meperidine and propoxyphene in elderly patients. Meperidine should never be used for long-term pain management (metabolite is toxic, accumulates, and can cause seizures).
      - Acetaminophen when used in combination with a narcotic may aid pain control. However, long-term use of acetaminophen should not exceed 3000 mg daily, as hepatotoxicity is

possible. Patients on concurrent warfarin therapy should not take more than 2500 mg of acetaminophen each day.
- Although the benefit of acupuncture or other complimentary therapies is uncertain, it may be appropriate to consider these treatments for some patients.
- Steroids may be beneficial for pain associated with nerve compression, bone metastases, or chronic pruritus.
- Xerostomia
  - Treat any mucosal infections (e.g., *Candida*).
  - Keep mucous membranes moist. Perform frequent mouth care with frequent applications of lubricating gels to lips. Use artificial saliva if indicated.
  - Encourage hard candies and cool, soothing liquids.
- Cough
  - Consider etiology and treat appropriately (e.g., GERD; postnasal drip; consider codeine if appropriate).
- Pruritus
  - See Chapter 3.
- Fluid overload
  - See Chapter 10.

Consultation/Hospitalization

- Consult with physician to discuss hospitalization or medical treatment for patients with bowel obstruction.
- Consultation with physician is recommended for pharmacologic therapy to treat pain, depression, anorexia, or other symptoms.
- Consultation with a pain management specialist may be indicated if the patient does not respond to pain control interventions.
- Consultation with hospice or pastoral services may be helpful for addressing spiritual concerns.
- Social worker consultation may be indicated if the patient or family is worried about financial issues.
- Consultation with physical therapist may be helpful for positioning techniques and modalities.

Complications

- Constipation
- Nausea/vomiting
- Pain
- Tenesmus
- Overflow incontinence
- Ileus

- Obstruction
- Fecal impaction
- Dyspnea
- Impaired quality of life

Education for Nursing Home/Rehabilitation Staff

- It is essential that the nursing staff understands the concept of palliative care and the need to respect the patient's and family's wishes. Careful and repeated education and discussion is invaluable to support the staff in dealing with these patients and their families.
- Educate staff about the patient's cultural background and how culture may influence a patient's and family's response to illness and death.
- Reinforce the importance of respecting each patient's dignity throughout the lifespan.
- Educate the nursing staff about the importance of assessing the patient's pain each shift (using a numeric rating scale or visual analogue scale) and documenting the response to pain management interventions.
- Discuss with nursing staff the importance of monitoring the patient for physical and psychosocial symptoms and reporting concerns to the primary care provider.
- Educate nursing staff about symptoms of pain in cognitively impaired patients (e.g., restlessness, agitation, anxiety).
- Explain to nursing staff the benefit of frequent mouth care and positioning.

Patient/Family Education

- If acceptable to the patient, frequent communication with the family is usually helpful to answer questions and offer support and guidance.
- Encourage patient and family to discuss concerns about pain, other symptoms, and questions regarding hospitalization.
- Reiterate to patients and families that addiction is not a concern when treating pain adequately.
- Explain to family that anorexia, cachexia, fatigue, weakness, constipation, and dyspnea are common end of life issues and explain treatments and other comfort measures.
- Prepare families for end of life changes (e.g., anorexia, decreased fluid intake, weakness, agitation, delirium, declining level of consciousness, or change in breathing patterns).
- Support family regarding end of life issues such as funeral arrangements.

Resources

- Center to Advance Palliative Care: *www.capc.org*

Bibliography

Crawley, L.M., et al. (2002). Strategies for culturally effective end-of-life care. *Annals of Internal Medicine, 136*(9), 673-679.

Frampton, K.K. Vital sign # 5: Pain assessment and management in LTC requires a thorough, team-oriented care plan. *Caring for the Ages, 5*(5), 26-35.

Gazelle, G., et al. (2001). The development of a palliative care program for managed care patients: A case example. *Journal of the American Geriatric Society, 49*(9), 1241-1248.

Victoria Hospice Society, et al. (2003). *Transitions in dying and bereavement: A psychosocial guide for hospice and palliative care.* Baltimore: Health Professions Press.

VANCOMYCIN

The increase in methicillin-resistant *Staphylococcus aureus* (MRSA) infections has affected patients and healthcare facilities throughout the world. The prevalence of MRSA is concerning because there are a small number of antibiotics available to treat MRSA infections. Currently, most MRSA infections are treated with intravenous vancomycin. In some instances, other antibiotics are indicated. Some MRSA infections may be sensitive to sulfamethoxazole-trimethoprim, tetracycline, or a fluoroquinolone. Quinupristin-dalfopristin, a streptogram; linezolid, an oxazolidone; and daptomycin are newer antibiotics that offer alternative pharmacologic treatment for MRSA. However, as vancomycin is still used for MRSA, coagulase-negative staphylococci, and other infections, familiarization with prescriptive and monitoring guidelines, is necessary.

History/Physical Examination

Before starting a patient on vancomycin therapy it is necessary to review the patient's history to determine appropriateness of therapy and potential risks. Allergies, medications, and past medical history should be reviewed and the patient's general health status determined.

Diagnostics

- Culture and sensitivity: possibly indicating need for vancomycin therapy
- BUN and creatinine: to assess renal function

Treatment

If intravenous vancomycin is determined to be the most appropriate antibiotic for the patient, it is necessary to calculate the correct dose and monitor the patient as follows:

Dose and Frequency Determination

- Dosing is based on body weight (15 to 20 mg/kg body weight with a maximum beginning dose of 1500 mg). The dose is prescribed to the nearest 250 mg increment, although for most adults, often the initial dose is 1 g IV, every 24 hours.
- Vancomycin dosing and frequency must be adjusted for patients with renal insufficiency and at risk for renal insufficiency. Frequency is usually based on serum creatinine clearance; renal function in some patients may be affected by other factors (e.g., liver dysfunction, hemodialysis).
  - Men: creatinine clearance (ml/minute) = 140 – age × weight (in kg)/serum creatinine (mg/dL) × 72
  - Women: creatinine clearance (ml/minute) = (140 – age × weight [in kg]/serum creatinine [mg/dL] × 72) × 0.85

Monitoring

- For patients with normal renal function requiring < 4 days IV vancomycin, but no other nephrotoxic or ototoxic medications, monitoring serum creatinine or vancomycin serum peak and trough level is not necessary.
- Oral vancomycin is given for patients with *Clostridium difficile* who did not respond to or who are allergic to metronidazole. For these patients, peak and trough monitoring is not indicated.
- Patients receiving intravenous vancomycin every 24 hours for > 4 days should have serum vancomycin peak and trough drawn at third dose; if vancomycin frequency is every 48 hours or more, obtain serum peak (one to two hours after vancomycin infusion is completed) and trough (30 to 60 minutes before the next vancomycin dose is given) concentrations after second dose.
  - The goal of the vancomycin peak is usually > 25 mcg/ml up to 40 mcg/ml. In some instances, a higher peak concentration is recommended, although the usefulness of peak concentration is unclear and debated.
  - The goal of the vancomycin trough is 5 mcg/ml to 10 mcg/ml, although higher troughs may be indicated for treatment of bacterial endocarditis, osteomyelitis, or severe illness.
  - If vancomycin peak and trough are within goal and the patient does not have renal insufficiency and is not on other nephrotoxic or ototoxic medications, a vancomycin trough can be checked weekly. However, many healthcare providers choose to monitor both peak and trough levels weekly.
  - If the vancomycin peak or trough is not within goal and dose is changed, the trough should be drawn before the third dose (of the adjusted dose).
  - The serum BUN and creatinine should be obtained whenever the peak or trough is drawn.

- Critically ill patients, patients with renal disease, obese patients, patients with fluid volume imbalance, and patients receiving other nephrotoxic or ototoxic medications should, if the vancomycin peak is within goal, have the trough rechecked every 3 days.
  - A midline or PICC line is preferred for intravenous vancomycin therapy.
- If the vancomycin peak is >40 mcg/ml (or higher than peak goal), the vancomycin dose should be decreased. A decrease in dose will decrease both the peak and trough concentration. In some cases, vancomycin may need to be held until vancomycin peak is within goal. The vancomycin can then be restarted at a lower dose.
- If the vancomycin trough is >10, the dosing frequency must be extended. This will also decrease the peak concentration. Dosing frequency is usually appropriate in 24-hour intervals (i.e., every 24 hours, every 48 hours, every 72 hours). Some patients may require more individual dosing frequency depending on peak and trough levels (e.g., every 30 hours).
- If the vancomycin trough is subtherapeutic (<5 mg), the dose should be increased or the dosing interval shortened.
- Close consultation with a pharmacologist is recommended for dose changes and scheduling intervals.

Consultation/Hospitalization

- Physician consultation is recommended before initiating intravenous vancomycin therapy to discuss appropriateness of therapy, dosing, length of therapy, and monitoring.
- Consultation with a nephrologist is recommended prior to starting vancomycin for patients with renal failure.
- Consultation with a pharmacologist is recommended for questions regarding vancomycin dosing.

Complications

- "Red man syndrome" related to rapid vancomycin infusion (the medication should be infused over 60 to 120 minutes)
- Hypersensitivity reaction (e.g., anaphylaxis)
- Bone marrow suppression
- Vancomycin resistant *S. aureus*
- Renal insufficiency
- Leukopenia
- Neutropenia
- Hearing loss
- Thrombophlebitis at IV site
- *Candida*

Education for Nursing Home/Rehabilitation Staff

- Discuss with nursing staff the importance of administering vancomycin as ordered and infusing over at least 1 hour.
- Discuss with nursing staff the importance of encouraging oral fluids to 2 liters/day to prevent renal insufficiency.
- Explain to nursing staff importance of monitoring patient for hypotension during medication infusion, as well as for wheezing, rash, or hearing loss.

Patient/Family Education

- Discuss with patient/family the reason for treatment, risks and benefits and potential side effects.
- Explain to patient the importance of reporting pharyngitis, fatigue, or other symptoms promptly to nursing and/or healthcare provider.
- Explain to patient the importance of adequate fluid intake (2 liters daily) to prevent nephrotoxicity.

Bibliography

Begg, E., et al. (1999). The therapeutic monitoring of antimicrobial agents. *British Journal of Pharmacology, 47*(1), 23-30.

Centers for Disease Control. (2004). MRSA. *www.cdc.gov/ncidod/hip/ARESIST/mrsa.htm.* Retrieved June 30, 2004.

Iwanoto, T., et al. (2003). Clinical efficacy of therapeutic drug monitoring in patients receiving vancomycin. *Biological and Pharmaceutical Bulletin, 26*(6), 876-879.

Launay-Vacher, V., et al. (2002). Clinical review: Use of vancomycin in hemodialysis patients. *Critical Care, 6*(4), 313-316.

Skidmore-Roth, L. (2004). *Nursing drug reference.* St. Louis: Mosby.

ANTICOAGULATION

Anticoagulation and antiplatelet therapy, along with thrombolytic agents, is used to prevent and treat thrombotic events. Patients with a deep vein thrombosis, pulmonary embolism, or increased risk of stroke (e.g., new onset atrial fibrillation) are often anticoagulated with intravenous heparin and warfarin to prevent embolus. Heparin and warfarin require careful laboratory and clinical monitoring to maintain adequate anticoagulation, but prevent bleeding. Low molecular weight heparin (LMWH), a newer anticoagulant, does not require intravenous therapy (it is given subQ) or laboratory monitoring and is as effective as heparin for some clinical conditions. New oral anticoagulants such as Ximelagatran (Exanta) may, in the future, replace warfarin. Exanta, for example, will have a fixed dose, is not affected by medications or foods, and will not require blood monitoring. However, the new anticoagulants are still under investigation.

The following guidelines for anticoagulation management are based on recommendations from the American Geriatric Society and the American College of Chest Physicians. (For more information, see Boxes 16-1 and 16-2).

- Heparin, 5000 units subQ BID preoperatively or prophylactically for bedridden patient until patient is ambulatory
- Anticoagulation for an orthopedic patient may consist of a daily aspirin, low–molecular-weight heparin, or Coumadin therapy with varying INR ranges and treatment duration. Some orthopedic patients may be on a fixed Coumadin dose, but for many orthopedic patients the INR goal is 1.5 to 2. It is essential to clarify anticoagulation orders as well as the duration of anticoagulation treatment with the surgeon.
- Anticoagulation is indicated for DVT prophylaxis, pulmonary emboli, acute coronary syndrome, unstable angina, left ventricular dysfunction, atrial fibrillation, mechanical prosthetic valves, and post–stent placement.
- Heparin
    - IV unfractioned heparin is not commonly used in postacute settings, but it is indicated for unstable anginas, acute coronary syndrome, and massive pulmonary embolism, and for use after coronary artery stenting. Frequent monitoring of PTT (every 4 to 6 hours) for dose regulation is necessary.
    - Start unfractionated heparin (UFH) bolus 5000 units IV (80 units/kg) followed by 1000 units/hour (18 units/kg) until PTT twice normal. Check PTT every 6 hours and regulate dose. Continue for 5 days. Check platelets every third day. Monitor carefully for heparin-induced thrombocytopenia (heparin should be discontinued if patient exhibits thrombocytopenia).
    - Heparin 5000 units subQ every 8 or 12 hours or LMWH in combination with Coumadin (see later) may be used for treatment of DVT instead of IV heparin.
- Warfarin (Coumadin)
    - Start within 24 hours of starting UFH or low–molecular-weight heparin (LMWH). Initial warfarin dose 2 to 5 mg PO daily. Elderly patients should be started on a lower dose. Obtain daily PT/INR.
    - Discontinue heparin when INR is 2 (or within therapeutic range) for 2 consecutive days (when used to prevent thrombosis, heparin and warfarin should be used concurrently for approximately 4 to 5 days).
    - Goal INR is 2.5 for DVT and AF with a range of 2 to 3; goal INR is 3 for mechanical heart valves, with a range of 2.5 to 3.5 (Table 16-1).
    - Check PT/INR daily for 2 weeks, then biweekly. When stable, check PT/INR monthly and correct dose as indicated (Box 16-1).
    - For patients on warfarin who require antibiotic therapy, recheck INR after second dose of antibiotic, adjust Coumadin dose as needed, and recheck PT/INR.
- LMWH: enoxaparin sodium (Lovenox) 1 mg/kg subQ BID or 1.5 mg/kg

TABLE 16-1   INR Goal and Routine Course of Anticoagulation

Condition	INR	Rotine Course
Fractured hip/orthopedic surgery	1.5-2	Treat for 6 weeks
1st DVT with reversible factors	2-3	Treat for 3 months
1st DVT with unknown cause	2-3	Treat for longer than 6 months
DVT, with persistent risk factors or metastatic cancer	2-3	Indefinitely
Prophylaxis DVT	2-3	Treat 6 months
Mechanical prosthetic valves	2.5-3.5	Long-term use
Atrial fibrillation	2-3	Long-term use
Recurrent TIA	2.5-3.5	3 months
If no TIA in 3 months	2-3	Long-term use
Pulmonary embolus	2-3	Long-term use

subQ QD *or* dalteparin (Fragmin) 100 units/kg every 12 hours [maximum dose 9000 units every 12 hours] deep subQ.
- Lovenox 30 mg subQ BID equals heparin 5000 units subQ BID.
- Decrease dose of LMWH by 25% in patients with poor renal function. **LMWH is contraindicated if there is a pork allergy or active bleeding.**

BOX 16-1   Management of INR

Management of INR Goal 2-3
- INR < 2: increase weekly dose by 10%
- INR 3-3.5: decrease weekly dose by 10%
- INR 3.6-4: hold 1 dose, decrease weekly dose by 10%
- INR > 4: hold 2 doses, decrease weekly dose by 10%

Prolongation of INR
- If INR > 4 but < 6 and patient not bleeding, hold Coumadin, check INR QD
- When INR 2-3, restart Coumadin and lower dose by 15%
- If INR > 6 and patient not bleeding, vitamin K 2.5 po or subQ in consultation with MD. Repeat INR next day, may repeat Vitamin K. When INR therapeutic, decrease dose by 15% and repeat INR in 1 week.
  - Oral Vitamin K is more effective than subQ Vitamin K when the INR < 9.
- If INR > 9 and no bleeding, hold Coumadin, Vitamin K 5 mg PO or subQ. INR QD.
- Vitamin K should be used cautiously with patients who have mechanical valves. Consult with MD. May need to give UFH and/or send to hospital.

Data from American Geriatric Society. (2002). The use of oral anticoagulation (warfarin) in older people. *Journal of the American Geriatric Society, 50(8), 1430-1445.*

- Check PT/INR daily and stop LMWH when INR 2 (or therapeutic) for 2 consecutive days, then monitor daily for 2 weeks, then biweekly. When stable, check INR every month.
- Anticoagulants and platelet inhibitors are commonly used together. Communication with the surgeon is necessary to discuss length of treatment.
- Patients receiving any anticoagulation therapy require special consideration (Box 16-2).

BOX 16-2   Special Considerations for Anticoagulation

- Knowledge of the target goal for the patient's problem is essential (e.g., if prophylaxis for DVT, goal INR would be 2.5; if patient has mechanical heart valves, goal INR would be 3).
- Coumadin schedule should be simple to insure compliance and minimize medication errors.
- Follow INRs closely when patient is on antibiotics or Tylenol, or if a new medication is added. Order Coumadin in 1 or 2 tablet sizes when writing discharge warfarin prescriptions to cover most dose changes.
- When administering Lovenox, the air bubble should not be expressed prior to injecting drug. Lovenox should be administered subQ in abdomen only.
- Anticoagulation and "Risk of Bleeding" should always appear on the problem list/care plan.
- Avoid IM injections when patient on anticoagulation.
- Age, liver function, heart failure, hyperthyroidism, pyrexia, diarrhea, dehydration, and Vitamin K deficiency can increase INR.
- Risk of thrombotic event increases if INR < 1.7.
- Risk of bleeding with Coumadin rises when INR > 5.
- Bleeding when INR < 3 is frequently associated with underlying problem.
- If risk of bleeding and elevated INR, consult physician for possible vitamin K.
- When patient is preoperative for surgical procedure or dental work, dentist or specialist may have protocol for stopping Coumadin. Discuss with patient/family/physican the risk related to discontinuation of Coumadin and need to start heparin or continue Coumadin with lower INR.
- When applicable, restart aspirin 24 hours after procedure if no active bleeding. When applicable, restart Coumadin day of surgery if no bleeding or bleeding is controlled and check INR QD until therapeutic.
- Common drugs that interact with Coumadin and may increase INR include Tylenol, β-blockers, corticosteroids, fluconazole, flu vaccine, darvon, antibiotics, tamoxifen, thyroid hormones, amiodarone, cimetidine, statins, proton pump inhibitors (PPIs), quinidine, loop diuretics, NSAIDs, mineral oil, Vitamin E, Vitamin C, trazodone, sucralfate, griseofulvin, carbamazapine, rifampin, spironolactone, and thiazides.
- Order NSAIDs cautiously in patients on anticoagulants.

Bibliography

Crowther, M., et al. (2002). Oral vitamin K lowers the international normalized ratio more rapidly than subcutaneous vitamin K in the treatment of warfarin-associated coagulopathy: A randomized controlled trial. *Annals of Internal Medicine, 137,* 251.

Hirsh, J., et al. (2000). The sixth ACCP guidelines for antithrombotic therapy for prevention and treatment of thrombosis. *American College of Chest Physicians, January,* 15-370S.

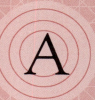
Common Locations of Skin Disorders

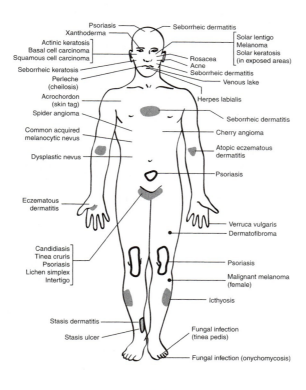

Psoriasis
Xanthoderma
Actinic keratosis
Basal cell carcinoma
Squamous cell carcinoma
Seborrheic keratosis
Perleche (cheilosis)
Acrochordon (skin tag)
Spider angioma
Common acquired melanocytic nevus
Dysplastic nevus
Eczematous dermatitis
Candidiasis
Tinea cruris
Psoriasis
Lichen simplex
Intertigo
Stasis dermatitis
Stasis ulcer

Seborrheic dermatitis
Solar lentigo
Melanoma
Solar keratosis (in exposed areas)
Rosacea
Acne
Seborrheic dermatitis
Venous lake
Herpes labialis
Seborrheic dermatitis
Cherry angioma
Atopic eczematous dermatitis
Psoriasis
Verruca vulgaris
Dermatofibroma
Psoriasis
Malignant melanoma (female)
Icthyosis
Fungal infection (tinea pedis)
Fungal infection (onychomycosis)

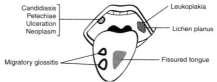

Candidiasis
Petechiae
Ulceration
Neoplasm
Migratory glossitis

Leukoplakia
Lichen planus
Fissured tongue

331

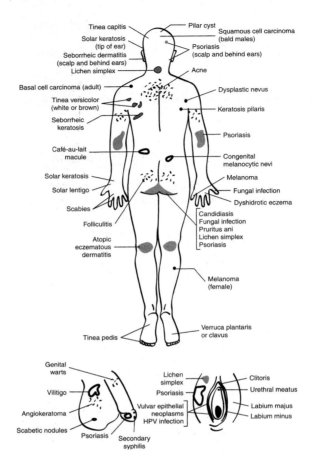

Tinea capitis
Solar keratosis (tip of ear)
Seborrheic dermatitis (scalp and behind ears)
Lichen simplex
Pilar cyst
Squamous cell carcinoma (bald males)
Psoriasis (scalp and behind ears)
Acne
Basal cell carcinoma (adult)
Tinea versicolor (white or brown)
Seborrheic keratosis
Dysplastic nevus
Keratosis pilaris
Psoriasis
Café-au-lait macule
Congenital melanocytic nevi
Solar keratosis
Solar lentigo
Scabies
Melanoma
Fungal infection
Dyshidrotic eczema
Folliculitis
Candidiasis
Fungal infection
Pruritus ani
Lichen simplex
Psoriasis
Atopic eczematous dermatitis
Melanoma (female)
Tinea pedis
Verruca plantaris or clavus

Genital warts
Vilitigo
Angiokeratoma
Scabetic nodules
Psoriasis
Secondary syphilis
Lichen simplex
Psoriasis
Vulvar epithelial neoplasms HPV infection
Clitoris
Urethral meatus
Labium majus
Labium minus

Osteoporosis

Older women, smokers, and patients with a history of vertebral fracture, chemotherapy, diabetes, kidney disease, liver disease, or prolonged history of steroid, antiseizure, or thyroid replacement therapy are at risk for osteoporosis. Men also may develop osteoporosis, usually at a later age than women but with even higher mortality rates 1 year after hip fracture: 31% of men versus 17% of women. Someone in the at-risk population who falls has a significantly increased risk for fracture. If the patient has not previously had a bone density measurement, one should be considered, particularly for patients admitted for long-term care. Patients admitted for rehabilitation can at least be counseled on the importance of bone density measurement after discharge.

Treatment Plan

- Kyphotic patients or patients with a history suggestive of osteoporosis require 1500 mg calcium (taken in divided doses with food) PO daily (if not contraindicated) and 800 IU vitamin D PO daily.
  - Calcium citrate may be better absorbed in older patients, who often have decreased gastric acid secretion.
- Biphosphonates are indicated for patients with osteoporosis.
  - Risedronate (Actonel), 5 mg PO daily or 30 mg PO once a week. Must be taken in morning before food with minimum 8 oz water. Patient must be upright for 30 minutes after medication is taken and cannot eat for 30 minutes. Dose must be adjusted if patient has renal disease.
  - Alendronate (Fosamox), 5 to 10 mg PO daily or 70 mg PO once a week. Must be taken in morning before food with a minimum of 8 oz water. Patient must be upright for 30 minutes after medication is taken and cannot eat for 30 minutes. Dose must be adjusted if patient has renal disease.

- Selective estrogen receptor modulator (SERM)
  - Raloxifene (Evista), 60 mg PO daily, is approved for prevention of osteoporosis, but efficacy in preventing hip fracture is unclear. Contraindicated if history includes thromboembolic event.
- Parathyroid hormone. Teriparatide (a new injectable parathyroid hormone), 20 mcg daily, may be indicated for some patients with a high risk for fracture, but long-term effects are unknown.

Bibliography

Campion, J.M., & Maricic, M.J. (2003). Osteoporosis in men. *American Family Physician,* 67(7), 1521-1526.

Formulas

Body Mass Index (BMI)

BMI = weight (kg) × height (m) squared

Normal weight = 18.5 – 24.9 kg/m^2

Underweight = < 18.5 kg/m^2

Overweight = > 30 kg/m^2

Corrected Calcium

Corrected serum calcium = serum calcium + 0.8 (4.0 – serum albumin)

Creatinine Clearance

Men: (140 – age) × ideal body weight (IBW)/serum creatinine* × 72

Women: ([140 – age] × ideal body weight [IBW]/serum creatinine* × 72) × 0.85

Erythrocyte Sedimentation Rate

Men = age/2

Women = (age + 10)/2

---

*Serum creatinine must be stable.

Serum Osmolality

$$2 \, (Na) + glucose/18 + BUN/2.8$$

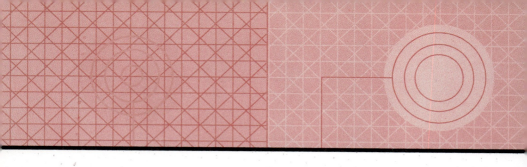

Index

Page numbers followed by f
indicate figures; t, tables; b, boxes.

Lungs (*Continued*)
  inflammatory response in, 51
  lung sounds, 51-53, 71, 182, 252
  transplantation of, 57
  volume reduction of, 57
LUQ (left upper quadrant), 121b,
    125
Lymphadenopathy, 123, 242,
    251-252
Lymphoma, 126, 176

M

Macrocytic (megaloblastic)
    anemias, 244, 246
Macules, 17-18, 22-23
Magnesium
  disorders of. *See*
      Hypermagnesemia;
      Hypomagnesemia.
  function and serum levels of,
      225, 227
  Slo-Mag, 228
Malignancy/cancer. *See also specific*
    tumors.
  chemotherapy for, 250-251, 256
  fever from, 249-251, 253
  hypercalcemia and, 222-223
  splenomegaly from, 252
Malnutrition, 250, 269, 289, 291
Managed care organizations
    (MCOs), 3
MAO (monoamine oxidase)
    inhibitors, 175, 270
Marinol (dronabinol), 293
Massage, 312
McBurney's point, 123
MDS-PAC (minimum data set-
    post acute care), 2-3
Medicaid Program. *See also* Center
    for Medicare and Medicaid
    Services (CMS).
  Balanced Budget Act (1997)
      and, 2
  reimbursement for subacute
      care, 11
Medicare Program. *See also* Center
    for Medicare and Medicaid
    Services (CMS).
  admission requirements of, 4,
      11
  Balanced Budget Act (1997)
      and, 2
  hospice benefits from, 314-315
  part A and B differences in, 11
  reimbursement for subacute
      care, 11
  reimbursement for subacute care
      from, 3
  single largest expense for, 98

Medication management. *See also*
    Drugs; IV (intravenous)
    therapy.
  absorption of drugs, 195
  at admission, 4-7
  adverse drug reactions, 89, 102,
      116-117, 250
  allergic reactions, 15-16
  allergic reactions and, 22, 48,
      323
  with anemias, 224
  blood glucose levels and, 175,
      181-182
  cardiotoxicity and, 265
  constipation and, 131b
  electrolyte imbalance and, 207,
      210-211, 215, 228
  falls and, 283, 285-286, 299,
      312
  feeding issues and, 289
  insomnia and, 300-304
  nephrotoxicity and, 146, 148,
      323-324
  ototoxicity, 323-324
  routes of administration for,
      312, 324
  titration in, 194
Megace (medroxyprogesterone),
    293
Melanoma, 19, 24
Melatonin, 304
Memory loss
  with anxiety and depression,
      264, 268
  with dementia, 164, 167-168
  with electrolyte imbalance, 175,
      217
  postoperative, 279
Mental health disorders
  anxiety, 263-266
  depression, 267-273
  obsessive-compulsive disorder
      (OCD), 263, 265, 302
  phobias, 263, 265
  post-traumatic stress disorder
      (PTSD), 263, 265, 302
Mental status
  alcohol/substance abuse and,
      268
  alteration in, 60, 66
  with dehydration or sepsis, 120
  fever and, 250-251
  with hypervolemia, 236
  with hypocalcemia/
      hypercalcemia, 217, 220
  with hypoglycemia/
      hyperglycemia, 173,
      175-178, 181
  with hyponatremia/
      hypernatremia, 202, 205

Mental status (*Continued*)
  personality changes, 164, 168,
      202
  with renal failure, 147
  sudden deficit with atrial
      fibrillation (AF), 75-76
  thyroid function and, 192
  with TIAs and strokes, 82
Mesentery, 123
Metabolic acidosis, 149-150,
    180
Metabolic syndrome, 180
Methicillin-resistant *Staphylococcus*
    aureus (MRSA) infections,
    322-324
Methotrexate, 25
Methylxanthines, 56
Microcytic anemias, 243-245
Micturition. *See also* Urinary tract
    infections (UTIs).
  frequency, 300-301
  hematuria, 251
  nocturia, 251, 283, 300-301
  polyuria, 181, 202
  prostate disease and, 300-302
Mild cognitive impairment (MCI),
    166
Milk-alkali syndrome, 220-222
Mini Mental State Examination
    (MMSE), 166
Mitral valve disease, 93
Mnemonic OPQRST, 89-91
Monoamine oxidase (MAO)
    inhibitors, 175, 270
Moraxella catarrhalis, 51
Morphine, 311, 317-318
Motrin (ibuprofen), 309
Mouth/oral care, 6, 18. *See also*
    Teeth/dentition.
Multisystem disorders
  fever, 249-257
  polymyalgia rheumatica (PMR),
      257-262
  rheumatoid arthritis (RA),
      253
  systemic lupus erythematosus
      (SLE), 253
Murphy's sign, 123-124
Muscles
  myalgia, 251
  PMR. *See* Polymyalgia
      rheumatica (PMR).
  spasm/tetany of, 217
  stiffness and aches in, 192
  weakness and atrophy of, 259
Musculoskeletal disorders
  falls and, 283, 285-286
  fractures, 250, 326-328
  polymyositis, 259
  treatment plans for, 96

Mycoplasma pneumoniae, 61
Myocardial infarction (MI)
  chest pain of, 87-88, 92
  as differential diagnosis, 57, 78, 125
  silent, 178, 184, 189
Myxedema, 192

N

Namenda (Memantine HCL), 169
Naprosyn, 260
Nasogastric (NG) feeding tubes, 293-296, 315
Nausea and vomiting
  fever-related, 251
  with hypoglycemia/ hyperglycemia, 174, 181
  treatment for, 313, 319
Nephrotoxicity, 146, 148, 323-324
Neuraminidase inhibitors, 67
Neuroimaging, 167
Neuroleptics, 162, 170
Neurologic deficits/neuromuscular signs
  with anemias, 242
  of delirium, 159-161
  of dementia, 164-169
  with fever, 253
  with hypervolemia, 236
  with hypocalcemia/ hypercalcemia, 221
  with hypoglycemia/ hyperglycemia, 174-175, 177, 182-183
  with hypokalemia/hyperkalemia, 214, 217
  with hypomagnesemia/ hypermagnesemia, 226, 228
  with hyponatremia/ hypernatremia, 202, 205
  symptoms of, 82-83
  of transient ischemic attacks (TIAs), 81-82
Neurologic disorders. *See also specific disorders.*
  delirium, 159-163
  dementia, 164-172
  as differential diagnosis, 269
  falls and, 283, 285-286
Neurontin (gabapentin), 304, 310
Neuropathic pain, 310
Neurotransmitters, 159
Nitrofurantoin (Macrodantin), 155-156
N-methyl-d-aspartate (NMDA) receptor agonists, 169
Nocturia, 251, 283, 300-301
Nocturnal hypoglycemia, 173

Nonketotic hyperglycemic hyperosmolar syndrome, 180-183, 185-186
Nonphysician providers. *See* Nurse practitioners (NPs)/physician assistants (PAs).
Nonsteroidal anti-inflammatory drugs (NSAIDs)
  for arthritis pain, 304
  avoidance of, 89, 102
  blood pressure and, 112
  examples of, 309-310
  for herpes zoster, 26
  nephrotoxicity of, 146
  side effects of, 307, 309, 319
Normocytic anemias, 244-245
Nurse practitioners (NPs)/physician assistants (PAs)
  certification of, 9
  Medicaid provider numbers for, 12
  patient visits by, 10-11
  reimbursement for, 11-12
  role in admission process, 4-5
Nursing homes
  admission to, 1-7
  anxiety and depression in, 263-264, 267-268
  Balanced Budget Act (1997) and, 2
  common infections in, 249
  CPT codes for, 11-12
  functional concerns in, 283-296
  hydration/dehydration issues in, 230-231
  physician visit CMS requirements in, 9-11
  regulations and reimbursement for, 9-14
  staff of. *See* Staff.
Nystatin (Mycostatin) cream, 27-28

O

O₂ sat (blood oxygen saturation), 52, 54-55, 71, 76, 102, 160, 252
Obesity
  blood pressure and, 112
  cardiovascular disease and, 81, 88, 99, 106
  diabetes mellitus and, 180, 183
  impact on healing, 31
  pulmonary disease and, 70
  skin and, 15
  sleep apnea and, 301, 303
Obsessive-compulsive disorder (OCD), 263, 265, 302

Obturator sign, 123
OCD (obsessive-compulsive disorder), 263, 265, 302
Online information
  about Alzheimer's disease (AD), 172
  about dementia, 172
  about sleep's effects on health and aging, 305
  about state nursing practice acts, 13
  for Medicare/Medicaid services, 13
Opioids, 310-312, 318-319
Orders from physicians, 5-7, 275
Organ systems, 13
Orthostatic hypotension, 231
Osteoporosis, 7, 261, 292, 333-334
Ototoxicity, 323-324
Over the counter drugs (OTCs), 241, 255, 260, 304
Oxycontin (oxycodone), 311
Oxygen
  administration of, 54-55, 62, 67, 72, 77
  blood saturation of (O₂ sat), 52, 54-55, 71, 76, 102, 160, 252

P

Pain
  abdominal and pelvic. *See* Abdominal pain.
  categories of, 308
  in chest. *See* Chest pain.
  classification of, 310-311
  delirium from, 160
  description/qualities of, 89-91, 122b
  documentation of, 313
  generalized
    acute versus chronic, 267, 306
    characteristics and risk factors for, 306
    complications of, 312-313
    consultation and hospitalization for, 312
    diagnostics for, 308-309
    differential diagnosis in, 308
    education about, 313
    history and physical for, 306-308
    treatment plans for, 309-312
  management of, 309-312, 319-320
  medications for, 95, 109
  neuropathic/nociceptive, 308
  nonpharmacologic measures for, 311, 313, 318-319